Family Health and Home Nursing

Doubleday & Company, Inc.
Garden City, NY

Library of Congress Catalog Card No. 78-72043
Printed in the United States of America

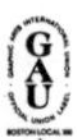

FOREWORD

For over half a century the American Red Cross has demonstrated its concern about home health care. Among its other services has been the offering of community education courses and instructional materials, including a textbook, to aid families in providing health care in the home.

In 1913, when the American Red Cross published its first health care textbook, medical and health care resources were not easily available to families. The Red Cross helped to meet the need for such resources by training nurses to give care to the ill at home and to teach families basic hygiene and home nursing skills. The first textbook was prepared to support that teaching. Red Cross home nursing service increased and became known as Town and Country Nursing Services. The value of the textbook also continued to increase, and the book gave growing support to teaching by the Red Cross and later by official public health nursing services, schools, colleges, and other groups.

To show the history of the textbook's development, a list of textbook titles and publication dates is given below.

1913	First edition	*Elementary Hygiene and Home Care of the Sick*
1918	Second edition	(Same title)
1925	Third edition	*American Red Cross Text Book on Home Hygiene and Care of the Sick*
1933	Fourth edition	(Same title)
1942	Fifth edition	*American Red Cross Textbook on Red Cross Home Nursing*
1950	Sixth edition	*American Red Cross Home Nursing Textbook*
1963	Seventh edition	(Same title)

At no time since the American Red Cross published its first home care textbook has national and international emphasis on family health and home care of the ill been as great as it is today. Disease prevention, nutrition, dental health, and control of costs are among the major areas in health care that have resulted in a renewed national interest in home health care. Concern regarding the quality, the humaneness, and the cost of institutional care is changing the type and the place of care for the mentally retarded, for those with muscular dystrophy and other developmental disabilities, and for other groups of persons who may require only the simplest personal care skills. Home nursing is one means of providing adequate care for many of these groups. In addition, many individuals and families have sought safer environments in which to live by moving away from cities. In doing so, they have often reduced the health resources available to them and have increased their need for knowledge and information regarding disease prevention and family health care.

Together with today's emphasis on home health care, there is an increasing emphasis on family and personal responsibility for health. To help people carry out this responsibility, the American Red Cross is committed to helping persons attain and maintain their highest possible level of wellness.

The content of this book has been expanded from that of the previous textbook in order to better meet the needs of persons concerned with family health and home nursing. This new textbook should be a valuable resource for families and persons of all age groups.

Alice M. Sundberg, R.N.
National Chairman
Nursing and Health Services
American Red Cross

ACKNOWLEDGMENTS

A textbook with information focused on the broad scope of family health and home nursing necessarily reflects the personal ideas and convictions of many people. In one way or another, literally hundreds of persons and many organizations have made valuable contributions to the general direction of this book and to the selection of specific content.

Special recognition is extended to Caroline White, Ph.D., R.N., and Mary Ellen Pendergrast, M.S., R.N., who at the time of writing were members of the University of Maryland School of Nursing and who volunteered their time and unusual talents to prepare an initial draft of this book. Their task was to preserve the unique qualities of the 1963 American Red Cross *Home Nursing Textbook* and to build a design to meet the challenges of the late 1970's and the early 1980's. To them the American Red Cross and the people it serves are greatly indebted.

Reviewing of the contents, individual chapters or in total, was done by many individual experts in the fields of nursing and health and particularly home health care. In addition, volunteer and paid staff of major organizations in the health field provided valuable assistance by their critiques and advice. To those persons and organizations mentioned below and to others who may not be mentioned, the American Red Cross and those who will benefit from this textbook owe much appreciation.

Lillian Adams, R.N., American Red Cross volunteer

American Cancer Society

American Hospital Association

American Medical Association

Joan Caserta, R.N., National League for Nursing

Gita Dhillon, R.N., American Red Cross volunteer

Mary Donovan, R.N., assistant director, Nursing and Health Services, American Red Cross National Capital Division

Pearl Dunkley, Ed.D., R.N., American Nurses' Association

Helen Dunn, Visiting Nurse Service of New York

Karyle Z. Fowler, M.D.

Margaret Gallen, R.N., American Red Cross volunteer

Cyrelle Gerson, American Pharmaceutical Association

Jack Kirby, Immunization Division, Center for Disease Control

Charlotte Kopelke, R.N., Johns Hopkins Hospital

Emily Kroog, Visiting Nurse Service of New York

Joan Marren, Visiting Nurse Service of New York

Helen Maule, R.N., American Red Cross volunteer

Nancy Mills, R.P.T., Visiting Nurse Association of Northern Virginia

Barbara B. Mortensen, Bureau of Dental Health Education, American Dental Association

Joan Olden, R.N., American Nurses' Association

Lillian G. Ostrand, R.N.

John Perrin, American Osteopathic Association

Eva Reese, R.N., Visiting Nurse Service of New York

Susan Ryerson, R.P.T.

Lois O. Schwab, Ph.D., American Home Economics Association

Eleanor Williams, Ph.D.

Judy Young, Visiting Nurse Service of New York

Appreciation and recognition are also extended to Upjohn Health-Care Services, Inc. (formerly Upjohn Homemakers Home and Health Care Services, Inc.) for its generous financial assistance in support of this project and to Lois and John Gorman for their editorial assistance.

Special gratitude is extended to all American Red Cross Nursing and Health Services staff, to the American Red Cross national headquarters staff of Disaster Services and Safety Services, and to American Red Cross administration and management for their support and assistance in this project. Marcia A. Dake, Ed.D., R.N., director, Program Development, American Red Cross Nursing and Health Services, was responsible for the coordination and development of materials for this project.

INTRODUCTION

The title of this textbook has been changed from that of previous American Red Cross home care textbooks in order to more accurately reflect the book's expanded content, focused on family health and the promotion of wellness.

The first several chapters provide information to help individuals as they strive for their highest level of wellness. Important information is provided regarding the health care system and its impact on individual and family health. Suggestions about sources of health care are also included.

Several chapters focus on understanding the family as a unit and the experiences of families as they grow and develop. Information about parenthood and how to prepare for it and how to promote and maintain high-level health of both the mother and the infant is presented in some detail. This information is followed by chapters that describe the physical, psychosocial, and emotional development of children as they grow from infants to young adults.

Adulthood is an important span of life, which may cover as many as 60 or more years. Information about the characteristics of the aging process, both physical and psychological, is presented in chapter 8 to assist the home nurse in the care of adults.

Chapters 9 through 14 contain information to help persons more fully appreciate the value of high-level wellness and to follow health habits that help to prevent accidents and disease. Chapter 9 has information on threats to health such as the use of drugs and tobacco and obesity.

The structure of the family has changed, and as a result, dealing with death and terminal illness often creates special demands on family members. Chapter 10 concerns dealing with death and dying as an important aspect of life and includes information about helping the dying person live more comfortably in the time remaining. The concept of hospice care for the terminally ill is also described.

Common illnesses, how to prevent them, and how to recognize symptoms when they occur are discussed in chapters 11 and 12.

Because many families must at some time cope with health care problems that cannot be cared for in the home, alternatives to home care such as hospitalization and nursing home care are discussed in detail in chapter 13.

What to do for common emergencies in the home is covered in chapter 14.

Chapter 15 describes community planning needed to prepare for disasters. It also includes information for individual and family use in preparing for disasters.

The last several chapters of this textbook include updated material that has been the significant strength of all previous American Red Cross home nursing textbooks: the philosophy, principles, and skills for providing home care for the ill. Emphasis is placed on the importance of evaluating the patient, planning the care, and recording and reporting the findings.

The term "health professional" is used throughout the book (with minor exception), rather than the identifying of the specific health practitioner who may be the source of primary health care or advice. This approach has been used because of the changes that are continually taking place in the roles of health care providers. A brief description of many of the primary health care providers is given in the Appendix to help clarify the scope of practice for each.

This textbook is designed as a major reference for the American Red Cross Home Nursing course as well as for the American Red Cross courses Parenting, Preparation for Parenthood, Mother's Aide, and Good Grooming. In addition, it is designed as a home reference for families.

CONTENTS

Chapter 1

Health and Wellness

WHAT HEALTH AND WELLNESS ARE

The World Health Organization defines health as follows: "Health is the state of complete physical, mental, and social well-being, not merely the absence of disease or infirmity." Or, to put it another way, health is an active state, a continual and dynamic balancing of physical, mental, and social requirements. Health includes the daily ability to function fruitfully and the knowledge to live in harmony with ourselves and our environment.

Although the goal of health is the complete well-being of each person, not all of us can achieve this goal for ourselves. But most of us *can,* through our own efforts, move upward on the scale of health in the direction of that goal. This type of active growth toward the goal of complete health is called high-level wellness. High-level wellness exists when the whole person—body, mind, and spirit—functions at the greatest potential for which the individual is capable, within the environment where he finds himself. Some persons enjoy high-level wellness even if they have a physical handicap. They have been able to adapt their way of doing things so that they derive satisfaction and function at their greatest capacity.

SIGNS OF HEALTH

Common signs of health that are easily recognizable include having—

- Energy more than adequate for daily activities
- Resistance to common colds and communicable diseases
- General happiness and positive attitudes
- The ability to cope with everyday stress without undue anxiety
- Skin that is firm and alive-looking, neither clammy nor dry, and free from rash, swellings, or blemishes
- Eyes that are bright, clear, and responsive, with eyelids free from inflammation
- Erect posture, with head, shoulders, and hips in good alignment
- Body weight evenly distributed
- Hair that is shining, and a scalp that is free from dandruff
- Teeth that are clean and without cavities or pain
- Gums of good color, without bleeding or tenderness
- Good muscle tone (ease in running and walking)
- The ability to relax, rest, and sleep well

- The ability to adapt to change
- Willingness to assume responsibility, with a feeling of satisfaction from doing both small and large jobs well
- Realistic short-term and long-range goals

MENTAL AND EMOTIONAL HEALTH

Mental attitudes play an important role in physical health. A person's personality (physical and mental actions and attitudes) develops throughout life. As a person grows older, personality characteristics are intensified. Each person needs to grow in self-understanding and self-acceptance, to better understand his own behavior and reactions. The person who understands himself can more easily make the effort to be friendly and outgoing and can enjoy a richer and more satisfying life.

Good mental health is easily recognized. It includes the ability to get along with oneself, the ability to get along with others, and the ability to adjust to changing situations. Although there may be a temporary upset in any of these areas, the ability for a person to make adjustments in his daily living is basic to his mental, and therefore physical, well-being.

All people want about the same things from life: something to do, someone to love, a place to live, health, and security. People experience great stress when they are lonely or have a deep sense of not being wanted, needed, or noticed. No one can escape some degree of stress, because it is a part of living. How a person reacts to stress, injury, or illness is often determined by training and habit, inherited tendencies, and past experience. Although there are no hard-and-fast rules for solving life's problems, the worry and tension these problems can bring can be lessened. Many people have found the following guidelines to be helpful:

- Take time for relaxation and play. There are many inexpensive hobbies and activities that provide relaxation.
- Keep physically fit. Mental and physical health are closely related, and your physical condition affects your overall outlook on life.
- Relieve feelings of tension, anxiety, or anger by physical activity that brings on relaxation or healthy fatigue. (Take a long walk, go swimming, dig in the garden.)

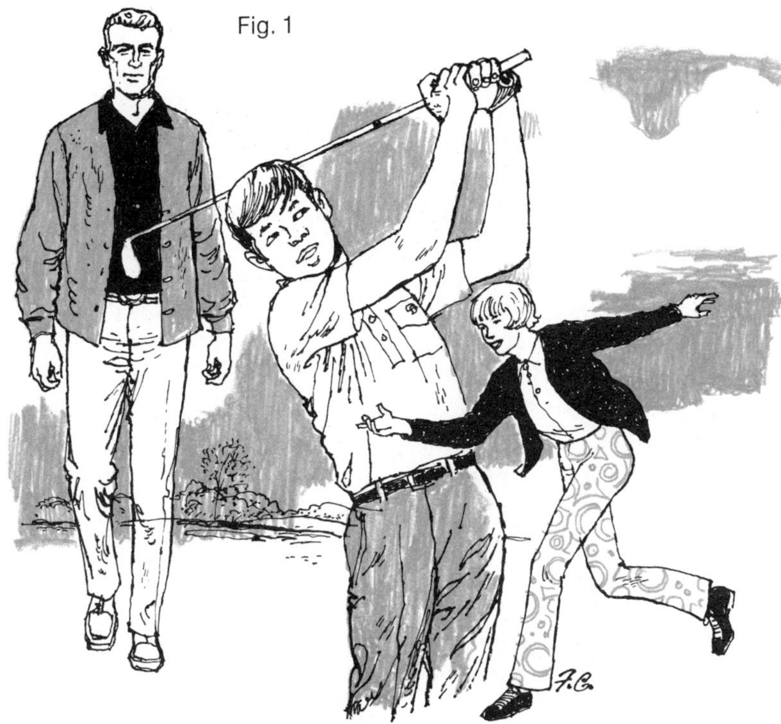

Fig. 1

- Share your troubles with someone. A good friend or a clergyman can often help to put your problems into proper perspective and to find a solution.
- Accept what cannot be changed. It is useless to fight against circumstances over which you have no control. It is also better for your mental health and social interaction to learn to understand and accept people as they are rather than to try to change them.
- Challenge yourself daily to improve your environment, living conditions, or health habits. (For example, stop smoking.)

THE ROLE OF THE INDIVIDUAL AND THE FAMILY IN MAINTAINING HEALTH

The primary responsibility for promoting and protecting health rests with the individual and the family. Every person should practice good health habits and should know the signs of illness that indicate the need for professional assistance. He should understand the effects of his own actions on the health of others (public health) and should be aware of health services available through the various levels of government and through voluntary health organizations.

The actions of individuals and families can affect the health of the entire community as well as their own health. People who fail to receive immunizations as needed not only risk disease themselves but add to the risk of an epidemic as well. People who are careless with garbage encourage the growth of harmful bacteria and rats and thus may cause disease throughout the whole community. Individuals and families should take the following steps to insure a high level of wellness for all:

- Know and practice the good health habits such as good nutrition, cleanliness, and exercise that are outlined in chapter 2.
- Know the signs of illness that demand treatment by a health professional. Changes in attitudes, feelings, and appearance, as well as physical symptoms, may indicate illness. See chapter 11 for more information on signs and symptoms that may call for professional health care.
- Use community health resources such as immunization programs to protect both personal and community health. Immunizations must be kept up to date in order to provide protection against the diseases, and all members of the family should receive them. (See immunization chart, page 139.)
- Participate in local efforts and political processes that influence the quality and availability of health services in the community.
- Get regular medical and dental checkups.

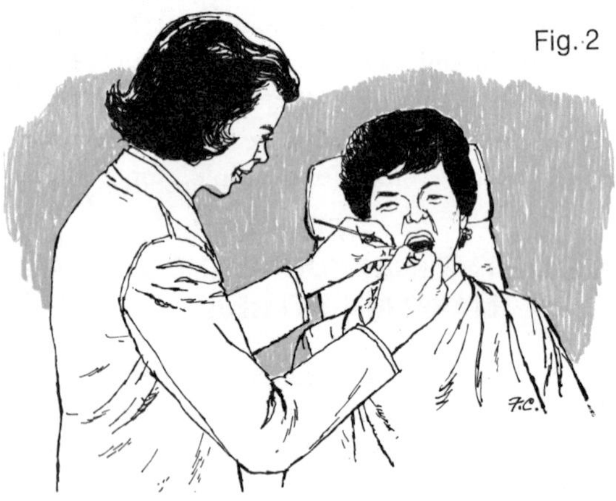

Fig. 2

Regular visits to health professionals provide the opportunity to ask general questions about maintaining good health. Some illnesses can be detected even before the individual is aware of any symptoms. Early treatment is easier and more effective and may prevent more serious illness later on. A yearly physical checkup by a health professional provides the occasion for checking blood pressure and doing tests to determine possible existence of such conditions as diabetes (done by testing for sugar in the urine or the blood), cancer of the cervix in women (done by Pap smear), cancer of the colon (by rectal examination), and glaucoma (by examination for tension in the eyes). The health professional will also assist the individual to obtain necessary immunizations on schedule. Every member of the family should have a regular source of health care. Dentists will usually advise how often each person should have a dental checkup.

THE HEALTH CARE SYSTEM

Individuals and families need the help of many persons, agencies, and institutions to promote and safeguard their health. All of these are considered to be parts of the health care system. In some way, each affects the individual's success in reaching his state of high-level wellness.

Health care professionals include physicians, nurses, dentists, pharmacists, psychologists, and other types of health specialists (see information on health professionals in the Appendix). Most health care professionals have special training and have to pass examinations that require knowledge and skill in their specialty. Health professionals* are licensed by the state, and a license can be taken away if a professional does not meet standards set for his kind of practice.

It is important for individuals and families to have a regular source of health care, to have a health professional who can give regular checkups and care when illnesses or accidents occur. Better health care can be given if the health professional knows the person's or the family's health history. If, for example, one health source has the records of a whole family, that health source can be sure that children have immunizations at the right age. If one family member has

*As mentioned in the Introduction, the term "health professional" will be used in this book when reference is made to doctor, nurse, pharmacist, or other, because the practice of health professionals is changing and may differ widely in some places.

diabetes, the health professional involved will be sure to advise other members on good habits and regular checkups.

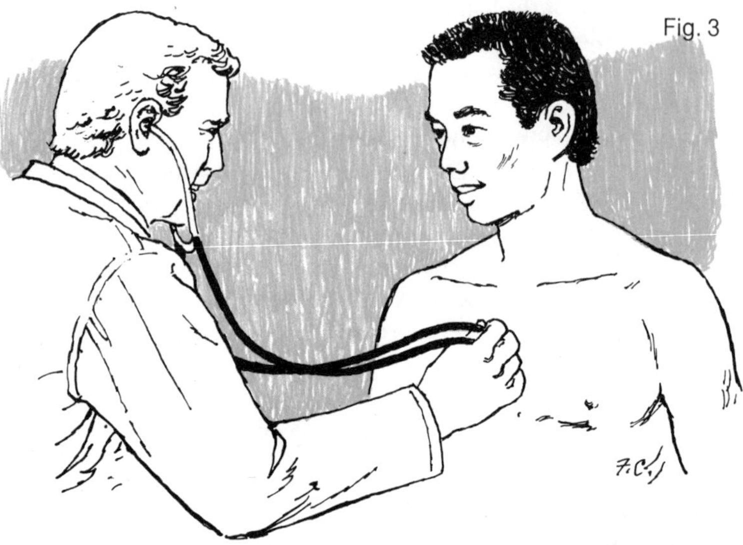

Fig. 3

The old idea of having a family primary health care provider is still sound. In some rural areas where there are not many physicians, one doctor or a registered nurse specialized as a nurse practitioner may serve an entire family. In other places, it is important to have contact with a primary health care provider, a physician (usually an internist), a nurse practitioner, or a specific clinic or group of health care professionals. The primary care provider or clinic will have the "whole picture" of family health and can make referrals to a specialist, such as a pediatrician, when needed.

How To Find a Primary Health Care Provider

Physicians, dentists, and registered nurse practitioners sometimes practice in individual offices, or they sometimes work together in groups of two or more health professionals. If they work in groups, all of the group may have the same specialty (such as obstetrics), or they may have persons with different specialties in the group (such as internist, obstetrician, or pediatrician). Group practice of health professionals is becoming more common.

Finding a physician, dentist, nurse practitioner, or other health care professional is a special job when a family or an individual moves to a new area. The primary care providers who have been caring for the family can often suggest someone in the new community. The local medical society or the local health department will usually give a list of health professionals who will accept new patients. The local hospital or a university medical or health center will also give suggestions. Remember that none of these agencies will give advice about a specific skill or ability; they will only assure the potential patient that the health professional is licensed in his specialty. It is sometimes helpful to ask friends, relatives, or neighbors about where they get their health care.

Health professionals may see patients in their office, in hospital emergency rooms, in outpatient departments, in ambulatory care centers, or sometimes in public health clinics. Health care may also be given in schools, at work, or at the offices of voluntary health organizations. In some cities, there are free clinics where service is given by volunteer health professionals.

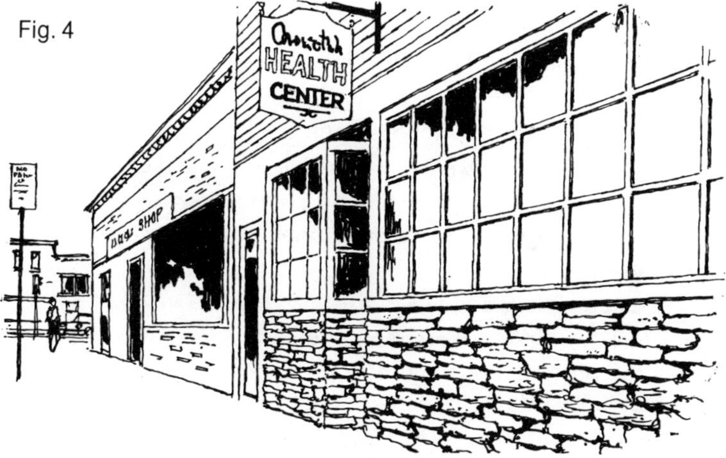

Fig. 4

Health care may also be given at home. Home health services began in the early 1880s with the establishment of the visiting nurse associations (VNAs). Today, referrals to home health service agencies or agencies that provide "meals on wheels" are made as appropriate at most major hospitals. These hospitals have a home health care coordination program, headed by a registered nurse or other professional and designed to plan and coordinate care in the home before a patient's discharge. In addition to VNAs, other agencies, established in the 1960s (with the advent of Medicare) to give skilled nursing care in the home, include a home health agency of a special area, nonprofit agencies, and proprietary home health agencies. City and county health departments are assuming more responsibility for community home care service under extended care. In addition, health maintenance organizations (HMOs) and some hospitals regularly employ community health nurses to give extended care in the home.

What To Look For in a Health Professional

Even after you have obtained the names of health care professionals or sources of health care, there are questions for you to consider before making a decision. A choice must be made, and it is helpful to have other facts:

- What kinds of services does the clinic or group offer?
- Is the doctor certified by a specialty board to practice as a specialist? (Certification of physicians means that they have a higher level of specialized knowledge and training than those who have the basic M.D. degree.)
- Does the clinic offer the services of a nurse practitioner?
- What are the office hours and what care is available other than during office hours for illness or injury?
- Will questions be answered over the telephone and during or outside office hours? Is there a charge for this service?
- Is there a registered professional nurse in the office who assists with health care?
- What are the costs and how must they be paid?
- In which hospital (if there is more than one in your community) does the physician or the health professional practice? Does the patient have a choice if there is need to go to the hospital?
- Can the physician make referrals when the patient is moving to a new location, and will the physician transfer the appropriate records?

These kinds of questions can be asked when you choose any kind of health care service. It is important to have this information about dentists, obstetricians, pediatricians, and other health care professionals.

Once you have chosen your health professional, do not think that you cannot change to another. It is important for a patient and a physician, a dentist, or a nurse practitioner to work well together toward the goal of high-level wellness. If such harmony does not exist, it may be a good idea to make a change. It is not wise, however, to change health professionals too often.

There are certain things you should expect of your health professional and there are certain things he should expect of you. You and the health professional together should have one common goal: the highest possible level of wellness for you, the patient.

One of the most important ways in which to help the health professional help you is through *honesty.* His success in treating you depends on his having all the facts. In fact, treatment can be very harmful if it is based on wrong or incomplete information. You should answer all questions and give any necessary information. Sometimes, asking questions yourself helps get to the real problem. *Always ask questions* if you do not understand what the health professional has said.

Health professionals should explain—

- Their opinion of your health problem
- The plan for your care
- The cost of the treatment
- What can be expected from the treatment, both good and possibly bad results
- What might happen if nothing is done

Common courtesies between individuals and health professionals include—

- Appointments kept on time or changed ahead of time if they cannot be kept
- Insurance information presented by the patient at the appointment so that health professionals can use it properly
- Itemized bills sent promptly and paid promptly
- Discussion taken place and agreement arrived at by both on the plan of treatment

Sometimes people have very serious questions about the plan of treatment that has been suggested. It is almost always reasonable to get the advice of a second specialist (a consultation), particularly if the treatment is very expensive or serious in nature. The health professional should be willing to share your personal record with other health professionals if you make the request. In the case of a problem between a patient and a health professional that seems hard to solve, the local medical society or the administrator of the hospital (if the problem occurs in a hospital) can usually be helpful.

The Government and Public Health

The Constitution of the United States defines certain areas of responsibility in which the federal government must protect the health and well-being of the nation's citizens. Any area of health and welfare that is not specifically assigned to the federal government is the responsibility of state governments.

It is the responsibility of the federal, state, and local governments to insure that there are safe and healthful conditions in every community and state, and in the entire nation. The government takes steps to protect the health of the public from the carelessness of the few, and it is especially concerned with preventing the spread of disease. Preventive measures include—

- Insuring that there is sanitary drinking water and sewage disposal
- Inspecting and regulating the quality of food and inspecting food establishments to insure that there is sanitary handling of food
- Requiring that new houses and buildings meet government health and safety standards for plumbing, electric wiring, and waste disposal
- Licensing physicians, nurses, dentists, and other health professionals
- Insuring that hospitals, nursing homes, and day-care centers meet standards of safe care
- Providing immunization programs
- Providing medical and financial assistance to people in special need of help, such as the poor, the elderly, the handicapped, and disaster victims
- Sponsoring research on illness
- Carefully controlling the use and safety of drugs
- Providing education on health matters through the schools and in special publications and courses
- Providing emergency assistance for a variety of problems through police and fire departments

Federal Government

In general, the federal government has authority and responsibility in three broad areas of public health:

- General concern for the health of the people of the nation
- Prevention of the spread of disease from one state to another
- Prevention of the introduction of disease from outside the United States

To carry out its responsibilities, the federal government studies national and international health problems. It conducts studies and research on all aspects of disease, including prevention. It helps control the spread of disease from one state to another by controlling the movement of animals, plants, fruits and vegetables, and infected persons. To prevent the entry of diseases from other countries, the government requires that goods and people meet certain health standards before entering the country. Legislation is also developed to promote health and prevent disease.

The federal government assists states in their public health programs in many ways. The purpose of federal assistance to states for health programs is to be certain that the basic health needs of all people are met. Since many states do not have enough tax money to provide good health programs for the protection of their citizens, federal grants help these states meet national standards in essential programs.

Participating Agencies

Most health activities of the federal government are carried out under the supervision of the United States Department of Health, Education, and Welfare (HEW). An important agency under HEW is the United States Public Health Service (USPHS), which is under the direction of the assistant secretary for health. The functions of the Public Health Service are to provide consultation to state health departments as well as to conduct and support research in health and allied sciences. The USPHS also serves as the federal agency that deals with other nations in international health matters. The operating agencies of the USPHS and their main functions are listed below:

- Food and Drug Administration (FDA)—The purpose of the FDA is to protect the health of the nation against impure and unsafe foods, drugs, cosmetics, and other potential hazards.

- National Institutes of Health (NIH)—The mission of the NIH is to improve the health of the American people by means of biomedical research into the causes, prevention, and cure of diseases. The NIH also shares biomedical information. Cancer and heart research, as well as mental health projects, are part of the agency's function.

Fig. 5

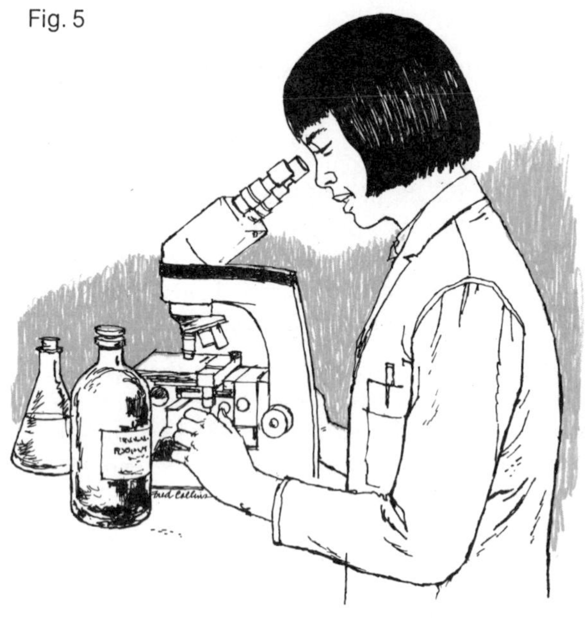

- Center for Disease Control (CDC)—The CDC administers national programs for the prevention and control of communicable diseases and other preventable diseases. The center also provides services and educational programs in special fields of health, such as smoking. It directs and enforces foreign quarantine activities and works with other departments to assure safe and healthful working conditions for working people.
- Health Resources Administration (HRA)—The HRA has responsibility for health manpower training, health planning and development, and the gathering and analysis of health statistics.
- Health Services Administration (HSA)—The HSA provides assistance to states and administers the Indian Health Service and public health clinics and hospitals for Coast Guard and Public Health Service Commissioned Corps personnel.

Medicare and Medicaid

Medicare and Medicaid are two major federal programs that are particularly important to individuals for payment of personal health services. Both programs were started in 1965.

Medicare and Medicaid are not static programs: their requirements have continued to be adapted to the economic, social, and political climate in each state. New programs and practices have been designed to meet special circumstances and needs, and some old programs and practices have been discarded. It is expected that future legislation affecting Medicare and Medicaid will be more and more concerned with meeting medical, nursing, and health needs for the nation's entire population at a reasonable cost.

Medicare

The Medicare program is administered by the Social Security Administration under the supervision of the U.S. Department of Health, Education, and Welfare. It is an insurance program that pays part, but not all, of hospital and posthospital costs (Part A) or medical costs, whether or not the insured is or has been hospitalized (Part B). Medicare is for persons aged 65 and over, for any permanently and totally disabled persons who have been getting social security disability benefits for 2 years or more, and for any person insured under social security who suffers from chronic kidney disease and needs a kidney transplant or dialysis treatment.

The hospital insurance part of the program (Part A) is financed mostly through social security payroll contributions paid by employees, employers, and self-employed people covered under social security. Under Part B, the supplementary medical insurance, a person may choose to buy outpatient medical insurance at a small monthly premium charge. Under both Parts A and B of Medicare, an annual fee is deducted from social security checks or sent to the U.S. Treasury by persons not on social security. A percentage of the bills from doctors, hospitals, and other health providers is paid by Medicare.

For further information on Medicare, especially on benefits, get a copy of *Your Medicare Handbook* from your local Social Security office or the post office. If you still have questions after reading the book, call the nearest Social Security office.

Persons who want to enroll in the program should apply for a Medicare card and investigate the benefits under Medicare 3 months before they turn 65. It may take several weeks to process an application. A birth certificate or other proof of age is needed when you make application. It is also possible to apply for a Medicare card by mail. If there is no Social Security office in your area, call the office in the nearest town. Collect calls will be accepted from areas that do not have Social Security offices.

Medicaid

Medicaid is a joint federal-state medical assistance program to help pay medical bills for four groups of low-income people: (1) the aged, (2) the blind, (3) the disabled, and (4) families with dependent children. States design and administer their own programs, consistent with the federal guidelines. County or city welfare, public assistance, or public health offices operate the programs for the state.

Eligibility requirements for Medicaid assistance vary from state to state. However, only the four groups of people are eligible for Medicaid. Others whose incomes and resources are large enough to cover daily living expenses but not large enough to pay for medical care may be eligible in some states. Information about eligibility can be obtained from local Social Security or welfare offices.

All state Medicaid programs pay according to federal guidelines for at least the following services to people of all ages who fit into the four categories:

- Inpatient hospital care and outpatient hospital services
- Laboratory and X-ray services
- Skilled nursing home services
- Physicians' services wherever provided
- Family planning services
- Home health care services
- Psychiatric services for those under 21 years of age

Some state Medicaid programs pay for the following services for the same groups:

- Dental care
- Intermediate care facility services
- Prescribed drugs and eyeglasses
- Clinic services

- Physical therapy
- Podiatrists' and chiropractors' services
- Care in mental institutions
- Any other medical or remedial care recognized under state law

For more information on Medicaid or on eligibility or how to apply for the program, call the local Social Security office. For services, call the local welfare department.

State Government and Public Health

State governments have the responsibility and authority to protect the health of the people in their state. States also have broad authority to organize their own governing bodies, usually called boards of health, to develop programs to meet the needs of their people.

Although there are some differences, laws regulating health matters are similar in most states. States must follow or meet federal guidelines and regulations for programs where there is federal funding or authority. State health departments set standards through licensing programs and through enforcing sanitary codes and health laws. State standards may be exceeded by some local health departments but must be met by all local health departments and agencies.

Most state health departments have highly qualified public health professionals as administrators who are assisted by staff prepared in various public health fields. Some state health departments provide direct services to local communities when there is a lack of local facilities or a scarcity of personnel.

Functions of state health departments change as health problems change. The health needs of citizens are analyzed as a basis of program priority. All state health departments keep statistics on births, deaths, and reportable diseases. These are known as vital statistics.

Local Government and Public Health

Any town, city, or county agency may function as the local health department, with authority and responsibility to protect and promote public health and high-level wellness. The health department gets money to run programs from local and state taxes. Federal funds are available to cover the cost of special programs. In most communities, the people decide how much health service and education they will support by approving or not approving taxes and by showing their feelings through other actions.

In general, all local health departments have the same broad responsibilities. Some services are routine, such as being sure the public water supply is safe. Other services are geared more directly toward the health of the total community, such as the inspecting and the licensing of restaurants and public eating places.

Local health departments are expected to enforce state and federal regulations to control communicable diseases. In the mid-1970s, studies showed that health officials had not been enforcing such regulations related to immunizations, and parents and school officials had become careless. Large numbers of preschool- and school-age children had not been immunized against measles, whooping cough, rubella, and polio; thus epidemics of these diseases were a threat. Preventable diseases had caused an unaffordable loss through human suffering, needless death, and dollars spent for care. This waste is a good example of a public health problem.

In some communities, health supervision of school children is a function of the local health department and includes physical examinations, vision testing, hearing testing, and general health counseling. Many local health departments also provide such services for the individual as diagnostic and treatment clinics, health screening clinics conducted by nurses for senior citizens, clinics that provide health supervision for well infants and children, prenatal and postnatal care, classes for expectant parents, and dental care, especially for children.

An important service offered by many health departments is health education. Facts about good health habits and suggestions to help young people and older people reach their highest possible level of wellness are provided without cost. Health hints and news may be shared by radio, television, newspapers, movies, posters, and pamphlets. Frequently, special speakers are provided for group meetings. The goal of health education is to get all people in the community to take actions that will keep them at a high level of wellness.

Almost all health departments at the local, state, and federal levels have some paid staff to carry out their functions. Most local departments have a health officer (usually a physician) and one or more nurses on their staff. If the staff is small, there may be only a registered nurse. Nurses make visits to homes to give advice about health and may teach how to care for babies or sick persons. Local programs are started and supported, depending on community involvement and interest, community health needs, local and state budgets, the leadership and vision of the professional staff, and staff availability.

Rural clinics under the direction of nurse practitioners and physician assistants were established in 1978 to bring health services to people who had none prior to the establishment of such clinics. The overall supervision of the staff is by a physician.

Population shifts have required that certain health programs and services be adapted, cut back, or strengthened. For example, since the child population tends to be centered in the suburbs today, more maternal and child health services are required there. Since an older age group tends to remain in the cities, there is often a need for more nursing homes and long-term home nursing services there. Also, the child population remaining in the cities tends to be mostly in low-income groups, who often have many health needs.

It is not certain what the future activities of health departments will be, but it can be expected that they will change to meet changing needs. What is certain is that there are more and more older people in most communities, and that there are more people with long-term illnesses.

Most older couples and families, older single persons without families, and persons with long-term or chronic illnesses need the help and support of the community and its agencies. The quality of health service and education programs in the future will depend on how well the government, the people, and all groups concerned with health work together.

National Health Planning and Resources Development Act

Like the health maintenance organizations, the National Health Planning and Resources Development Act (NHP&RDA, 1975) was designed to provide for the two major trends in health care today: comprehensive care for all people and protection of the rights of consumers.

The task of providing comprehensive health care for everyone and the involvement of the consumer in decisions about his care includes assuring (1) that all people have access, without financial or other barriers, to the whole spectrum of health services and (2) that they have access to a meaningful personal relationship with at least one health professional in order to provide continuity of service. This relationship may be with a physician, a nurse practitioner, a paraprofessional, or a member of a team of health professionals having different specialties, through which coordination and referral to appropriate resources would be instituted. For people in the United States who receive insufficient health services, the further need for personal or family relationship to health professionals and primary care services should be emphasized.

Payment for Health Care Services

Because health care services are so expensive, few people can pay their health care bills without assistance from an outside source. Being prepared to meet health care costs through insurance is similar to having insurance protection against other kinds of disasters, such as home fires and automobile accidents. The Medicare and Medicaid programs of the federal government are one source of health care assistance. Health maintenance organizations (HMOs) are another source. The HMO approach includes an insurance type of program along with a plan of care (see page 22).

The majority of Americans are financially protected against the cost risks of illness by insurance coverage provided by, or at least through, their employer's group health insurance plan. For those persons who do not have the advantage of insurance through their employer, there are professional, social, occupational, and other groups that offer the opportunity to obtain such insurance through a group plan. For example, the American Association of Retired Persons, some banks, and the American Automobile Association are different types of organizations that have group health or hospital insurance plans available to their members. With hospital costs ranging in the hundreds of dollars per day, having an inpatient insurance protection is a near necessity.

It is important for individuals and families to check their insurance plans carefully for the types of care that are covered. Is nursing, dental, or home health care covered? Are the costs of maternity, labor, and delivery covered? Does the policy provide full coverage of the cost or are there limits to the money that will be paid for certain types of care? It is wise to know what your insurance will cover before an emergency occurs. It is also wise for you to carry information about your insurance with you at all times. Usually, a small, wallet-size identification card is provided by the insurance company.

Voluntary Organizations and Agencies

Although most major public health programs are funded by tax dollars, the American way of life includes being a good neighbor. This means that there will always be private voluntary health organizations through which individuals can share their experience, talents, and money to help others. Voluntary health organizations educate people in good health habits, in the prevention of disease, and in the care necessary for those who suffer from specific diseases or injuries. They help to draw attention to major health problems. These organizations are not supported by taxes but by money donated by private individuals or groups in local communities. Both public (tax) and private (nontax) dollars are required to provide services needed to fight certain diseases. For example, the American Cancer Society helps persons privately who have cancer and provides funds for research, while the federal government carries out such research at the National Cancer Institute and provides funds to institutions and individuals to do research.

Although money in the form of private gifts and donations is received from people in local communities, many organizations are national in scope. The control that the national office has over local programs and services varies.

There are two important facts to be remembered about most voluntary health organizations: (1) their work is financed by privately donated dollars and (2) the major leadership and service is given by volunteers. Although many organizations, such as the American Red Cross, do have a paid staff in their national and local offices, the volunteers give the actual, direct leadership and service to millions of people—such as teaching people to take blood pressure or to give care to sick family members at home.

Other kinds of organizations, often started by persons interested in a specific disease or health problem, include the American Heart

Association, the National Society for the Prevention of Blindness, the National Multiple Sclerosis Society, and the National Foundation–March of Dimes (see Appendix for others).

Special Groups

There are special groups, such as those with primarily a religious affiliation, that carry out a wide range of health-related activities. Though the parent organization may be of a specific religious denomination (Catholics, Latter-Day Saints, Methodists, etc.), its activities may serve all persons. Special hospitals or nursing homes are a good example of one such type of activity. Other groups (Amish, Menonites, Seventh Day Adventists, Baptists, etc.) make a great contribution through their education and direct health care programs.

Insurance companies have also long been active in the field of education to promote health. They have made available many excellent booklets and other teaching materials to help the public learn about health.

Health Maintenance Organizations

Health maintenance organizations (HMOs) reflect two major trends in medicine and in the official approach to health care: toward comprehensive health care for all people and toward emphasis on the rights of consumers. An HMO differs from other clinics by requiring an annual payment whether or not the service is used. Payment is not based on "fee for service."

HMOs provide a defined range of health care services to their members. These services usually include preventive services, which are important to all members, young and old. Individuals and groups contract with an HMO, which then becomes their "health care delivery system." Members pay a premium, for which they receive complete hospital and medical care services as needed, usually at little or no additional cost.

The role of the health care consumer is expanding from that of patient to include the roles of planner, implementer, and assessor of the evolving health care system. Patients are having a stronger and stronger voice and vote in influencing medical technology advances, health programming, and services–developing, implementing, evaluating, coordinating, setting priorities, and making decisions.

Consumers are now playing an active advisory role within health maintenance organizations. The management of these organizations is accountable legally, fiscally, publicly, and professionally.

Although HMOs generally prefer to have people enroll early in life, so that their health care can be handled continuously by one group of health practitioners, some HMOs do accept new enrollees who are 65 or older. In addition, not all HMOs will cover treatment for chronic conditions, such as diabetes and heart disease, if the person had the disease before becoming a member. Check with the HMO in your area to determine whether you are eligible to join.

The relationship of Medicare and Medicaid to the local HMO should be checked out by eligible persons. In some areas, the small HMO premium will cover those costs that Medicare's hospital insurance will not pay, plus all the services offered by Medicare's medical insurance plan. In other words, in some areas it might be less costly for a Medicare recipient to join an HMO rather than pay the monthly premiums for Medicare's medical insurance plan.

Each person should check with the local HMO for eligibility requirements and information about coverage. Compare the local HMO plan with Medicare or Medicaid coverage so that the best possible coverage at the lowest possible cost can be selected. Information about HMOs can be obtained from Group Health Association of America, 1717 Massachusetts Avenue, N.W., Washington, D.C. 20036. Ask for the address of the HMO nearest you.

INTERNATIONAL HEALTH

The outbreak in the United States of a disease called Russian flu should serve as a reminder that the level of wellness throughout the entire world affects persons in all parts of the world. The fact that man has walked on the moon adds to the reality that geographic separation of countries no longer separates man from man in any part of the world. These facts increase the need for persons to be concerned about world health. The federal government has responsibility for world health as it affects the people of the United States. There are also international agencies and organizations that have as a major part of their function activities to promote health, especially in underdeveloped countries.

The World Health Organization, organized in 1948, and the Pan American Health Organization, organized in 1924, are the two major international organizations through which the federal government joins with governments of other countries to promote health of all people. The activities of these organizations are focused on problems of health and disease that affect people of the whole world or of several countries. For example, the control of malaria or diphtheria is a worldwide problem. Smallpox has been eliminated throughout the world.

A voluntary international health association known by both children and adults in the United States is the United Nations International Children's Emergency Fund (UNICEF). It has now become the custom to encourage children to help provide food and health care to children of the world by collecting "pennies for UNICEF" rather than "treats" for themselves at Halloween. Project HOPE and Cooperative for American Relief Everywhere (CARE) are less well known but no less important. CARE, established in 1945, is a good example of a joint effort between governments and concerned people to provide support for education and services that affect the health and welfare of people. Medical International Cooperation Organization (MEDICO), founded in 1958, is a service of CARE that provides the system through which volunteer physicians provide medical care in underdeveloped countries.

Many national voluntary health organizations work with similar organizations in other countries through an international organization. For example, the National Multiple Sclerosis Society is a member agency of the International Multiple Sclerosis Society. The American Red Cross is a member of the League of Red Cross Societies and the International Committee of the Red Cross. The International Committee of the Red Cross, with headquarters in Geneva, Switzerland, was founded in 1863 and contributes to the improvement of international humanitarian law. The League of Red Cross Societies is a world federation of Red Cross societies. It was founded in 1919 and is also located in Geneva. The League's primary role is to promote cooperation among its member societies and coordinate their efforts, particularly in meeting the needs of victims of great natural disasters and refugees from war situations. The American Red Cross cooperates with other countries through sharing information about its services and sharing its educational materials. Some Red Cross instructional material, such as the home nursing textbooks of the past, have been translated into as many as 15 or 20 different languages.

MIRACLE CURES AND QUACKS

Be on guard against those who promise miracle cures. Useless treatments waste a lot of money. They may also keep a person from getting good medical help when needed, while the condition may become worse. Be careful of persons who—

- Advertise in or are promoted by popular magazines
- Use people's words of praise to support their expertise
- Say the medical profession is against them, trying to cover up their "great cure"
- Promise instant and certain results

If a health care professional has been selected from a list of names given by the sources mentioned earlier, he will be licensed.

FINDING OTHER HEALTH RESOURCES

The help you need is often other than medical care, such as medical supplies or equipment for the home or major extended nursing care outside the home. Remember that most health professionals are good sources of general health information. The local health department is also prepared and willing to answer general questions. In large cities, the health department has many different offices and provides a variety of services.

Chapter 2

How To Stay Healthy

Health is one of the most valuable human possessions. Most persons can maintain it by carrying out sound health practices. Eating the right kinds and amounts of foods will usually assure having a smoothly functioning body and enough energy for everyday activities. Adequate exercise improves the functioning of all systems of the body—digestive, nervous, muscular, and circulatory. Maintaining the body and the environment in ways that control the growth of bacteria or virus, the spread of infection, and the possibility of accidents will do much to develop a high level of wellness.

Good health habits in regard to nutrition, exercise, cleanliness, and safety do much to prevent weight-gaining, poor teeth and gums, constipation, frequent colds, and many other conditions or illnesses that threaten health or life. Suggestions in this chapter, if carried out, can help a person live a healthier, happier, and longer life.

FOOD AND NUTRITION

The human body in its functioning is more amazing than the finest watch or the most intricate machine. But like a machine, the body needs fuel to maintain its operation. Every breath, every heartbeat, every movement of the body requires energy, and that energy is supplied from only one source: food. Unlike a machine, however, the body can often repair itself if conditions are favorable.

Foods are composed of nutrients, and each nutrient has its own special function. Proteins, fats, sugars and starches, vitamins, and minerals are used in building, maintaining, and repairing body tissues, providing warmth and energy, and regulating the body processes. Each day, a person should choose those foods that will supply the nutrients needed by the body. No single food can furnish all the nutrients needed. If a person understands the food needs of the body and the composition of the more common foods, it is easier to plan meals that are both adequate and varied, taking into account what foods are available, personal choice, and cost.

A person who feels run down, tired, and unable to work may simply be suffering from an inadequate diet. Sometimes illness occurs because of a serious lack of one or more of the specific nutrients that the body must have to function properly. On the other hand, the most serious diet-related illnesses in the United States are more closely linked to overeating of food or of certain food components than to undereating. Overeating of fat, particularly saturated fat, and cholesterol contribute to high blood lipid levels, which, in turn, increase the risk of coronary heart disease. High salt consumption contributes to hypertension in persons who are genetically predisposed to this disorder. High caloric intake from too much food contributes to obesity, and high sugar intake contributes to tooth decay.

Nutrients—Their Functions and Sources

Since the choice of foods should be based on the body's needs, a person should become familiar with the essential nutrients, their functions in the body, and their most common sources in foods.

Sugars and Starches

Sugars and starches (carbohydrates) are important sources of energy. How much energy a given food will produce when oxidized in the body is measured in calories. Sugars occur naturally in fruits; refined sugar is a principal ingredient in candy, soft drinks, and desserts. Refined sugar contains only calories but no nutrients; its use should be strictly limited. Starches are found principally in bread and baked goods, cereals, rice, and macaroni.

Fig. 6

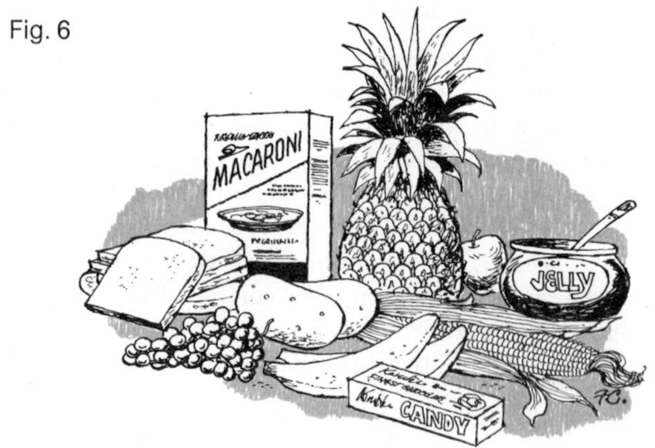

Fats

Fats are also needed for energy. They move more slowly through the digestive tract than other foods and they tend to delay feelings of hunger. Fats are higher in calories than starches, sugars, or proteins; thus, small amounts can greatly increase the calorie intake. Eating lean meats and preparing meats by broiling or roasting rather than by frying helps to reduce the amount of fat eaten. Foods high in saturated fats tend to increase blood cholesterol levels. Foods high in saturated fats include beef, pork, lamb, whole milk, cream, cheddar cheese, and cream cheese. Fish, poultry, and salad oils (corn, soybean, and safflower oils) tend to be high in polyunsaturated fats and low in saturated fats.

Fig. 7

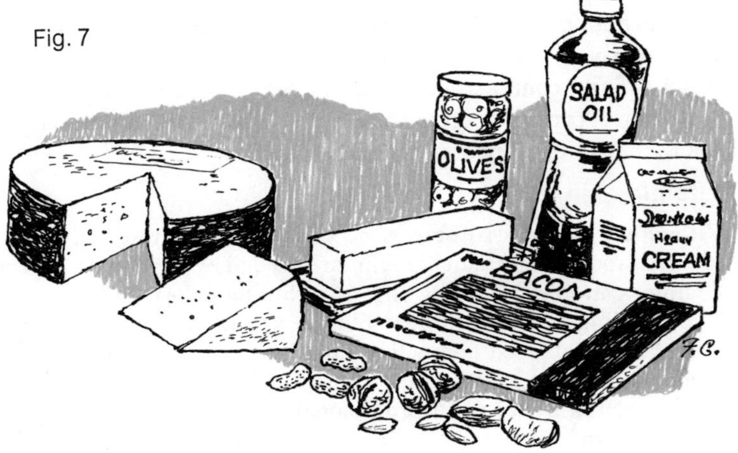

Proteins

Proteins are essential to the growth, maintenance, and repair of body tissue. If not enough calories are supplied in the diet from sugar, starch, or fat, proteins will be oxidized for energy. This is an expensive use of protein. Proteins are essential in the diet for building and maintaining body tissues; no other nutrient can perform this function. Proteins form a structural part of skin, hair, nails, muscles, connective tissue, and all the body organs.

Proteins are made up of amino acids. Of the more than 20 amino acids, some are essential to the body because the body cannot manufacture them. Proteins that contain all of the essential amino acids are known as complete proteins. Animal foods such as meat, poultry, fish, eggs, milk, and cheese contain complete proteins (Fig. 8).

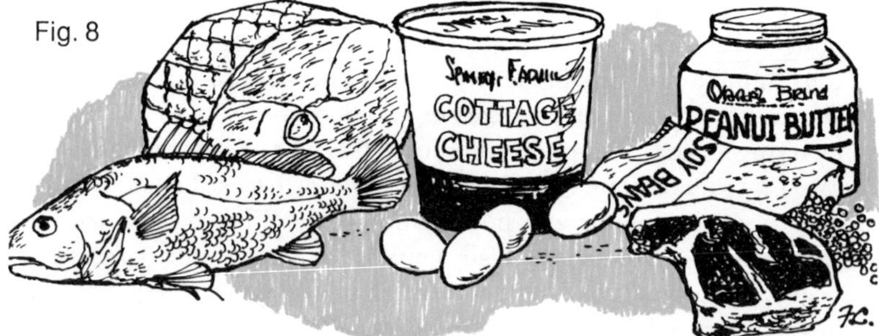

Fig. 8

Incomplete proteins are those that are low in one or more of the essential amino acids. Most plant proteins are incomplete; however, one plant source can be combined with another to form a complete protein. Thus, combinations such as rice and beans and corn and beans form complete proteins. Breads, cereal grains, and dried beans, therefore, contribute protein to the diet.

Vitamins

Vitamins are organic substances necessary for regulating body processes. Although only small amounts are needed by the body, a lack of vitamins can have crippling effects, including deformed bones, delayed healing of wounds, night blindness, and even severe depression. A well-balanced diet will usually insure a sufficient supply of vitamins for good health. Supplemental vitamins should be taken *only* if ordered by a health professional; excesses of some vitamins may be harmful.

Vitamin A contributes to the normal development of bones and teeth and enables a person to see well in dim light. Rough, dry skin and night blindness may be signs of a vitamin A deficiency. Foods rich in vitamin A include fish, liver oils, liver, whole milk, butter, margarine, cheese, eggs, apricots, and dark green and yellow vegetables such as carrots, squash, pumpkins, and spinach.

The B Vitamins are responsible for many body functions affecting both physical and mental well-being. They affect appetite, vision, skin, cell functioning, and the nervous system. Lack of B vitamins can result in depression; a severe shortage can lead to mental confusion and anxiety. Foods rich in B vitamins include lean and organic meats (liver, heart, and kidneys), milk and eggs, whole-grain and enriched products such as bread, cereals, and wheat germ, and brewer's yeast, nuts, mushrooms, and peas and lima beans.

Vitamin C (ascorbic acid) binds cell tissues together, helps resist infection, and aids healing. It also strengthens the blood vessels. Lack of enough vitamin C may result in easy bruising or in bleeding gums. Vitamin C is found especially in citrus fruits (oranges, lemons, limes, grapefruit), cantaloupe, fresh strawberries, potatoes, tomatoes, and raw cabbage. Fresh cabbage served as coleslaw may be the cheapest source of vitamin C when fresh citrus fruit is scarce or expensive.

Vitamin D is needed by the body in order for the body to use calcium and phosphorus to form strong bones and teeth. This vitamin is critical in the diets of infants and children. Lack of it in infancy can lead to rickets, a condition characterized by bowed legs. Vitamin D is produced in an unusual way: by the skin cells when they are exposed to sunlight. Other good sources of vitamin D are cod liver oil and some types of fish, including tuna and salmon. Milk and margarine are often artificially fortified with vitamin D. Since vitamin D is stored by the body, care must be taken to avoid excessive intake, which can be harmful.

Minerals

Iron is needed to form red blood cells. Iodine regulates the rate of growth and other body processes. Calcium and phosphorus are crucial to bone development. Copper, fluorine, potassium, magnesium, sodium, chromium, and zinc are needed in small amounts to maintain body functions. Fluoride strengthens the tooth enamel against decay. Good sources of minerals include fresh and dried fruits, leafy green and yellow vegetables, milk, eggs, seafood, and meats such as liver (Fig. 9). Milk is a particularly good source of calcium. Because it is essential for the development of strong bones, children and pregnant or nursing women need more than the 2 cups of milk a day that are recommended for all adults.

Fig. 9

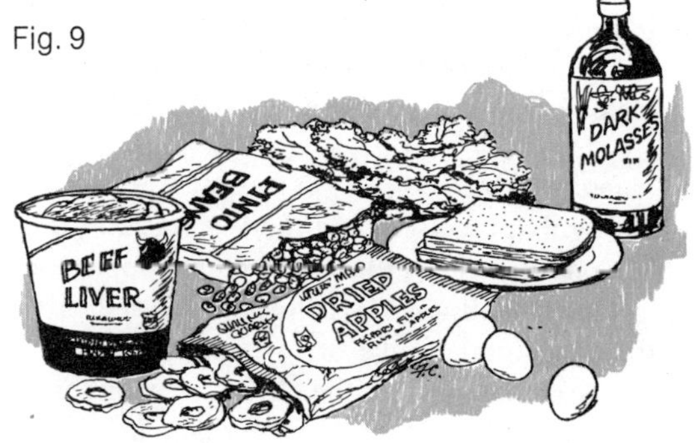

Water

Water makes up about two thirds of the body weight. It serves to move nutrients to all parts of the body and regulates body processes and body temperature. It helps the kidneys remove wastes from the blood and intestines. The body cannot function without water. Man can go without food for weeks, but he cannot live more than a few days without water.

The average adult needs a minimum of from six to eight glasses of liquid daily and even more in warm weather. Large amounts of water are contained in many fruits and vegetables.

Roughage

Roughage includes substances in foods that the body cannot digest. It provides bulk that pushes foods through the digestive tract. Lack of roughage leads to constipation and perhaps to diverticulitis (see Glossary). Foods high in roughage include fruit skins and seeds, raw vegetables, whole grains, bran cereals, and edible seeds such as sunflower and pumpkin seeds.

Choosing Foods for Health

Since no one food can provide all the nutrients required daily by the body, a variety of foods must be chosen to maintain good health. Meal planning and food selection are easier when a simple food guide is used. One easy-to-follow pattern is given in "Food for Fitness: A Daily Guide," on page 35. The guide includes the "Basic Four": the milk group, the meat group, the vegetable-fruit group, and the bread and cereal group. The foods that are grouped together have almost the same nutrients but they vary in nutrient value per serving and in mineral content. Pork, liver, and fish, for example, are good sources of protein; however, liver is a better source of iron, pork a better source of vitamin B, and fish a better source of iodine.

"Food for Fitness: A Daily Guide" is easiest to follow if the foods chosen are not highly processed. It should be noticed, however, that the guide makes no mention of fat, cholesterol, sugar, or salt in the diet. For high-level wellness, it is recommended that foods be selected so that the total intake of fat, saturated fat, cholesterol, sugar, and salt is as low as possible. Many persons in the United States need to increase the amount of roughage in their diet.

FOOD FOR FITNESS: A DAILY GUIDE*

Meat Group

Foods Included

Beef, veal, lamb, pork, variety meats, such as liver, heart, kidney.
Poultry and eggs
Fish and shellfish
As alternates—dry beans, dry peas, lentils, nuts, peanuts, peanut butter

Amounts Recommended

Choose 2 or more servings every day.

Count as a serving: 2 to 3 ounces of lean cooked meat, poultry, or fish—all without bone. One egg; ½ cup cooked dry beans, dry peas, or lentils; 2 tablespoons peanut butter may replace one-half serving of meat.

Vegetable-Fruit Group

Foods Included

All vegetables and fruits. This guide emphasizes those that are valuable as sources of vitamin C and vitamin A.

Sources of Vitamin C

Good sources—Grapefruit or grapefruit juice, orange or orange juice, cantaloupe, guava, mango, papaya, raw strawberries, broccoli, Brussels sprouts, green pepper, sweet red pepper

Fair sources—Honeydew melon, lemon, tangerine or tangerine juice, watermelon, asparagus, cabbage, collards, garden cress, kale, kohlrabi, mustard greens, potatoes and sweet potatoes cooked in the jacket, spinach, tomatoes or tomato juice, turnip greens

Sources of Vitamin A

Dark green and deep yellow vegetables and a few fruits—namely apricots, broccoli, cantaloupe, carrots, chard, collards, cress, kale, mango, persimmon, pumpkin, spinach, sweet potatoes, turnip greens and other dark green leaves, winter squash

*U.S. Department of Agriculture, *Nutrition: Food at Work for You* (Washington, D.C., 1975).

Amounts Recommended

Choose 4 or more servings every day, including—

1 serving of a good source of vitamin C or 2 servings of a fair source.

1 serving, at least every other day, of a good source of vitamin A. If the food chosen for vitamin C is also a good source of vitamin A, the additional serving of a vitamin A food may be omitted.

The remaining 1 to 3 or more servings may be of any vegetable or fruit, including those that are valuable for vitamin C and for vitamin A.

Count as 1 serving: ½ cup of vegetable or fruit; or a portion as ordinarily served, such as 1 medium apple, banana, orange, or potato, half a medium grapefruit or cantaloupe, or the juice of 1 lemon.

Milk Group

Foods Included

Milk—fluid whole, evaporated, skim, dry, buttermilk
Cheese—cottage, cream, Cheddar-type, natural or process
Ice cream

Amounts Recommended

Some milk every day for everyone.

Recommended amounts are given below in terms of 8-ounce cups of whole fluid milk:

Children under 9 . . .	2 to 3	Adults	2 or more
Children 9 to 12	3 or more	Pregnant women	3 or more
Teenagers	4 or more	Nursing mothers	4 or more

Part or all of the milk may be fluid skim milk, buttermilk, evaporated milk, or dry milk.

Cheese and ice cream may replace part of the milk. The amount of either it will take to replace a given amount of milk is figured on the basis of calcium content. Common portions of cheese and of ice cream and their milk equivalents in calcium are—

1-inch cube Cheddar-type cheese	= ½ cup milk
½ cup cottage cheese	= ⅓ cup milk
2 tablespoons cream cheese	= 1 tablespoon milk
½ cup ice cream or ice milk	= ⅓ cup milk

Bread-Cereal Group

Foods Included

All breads and cereals that are whole grain, enriched, or restored. *Check labels to be sure.*

Specifically, this group includes breads, cooked cereals, ready-to-eat cereals, cornmeal, crackers, flour, grits, macaroni and spaghetti, noodles, rice, rolled oats, and quick breads and other baked goods if made with whole-grain or enriched flour. Bulgur and parboiled rice and wheat also may be included in this group.

Amounts Recommended

Choose 4 servings or more daily. Or, if no cereals are chosen, have an extra serving of breads or baked goods, which will make at least 5 servings from this group daily.

Count as 1 serving 1 slice of bread, 1 ounce ready-to-eat cereal, ½ to ¾ cup cooked cereal, cornmeal, grits, macaroni, noodles, rice, or spaghetti.

Other Foods

To round out meals and meet energy needs, almost everyone will use some foods not specified in the four food groups. Such foods include: unenriched, refined breads, cereals, flours; sugars; butter, margarine, other fats. These often are ingredients in a recipe or added to other foods during preparation or at the table.

Try to include some vegetable oil among the fats used.

Food intake and exercise are the two factors that control body weight. When the foods eaten provide more calories than the body needs, the excess calories are stored as fat. If this occurs regularly, the body gains weight. If the foods eaten provide fewer calories than the body needs, the body uses previously stored fat, or even robs tissue from the body. It is wise for persons of all ages to maintain a desirable weight for their height. (See height and weight chart, which follows.) People who are overweight should carefully consider the following facts:

- The body is hampered in its functions when it is carrying too much weight.
- Sudden, unusual, or excessive weight gain calls for consultation with a health professional before starting a major dieting program.
- A good reducing diet includes food from each of the four basic

DESIRABLE WEIGHTS FOR MEN AND WOMEN

According to Height and Frame, Ages 25 and Over

HEIGHT (In Shoes)*	Weight in Pounds (In Indoor Clothing) SMALL FRAME	MEDIUM FRAME	LARGE FRAME
Men			
5′ 2″	112–120	118–129	126–141
3″	115–123	121–133	129–144
4″	118–126	124–136	132–148
5″	121–129	127–139	135–152
6″	124–133	130–143	138–156
7″	128–137	134–147	142–161
8″	132–141	138–152	147–166
9″	136–145	142–156	151–170
10″	140–150	146–160	155–174
11″	144–154	150–165	159–179
6′ 0″	148–158	154–170	164–184
1″	152–162	158–175	168–189
2″	156–167	162–180	173–194
3″	160–171	167–185	178–199
4″	164–175	172–190	182–204
Women			
4′ 10″	92– 98	96–107	104–119
11″	94–101	98–110	106–122
5′ 0″	96–104	101–113	109–125
1″	99–107	104–116	112–128
2″	102–110	107–119	115–131
3″	105–113	110–122	118–134
4″	108–116	113–126	121–138
5″	111–119	116–130	125–142
6″	114–123	120–135	129–146
7″	118–127	124–139	133–150
8″	122–131	128–143	137–154
9″	126–135	132–147	141–158
10″	130–140	136–151	145–163
11″	134–144	140–155	149–168
6′ 0″	138–148	144–159	153–173

*1-inch heels for men and 2-inch heels for women.

Prepared by the Metropolitan Life Insurance Company. Derived primarily from data of the *Build and Blood Pressure Study, 1959*, Society of Actuaries. Reprinted with permission.

food groups. Fad diets, such as eating only grapefruit or beef, often do not contain the necessary nutrients for the body and can be very harmful, even though signs of illness may not appear at the time.

- Dieting can be very difficult. Some people have more success if they join programs with other persons who are trying to lose weight.

In general, to maintain a desirable weight, a person must remember that exercise and activity use up energy or burn calories. If activity is cut back but the amount of food stays the same or increases, weight will increase. As adults get older or reduce activity, their bodies need less food.

Meal Planning

Planning the Menu

The number of meals per day may be varied. However, having fewer meals than three per day is not recommended. Many people prefer smaller, more frequent meals. Older persons often find smaller meals easier to digest. Young children may be too active to sit still for long periods of time to eat. Some people like a light breakfast and lunch and a larger meal in the evening, while others prefer to have a large meal at midday. It is important, however, to provide the body with enough nutrients and energy in the morning to sustain it throughout the activities of the day. Breakfast should include foods that contain carbohydrates and proteins. Throughout the day it is important to eat foods from all four basic food groups.

Special challenges in meal planning are brought about by the relative availability of foods, geographic location, religious beliefs, lifelong eating habits, and simple likes and dislikes. If a vegetarian diet is necessary or preferred, it is possible for such a diet to be adequate if the calorie intake is adequate to maintain normal body weight and if a wide variety of vegetarian foods are eaten each day. Vegetarians who consume no animal foods should take vitamin B-12 either in tablet form or in a fortified food such as soybean milk.

It is a good idea to let the whole family help in menu planning; not only will each person have a better chance of getting favorite foods, but all family members will learn more about making selections from the four basic food groups.

Planning a week's menu before going shopping, using a list, and buying only the items on the list helps the shopper avoid the temptation to pick up "junk" foods (calories without nutrients), such as candy and potato chips, and otherwise run up the food bill. Planning also makes it possible to take advantage of sales. Meals should include a variety of foods, and costs can be cut if a definite plan is followed for the use of leftovers.

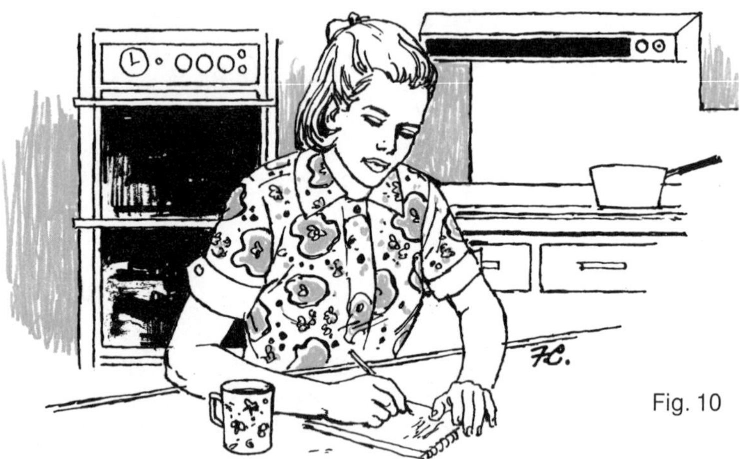

Fig. 10

Buying and Storing Food

The wise food buyer—

- Knows prices for certain foods at various stores.
- Uses the week's menu as a guide for purchases.
- Selects foods carefully to get the most value by size of can, box, or bottle that best serves individual or family needs.
- Uses unit pricing when it is provided in a store. (Labels on the shelves give the price per pound or other unit of measurement.)
- Reads labels. (The first ingredient listed on the label is present in the largest amount by weight. A breakfast cereal with sugar listed as the first ingredient has more sugar than cereal.)
- Stores the food properly.

The Food and Drug Administration requires that food containers list the nutrients contained in the food and give any other information to aid in more effective use. Labels must give the following information:

- Number of average-size servings in the container

- Nutrition information per serving
- Number of calories per serving
- Number of grams of protein, carbohydrates, and fat per serving
- Percentage, per serving, of the body's daily need for protein, vitamins, and minerals
- Last date by which the food should be sold or eaten

A smart shopper will make use of nutrition labeling to plan adequate meals, to find the best sources of certain nutrients, to more accurately count calories eaten, and to avoid nutrients that must be restricted on special diets (such as cholesterol and sodium).

Careful selection of foods means looking for quality and price. Day-old breads, for example, usually cost less but are still good. Shoppers can now take advantage of a new system called unit pricing to determine the relative savings or loss in buying a particular size package of food. The unit price label on the shelf shows the price per quart, pound, or other unit of measure for products in different-sized containers. Although the larger sizes are generally more economical, small sizes could be cheaper in the long run if the time it would take to use the whole package and the time before the food would spoil were considered.

Food labeled "low calorie" must contain no more than 40 calories per serving. A food may be called "reduced calorie" if its caloric content is at least one third lower than a similar food for which it can substitute.

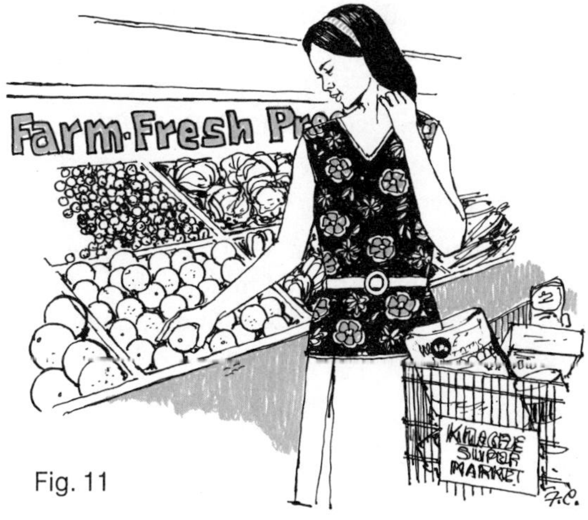

Fig. 11

Shopping for food should be the last task before going home, so that perishable foods can be refrigerated as quickly as possible. It is wise to have all frozen foods packed in one bag so that they may be unpacked directly into the freezer. When a person is unpacking food, the week's menu should be close at hand, to serve as a guide for storing food purchases. Large packages of meat, such as ground beef, can be divided into individual or meal-size servings before wrapping and freezing. Care should be taken to wrap foods well so that they are airtight, to prevent moisture loss or freezer burn.

Preparing Food

How food is prepared makes a difference both in its nutritive value and in its taste. Improper storage or unsanitary handling can make the food unsafe to eat.

The person preparing food should observe the following rules:

- Always wash hands before food is prepared.
- Keep the kitchen and the utensils clean. Wash the cutting board, table, and counter top thoroughly after raw meat, fish, turkey, or chicken has been cut or prepared on them. Meat and poultry, especially chicken, may have germs that would cause illness if they got on food to be eaten raw.
- Wash fruits, vegetables, and whole fish before they are prepared. Meat should not be washed but can be wiped with a dry paper towel.
- Keep any foods that will be served cold in the refrigerator.
- Steam vegetables or boil them in a very small amount of water in order to prevent dissolving vitamins and minerals in the cooking water.
- Do not overcook foods. Overcooking destroys nutrients and taste.
- Keep garbage covered, in order to avoid attracting flies and other disease-carrying insects.

Some foods breed harmful bacteria very quickly if they are not kept refrigerated. Examples are milk and milk products, fish, meat, custards, mayonnaise, and salads made with mayonnaise, such as potato, egg, or chicken salad.

Family Mealtime

Unless a high value is placed on the benefits of family mealtime, the pressures of the day may prevent a genuine family meal. Shifting patterns of family life (more women with full- or part-time jobs; busy schedules involving church, school, and social activities, etc.) may conflict with mealtime. Family mealtime has thus become almost a thing of the past for some families. For many families, school and work schedules prevent having a family meal at breakfast, except on weekends. These kinds of problems tend to increase the use of fast-food products and the "catch as catch can" approach, regardless of the cost in dollars or poor diet.

Mealtime is an opportunity for communicating, exposing children to a greater variety of foods, and practicing good manners. Without a family meal, special efforts are required to demonstrate this positive behavior. It may be worthwhile for even busy families to attempt to bring everyone to the table at the same time at least once during the day. Single persons may also want to plan to share mealtime with others once a day in a pleasant setting.

Special Diets

People who have serious chronic illnesses may have to follow special diets. Kidney disease, ulcers, diabetes, high blood pressure, and high levels of blood cholesterol or triglycerides are conditions that require specific and rigid diets. The labels of food packages should be checked for nutrients and contents that are important for special diets.

Voluntary health organizations are a good source for additional information and hints for special diets. The American Diabetes Association, for example, has menu plans for persons with diabetes, while the American Heart Association has detailed menu plans and recipes for people with high blood pressure or elevated blood cholesterol or triglycerides. Addresses and telephone numbers of these and other such organizations are in the telephone directory, or an inquiry can be directed to their national headquarters. (See the list of organizations in the Appendix.)

Special Food Programs

The information in this book and in courses offered by the American Red Cross, as well as in books and pamphlets published by local, state, and federal governments and other organizations, can provide much-needed information on nutrition.

Although the United States has been labeled the land of plenty, many people have inadequate diets or know little or nothing about good nutrition. The level of nutrition of the nation's people is of particular concern to the federal government. Many people do not have the money to buy adequate food, even though they may know what foods they should have. To counteract these circumstances, the federal government sponsors programs that are aimed at meeting nutritional needs. These federal programs change from time to time in an attempt to better serve people, especially those who risk major health problems if dietary needs are not met. Everyone should be aware of the possible ways in which the dietary needs of people in their communities can be met through federal, state, and local planning.

The Special Supplemental Food Program for Women, Infants, and Children (WIC) makes money available to the states to provide for women, infants, and children who otherwise would not have balanced diets. Through food coupons or direct distribution of food supplements, the program promotes good nutrition for pregnant and nursing women, in order to assure the health of babies, and provides balanced diets for infants and children up to 5 years of age so that they may grow to be healthy adults. State health departments can provide further information on this program.

The food stamp program makes money available to states to be used for lower-income families. The lower a family's income, the less the family has to pay for its allotted amount of food stamps. County social service departments can provide further information on the program. The school meal program makes free meals available within schools for certain eligible children.

Lack of money or of knowledge of nutrition are not the only reasons why some people do not have adequate diets. Many older people do not eat enough food or the right kind. Although poor appetite or poorly fitting dentures contribute to this situation, often older people living alone are simply not motivated to prepare meals that they will eat alone. Many older people cannot get out to a store to buy food and other essentials. Many communities have "eating together" programs for senior citizens that provide one complete hot meal per day in a community-sponsored facility (Fig. 12). This kind of activity also gives the older person an opportunity to get together with others who have similar interests and needs. One organization may provide the meals while another group such as the American Red Cross may provide transportation for persons who need it.

In some communities, a "Meals on Wheels" service is also available. Through this service, one full hot meal and sometimes another

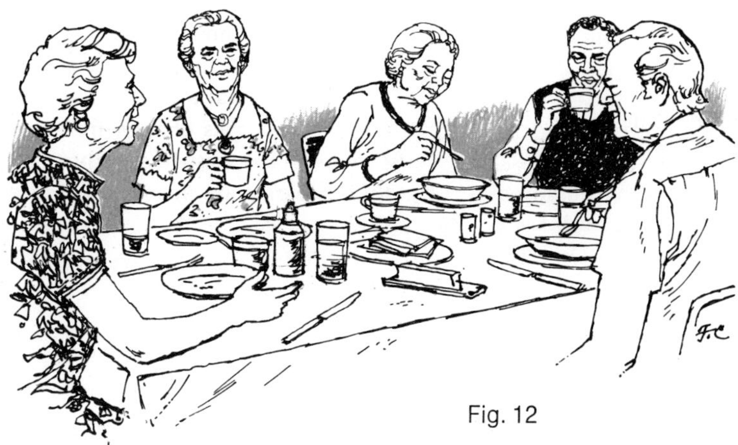

Fig. 12

lighter cold meal are brought to the homes of the elderly or of persons who are ill and cannot prepare their own meals or get out to eat with a group. With programs such as these, many older and infirm persons can avoid going into nursing homes or hospitals. Information on various eating programs for the elderly may be obtained through local health departments, churches, and the American Red Cross.

PERSONAL HYGIENE

Personal hygiene is a term that has been used for many years to refer to basic habits of cleanlinesss and grooming, patterns of sleeping and elimination, and similar activities. Personal hygiene measures strengthen the body and lessen the danger of infection and disease, making possible a high level of wellness.

Hand Washing

Hand washing is one of the most important personal hygiene habits. Every day we touch things that have disease-causing germs, and we also touch food. Thus, unless we have a regular habit of washing our hands, we unnecessarily expose ourselves to diseases. Hands should be washed—

- Before eating
- Before handling or preparing food

- After handling soiled articles
- After using the toilet
- Before and after caring for a sick person

When the hands are washed, care should be taken to—

- First rinse the hands in warm water to soften dirt and grease
- Soap thoroughly and rub lather over the tops of the hands and wrists, as well as over the palms
- Clean under the fingernails, where dirt and bacteria are especially likely to get trapped
- Repeat the lathering
- Rinse thoroughly
- Dry with a clean towel

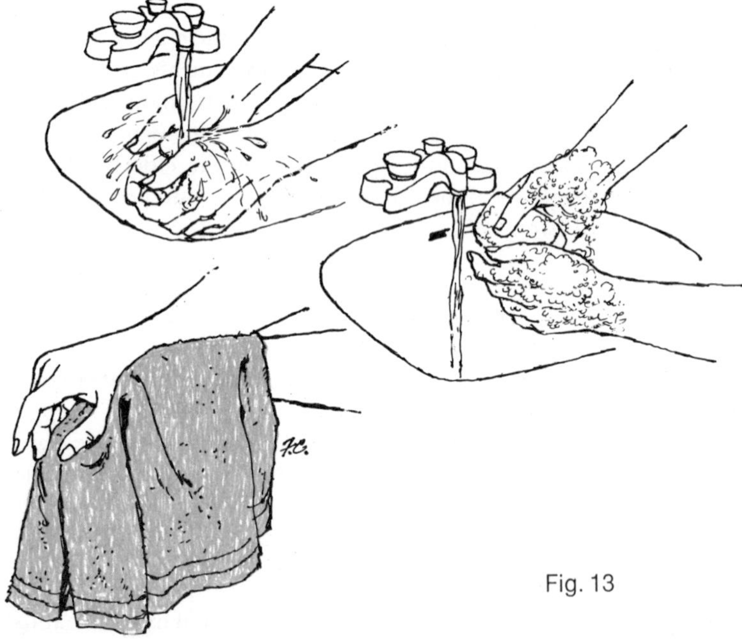

Fig. 13

Each person should, if possible, have his own towel and washcloth and a separate place to hang them. In the kitchen, there should be one towel for drying hands and another for drying dishes or food. In cases of known illnesses or communicable diseases, greater precautions are required in hand washing (see chapter 17).

Bathing

In addition to the removal of dirt, germs, and body secretions (perspiration, oil), bathing the entire body serves several other purposes. A bath or shower refreshes and relaxes the body and is therefore a time of pleasure. It also provides minor exercise and, if warm water and brisk rubbing are used, can stimulate circulation. At bath time, the body may be inspected for rashes, bruises, or moles that may be changing shape or color.

Frequency of bathing depends on the accessibility of bathing facilities, on the condition of the skin, and on the personal need to be clean. It is not necessary to bathe the whole body daily; however, the genital and rectal areas should be washed daily to prevent odor and infection. Although most soaps are effective cleaning agents, some soaps are less likely to dry out the skin. Lotions may also be used to prevent dry skin.

Special care should be taken to dry the area between the toes. Warm, moist areas that do not get air are especially susceptible to the growth of bacteria. Since feet are usually kept warm and moist in shoes, "athlete's foot" (a fungus infection) is fairly common; for the most part, it can be prevented by keeping the area between the toes clean and dry.

SAFETY NOTE. Never leave an infant, toddler, or handicapped or weak person alone in the tub or shower. When assisting with a bath, plan to stay with the person. Turn off the stove, take the telephone off the hook, and do anything else that will insure that there will be no interruptions. If you must leave, make sure the person you are assisting is not in the water and cannot fall or otherwise be injured.

Examination of the Breasts

Breast self-examination for cancer should be part of the routine personal care for all men and women. This procedure was once advised only for women, but breast cancer occurs in men also, although less frequently. Women are advised to examine their breasts after the time of menstruation, when the breasts are smaller and less knotty in consistency. The procedure is as follows:

1. Begin the examination in the shower or tub or when the breasts are wet. (This allows the hands to move more easily over the skin.) Check for any lump or thickening by moving the hands across and around the breasts.

2. After the bath, stand before a mirror. Place both hands on the hips and look in the mirror for any dimpling or change in size or shape of the breasts. Then place the hands over the head and look for changes in the breasts.
3. Lie on the back with a pillow under the right shoulder and the right hand under the head. Using the left hand with fingers flat, press gently on the right breast with a small circular motion, beginning at the nipple and working over the entire breast. When the entire breast has been checked, repeat the same process for the left breast.
4. Squeeze each nipple gently to check for discharge.

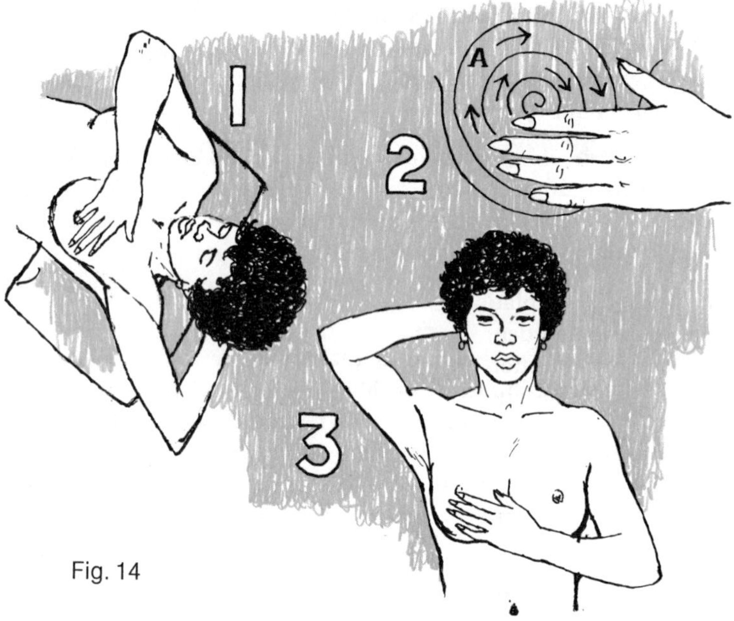

Fig. 14

Anything unusual about the way the breast looks or feels, and especially any changes, should be evaluated by a health professional.

Most problems found by breast self-examination are not cancer, but it is always good to have an expert opinion.

Teeth, Gums, and Dentures

Thorough, daily care of teeth and gums prevents loss of teeth due to decay of the tooth itself or due to infection and damage to the gums. A clean mouth that is well cared for makes a person feel and look better and makes food taste better.

A well-balanced diet that includes foods from all four basic food groups is necessary for a healthy mouth. Eating sweets often and eating sticky sweets are very dangerous for dental health. Cutting down sugar intake, particularly by cutting down on soft drinks, candy, and sweetened gum, can help prevent tooth decay. If it is necessary to chew on something, fruits and fresh, raw vegetables are a better choice; they have the added advantage of not promoting plaque formation.

It is good practice to brush the teeth after each meal, but few people can do so. If brushing is not possible, it is wise to rinse the mouth with water after eating, using as much pressure as possible. This will remove food particles from around the teeth even though it does not remove plaque.

Brushing the teeth and gums and using dental floss to clean the spaces between the teeth removes plaque, a sticky, colorless layer of bacteria that constantly forms on the teeth. If the plaque is not removed *daily,* it will build up into a hard material called tartar, which only a dentist or dental hygienist can remove. If the teeth are not kept free of plaque, gum infection and tooth decay occur. Regular trips to a dentist or dental clinic will allow early detection of decay and infection and the removal of any buildup of plaque that may occur despite efforts to brush and floss regularly.

Most dentists recommend a straight-handled brush with a flat brushing surface and soft, rounded-end bristles. Soft bristles are less likely to injure gum tissues. The head of the brush should be small enough to reach all areas of every tooth. Children need smaller brushes than adults. The dental professional may also suggest a toothpaste with fluoride to help prevent tooth decay. The dentist may suggest either waxed or plain dental floss; otherwise, it is a matter of personal choice.

American Dental Association Recommendations

The American Dental Association (ADA) evaluates therapeutic dental products such as fluoride toothpastes. If the ADA finds a certain product effective, the manufacturer is permitted to carry the ADA statement to that effect on the box or the product label. Toothpastes that carry the ADA seal have been proven effective. Look for the seal on the carton or tube.

In addition, the American Dental Association, through its Council on Dental Materials and Devices, recognizes some electric toothbrushes and some irrigating devices as being effective in cleaning the teeth and gums. Look for the authorized Council statement on the carton.

Providing good care to the teeth and gums requires at least one daily session of brushing and using dental floss (Fig. 15). It may be helpful to plan a regular time for brushing and flossing, a time that is most often convenient. The important goal should be to completely remove the plaque each day. Sometimes it is suggested that a special solution or tablet be used that will make the plaque visible. Both tooth decay and gum (periodontal) disease *can be prevented.* Most dentists recommend that you—

- Brush and floss thoroughly at least once every day, to remove the plaque and irritants

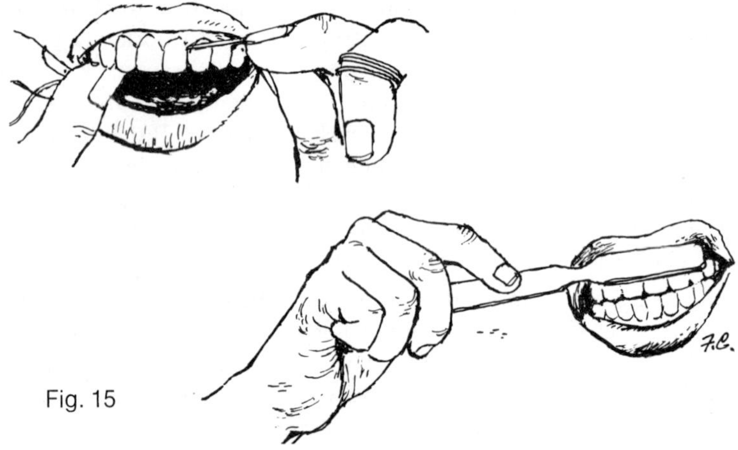

Fig. 15

- Use fluorides daily, to strengthen the tooth enamel against decay
- Eat a varied and balanced diet
- Avoid sweet snacks
- Have dental examinations regularly

A regular pattern for reaching each part of the mouth when brushing assures that each tooth will be reached. One way is to think of the mouth as being in four sections: upper right, lower right, upper left, and lower left. Follow the same pattern each time. The procedure described below is recommended:

1. Use the toothbrush at a 45-degree angle against the gum.

2. Using a gentle, scrubbing motion, move the brush back and forth with short strokes (one half a tooth wide).
3. Brush the outer surface of each tooth.
4. Brush the inner surface of each tooth. (For the front teeth, hold the brush so that the bristles are vertical to the gum.)
5. Brush the chewing surfaces of the teeth.
6. Rinse with plenty of water to clean out loosened food particles.

Practice makes the process easier and more effective. Replace the toothbrush when it is worn. A worn brush will not clean teeth well.

Flossing removes plaque from between the teeth, especially near the gum line, where a brush cannot reach. When flossing is first started, there may be bleeding from the gums, but removal of plaque and the stimulation of blood circulation will promote healing, and the gums will become more healthy. If bleeding should continue, consult a dentist. The following procedure is recommended:

1. Use about an 18-inch (about 46 centimeters) length of floss.
2. Wind most of the floss around the middle finger of one hand and wind the rest around the middle finger of the opposite hand so that 3 or 4 inches (about 7 or 10 centimeters) of floss extends between the fingers.
3. Grasp the floss tightly between the thumb and index finger of each hand.
4. Leave about 1–2 inches (2.5–5 centimeters) of floss between the hands.
5. Insert the floss between the teeth with a gentle sawing motion. (Do not snap the floss against the gums—doing so may injure the gums.)
6. When the floss reaches the gum line, curve it into a C shape against one tooth and gently slide it into the space between the tooth and the gum until resistance is felt.
7. While holding the floss tightly against the tooth, move the floss away from the gum by scraping the floss up and down against the side of the tooth.
8. Repeat for all the spaces and teeth, winding the floss from one hand to the other as it becomes soiled.

A mouthwash can temporarily freshen the mouth and breath. However, the American Dental Association warns that bad breath may indicate poor oral health or other body disorders. If bad breath or a bad taste in the mouth persists for more than a day or two, check with a dentist or other health professional. Medicated mouthwashes should be used only when ordered by a dentist.

Dentures

A clean mouth and teeth are also important to the health of those who wear dentures (false teeth). Dentures should be brushed with a special denture brush or a soft brush not used on natural teeth, and warm water should be used. (Hot water tends to warp plastic.) Special cleaning agents, peroxide, or baking soda and water will usually clean the dentures and make them more pleasant in the mouth. Dentures should be stored in liquid, because they may warp if they become dried out. To avoid accidental breaking while cleaning dentures, it is wise not to wash them near a hard surface. They can be washed over a basin with water in it to avoid breakage if they fall (Fig. 16).

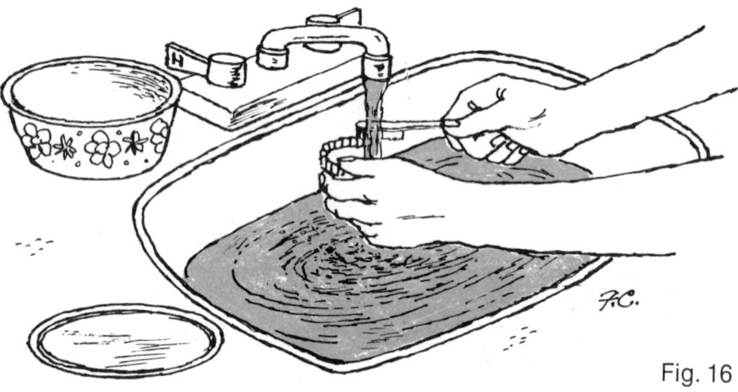

Fig. 16

It is important that dentures fit well and be generally comfortable in the mouth. If dentures do not fit well enough so that meats and raw vegetables and fruits can be chewed with relative ease, a person's nutrition may suffer. If dentures cause sores in the mouth, they do not fit properly and should be checked promptly by the dentist. Tissues in the mouth tend to change as persons age, and it may be necessary to have dentures refitted. Dentists should advise as to whether dentures should be worn at night.

Hair Care

Care of the hair is important. Hair can reflect a person's state of health and state of mind. Good health and nutrition contribute to attractive hair. Although the wisdom of brushing the hair 100 strokes a day is now being questioned, it is suggested that the hair and scalp be brushed well, at least before washing, to stimulate circulation. A natural bristle brush is usually recommended.

Styling of hair is a matter of culture, fashion, or personal preference; however, overuse of chemicals on the hair may damage both the hair and the scalp. If dandruff (a condition in which there is flaking of the skin and itchiness of the scalp) is present, more frequent washing or brushing or a milder shampoo may control the problem. If dandruff continues, it is wise to check with a health professional.

Hair should be washed whenever it looks or feels oily or dirty. Washing should include one or two applications of shampoo, depending upon how often the hair is washed. The hair should be lathered thoroughly for several minutes with each application. The whole scalp should be massaged with the fingertips. Rinsing should be thorough enough to remove all soap.

Elimination

Under normal conditions the lower bowel of the healthy person is emptied at regular intervals. Waste material (bowel movement) passes through the intestines by means of muscular contractions that are set in motion by the intake of food. When the waste material reaches the rectum, the nerve endings are stimulated, and the person feels the need to have a bowel movement (BM).

Bowel habits vary from individual to individual. Some persons have a bowel movement every day, while others normally have one only once in two or three days. If the BM is soft and formed, it can usually be assumed that elimination is normal. A hard, dry BM indicates constipation. Older people are more likely to experience this condition, in which the dry, hardened BM cannot be expelled. Sometimes the constipated patient with a fecal impaction may experience frequent passage of small amounts of fluid BM (diarrhea) that bypasses the impaction. Suppositories (see chapter 19) or an enema (see chapter 23) may be required to empty the lower bowel of a constipated person. Regular use of laxatives or frequent enemas, however, is not good practice for most people; it tends to destroy the normal muscle action of the bowel.

The following routine practices may be helpful to persons who tend to have irregularity of bowel movements:

- Drink from 6 to 8 glasses of fluid a day.

- Every day, eat foods that supply roughage, such as raw fruits and vegetables and whole grains.
- Establish a usual time of day for toileting, and allow sufficient time to avoid hurrying.
- Have some daily exercise and increase it if necessary.
- Drink warm fluids before toileting to relax the bowels.
- Read, even a litte, to relax.

CLOTHING AND SHOES

Clothing should fit well. An easy fit is preferred for work, physical activity, and the active play of children. Undergarments, stockings, or socks (especially stretch socks) that constrict any part of the legs should not be worn. Clothing that fits feels and looks better.

The fiber content of clothing can influence comfort. In general, cotton fabrics absorb more body moisture than synthetics, and they may "breathe" more in warm weather. Wools or synthetics irritate the skin of some people. In addition to comfort, durability and ease of care may influence the choice of fabrics.

Shoes can have a major impact on how a person feels and on whether he can stand and move about with ease and comfort. Some styles contribute more to comfort and stability of balance than others. Heels aid in balance and posture, but very high heels are dangerous. Rubber heels and soles are less likely to skid on wet or highly polished surfaces than others and may aid in maintaining stability and balance. The weight of shoes may affect ease of movement for a weaker person. Cloth linings absorb moisture and perspiration.

Improperly fitting shoes can contribute to a number of foot problems. A person should never be pressured into buying shoes that need to be broken in so that they will fit properly; it takes time and patience to find shoes that fit. Shoes should have few seams to rub on the foot. The back of the shoe should fit snugly but not tightly. When a person stands wearing the shoe, the tip should be from ½ to ¾ of an inch (1.3–1.9 centimeters) beyond the end of the longest toes. If the shoe is too short, it leaves no space for the toes to grip in walking. If the shoe is too long, there is not enough support. The arch of the foot should fit snugly into the narrow part of the shoe between the heel and the ball (wide part) of the foot. There should be enough space in the shoe over the widest part of the foot to make a small pinch of leather. It is particularly important that children's shoes be large enough, because their feet grow rapidly. Feet change in size as a result of large amounts of gain or loss in weight, especially in older persons. Foot problems may occur if shoes are not changed when foot size changes.

EXERCISE AND PHYSICAL FITNESS

Modern conveniences, such as the automobile, and reduced physical activity in most jobs and household chores present many Americans with a challenge to keep fit. Daily work once provided adequate exercise for all family members, but now most people must make a special effort to include physical exercise in their daily routine. Exercise is an important part of any daily program to maintain a high level of fitness. It benefits both physical and mental health.

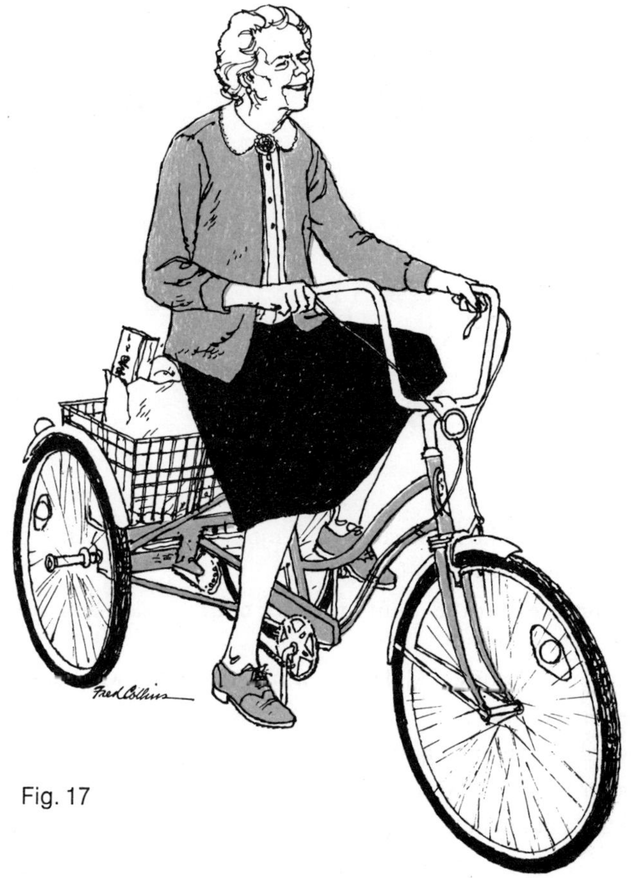

Fig. 17

Exercise comes in many forms: walking, running, cycling, swimming, yoga, home or group exercise programs, tennis, dancing, gymnastics, team sports, etc. Exercise groups for children and adults can be found at schools, places of work, community recreation centers, and the Ys. Exercise provides a change of pace and diversion from daily problems. It may be a time to be alone or a time to be with others, according to a person's preference. There is also the pleasure of mastering skills or achieving personal goals.

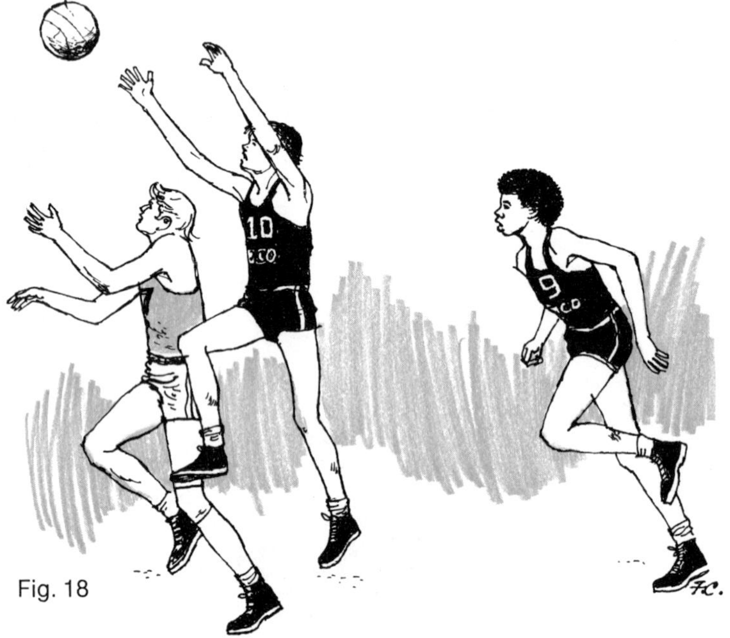

Fig. 18

Benefits

An individual who is physically fit enjoys many benefits:

- Muscular strength and vigor
- Endurance and the ability to carry out necessary activities with energy to spare
- Improved posture and decreased frequency of lower back pain
- Better appetite
- Coordination and agility
- Easier weight control
- Relief from mental tension, strain, and boredom

- A feeling of relaxation after exertion
- More efficient action of heart and lungs
- Reduced risk of heart (cardiovascular) disease

Beginning a Program

The following points should be kept in mind when a person is planning to begin an exercise program:

- Check with a health professional regarding the proposed plan.
- Strive for balanced exercise in which all muscle groups are used.
- Warm up gradually to prepare the body for more vigorous activity; start with continuous rhythmical activities such as easy stretching and pulling or rotating of the torso, arms, and legs.
- Alternate periods of vigorous activity with less stressful ones. For improved fitness, it is necessary that the body work hard at some point during the routine.

Publications from the President's Commission on Physical Fitness are highly recommended. *The Fitness Challenge in Later Years* is suitable for all ages and is very clearly written. It includes tests for determining the beginning level of exercise, it provides adequate challenge to maintain fitness, and it gives progression in routine as fitness increases.

Posture

The way a person holds his body while standing, walking, sitting, or lying down is referred to as posture. Good posture allows for deeper breathing, helps prevent fatigue, and avoids unnecessary strain on the muscles. Holding the head up and the shoulders back makes breathing more efficient by enlarging the chest area. Exercises that throw the shoulders back and tighten the abdominal muscles are especially helpful for good posture and do much to prevent back problems.

If kitchen sinks and counters are at a convenient height, harmful stooping will be unnecessary. When lifting a child or a heavy object, a person should not bend from the back but at the knees. Proper posture while resting requires a fairly firm mattress; sleeping on an overly soft or sagging mattress may contribute to an aching back. While in bed, it is good to avoid staying in one position for a long period of time.

HOME CLEANLINESS, COMFORT, AND SAFETY

The practice of hygiene in the home should result in a clean, comfortable, and safe living environment. Cleanliness helps to prevent the growth of harmful organisms, unpleasant odors, and annoying insects. Adequate ventilation and proper humidity make the home more comfortable and promote better health. Accidents and injuries can be avoided in a safe home.

Housekeeping

It is especially important to keep bathrooms and kitchens clean to control possible sources of infection. Specific suggestions regarding kitchen cleanliness are outlined in the section on food preparation. The brush and cloth for cleaning the toilet should be used only for that purpose and should be kept separate from washcloths and other cleaning items. Toilet seats should be cleaned regularly to avoid their becoming a source of infection.

Pets pose special problems with respect to cleanliness and health. Children must be taught not to play with animal "droppings," litter boxes, and pet food. Litter boxes should be cleaned frequently to avoid odor and to control a possible source of illness.

Additional housekeeping precautions are required when there are communicable diseases in the family (see chapter 12).

Ventilation and Humidity

Good ventilation in a home provides a change of air, and fresh air tends to slow the growth of bacteria. Good ventilation is particularly important when a person has a communicable or upper respiratory disease such as a cold. The windows should be open for at least a short time every day.

The amount of moisture in the air (humidity) greatly influences comfort and may affect health. If there is too little moisture in the air, many persons experience discomfort from sore throat, dry mouth, or dry nose, particularly upon waking in the morning. Central home heating systems that circulate hot air tend to dry the air greatly. A humidifier placed in a central location of the home can increase the amount of moisture and make the air more comfortable. Sometimes it is possible to attach a humidifier to the central furnace.

There are several kinds of electrical appliances designed to add moisture to the air of a room. Most of these are fairly low in cost and can be bought at drugstores. One type of vaporizer brings water to a boil and releases a flow of steam into the room. The newer type, generally preferred because there is no heat or steam that can cause burns, is a cool-mist humidifier (Fig. 19). This type contains a pump that throws a stream of unheated water onto a paddle wheel or screen to break the water into tiny droplets that can then be blown

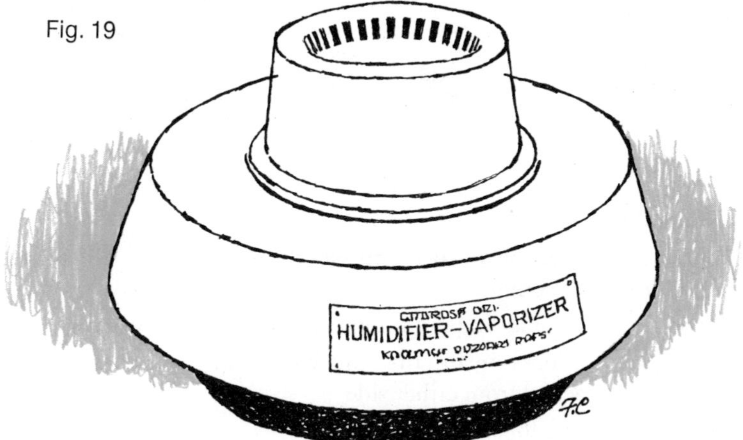

Fig. 19

out into the room. Whichever type of humidifier is used, the following precautions should be taken:

- Carefully read the directions that come with any vapor appliance.
- Keep the electric cord safely out of the way to prevent tripping.
- Unplug the appliance before moving, cleaning, or refilling it.
- Clean the humidifier frequently to remove buildup of mineral deposits from the water.
- Add disinfectant or chlorine bleach to the cold water tank and paddle wheel or screen device (½ tsp. to 1 gallon of water).
- Refill the container every few hours to be sure it does not run dry.

Safety

Safety features in a home include—

- Handrails and good lighting for stairways (Fig. 20)
- Hand grips in the bathtub and shower and nonskid strips in the bottom of the tub or shower (Fig. 21)

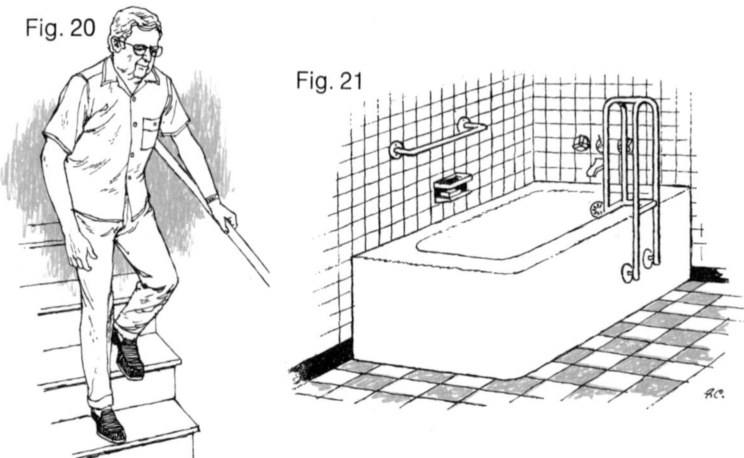

Fig. 20

Fig. 21

- Nonskid flooring
- Changes in levels between rooms clearly marked by a different color of floor covering
- Good lighting, including night lights in halls and bathrooms
- Safety release locks on interior and bathroom doors that allow them to be opened from either side
- Secure screening for windows and doors
- A safety screen in front of any fireplace

Careful placement of items that can be safety hazards is very important:

- Keep sharp or dangerous tools, medications, and dangerous cleaning substances in a safe place when not in use.
- Keep knives and sharp implements in a special rack, out of the reach of small children.
- Do not allow toys or other items to clutter heavily traveled areas (Fig. 22).
- Avoid the use of loose scatter rugs. Tape them to the floor or use nonskid or rubber backing.
- Keep drawers and cupboard doors closed.
- Keep curtains or other flammable items away from stoves, candles, or other open flames.
- Turn pot handles inward when cooking so that pots are not likely to be bumped or pulled over by children, causing burns or dangerous spills.

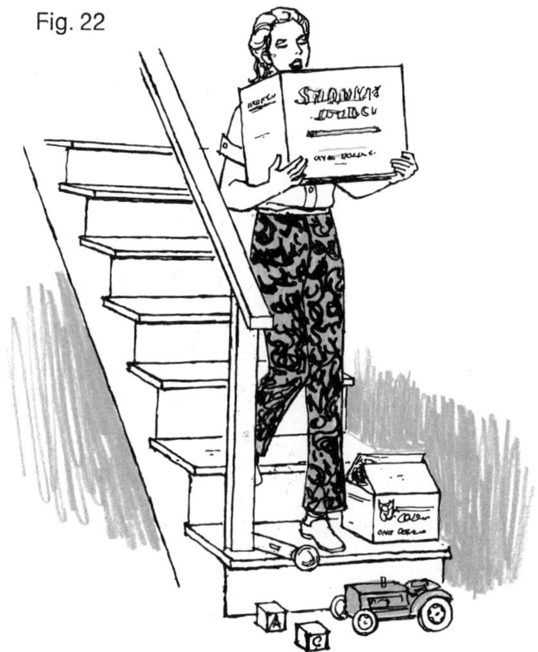

Fig. 22

- Disconnect electrical appliances such as toasters and can openers when not in use.
- Do not use electrical cords that are frayed or cracked or that fit loosely into the outlet.
- Run electrical cords along walls (preferably taped down), not across heavily traveled areas, under rugs, or where they would be exposed to moisture.
- Cover unused electrical outlets if children are present.
- Follow the directions of the manufacturer when using appliances and dangerous cleaning substances.

Cleaning agents, medications, and poisonous substances need very special care. Keeping them out of the reach of children and in locked cupboards may be a matter of life or death. Anyone who uses such material should be sure to read the labels carefully and follow instructions. Spray products such as cleaning supplies, deodorants, and cosmetics may be a health hazard because of harmful substances that they contain. Most products are available in nonspray forms, which are considered safer and are often less expensive.

Chapter 3

The Family

It has often been said that if you have everything but don't have your health, you have nothing. The value of this statement is nowhere more obvious than in the family setting. Today, more than ever before, society needs strong, healthy families, families who can interact meaningfully among themselves and with others and who work for the healthy physical, mental, and emotional growth and support of each member of the family. This is not the easiest task to accomplish, and there is no such thing as a perfect family. There are problems in family life as in any other aspect of life, and people do not change because they marry or because they become part of a group. Each person has his own unique personality, likes and dislikes, and special talents.

A happy family life is one of the most rewarding goals sought by most persons. What most families seek is to promote, and to depend on, the mental, social, emotional, and physical growth of other human beings in an atmosphere of mutual affection, trust, loyalty, and respect for individual differences.

Since all of us, at one time or another, are part of some kind of family unit, we all have the challenge of family tasks and responsibilities. Every relationship from infancy to old age is affected by family relationship in the common experiences of life, in the respect for the person and the courtesies upon which civilization is based, and in loyalties to culture, community, and country.

Several of the following chapters give more detailed information about the various phases of the life cycle—pregnancy, infancy, childhood, adolescence, adulthood, and dying. This chapter is concerned mainly with the impact of the family on the individual and of the individual on the family.

WHAT CONSTITUTES A FAMILY

A family traditionally is a social unit related by ties of marriage, birth, or adoption. The smallest family unit (or *nuclear* family) consists of husband, wife, and children. The broadest family unit (or *extended* family) includes grandparents, grandchildren, aunts, uncles, and cousins who are related either by blood or by marriage. The nuclear, or immediate, family tends to live under the same roof until children are ready to either leave home or begin families of their own, or do both. Interaction and communication in the immediate family are constant and daily, and each member contributes in some way to the family's goals and is an essential part of the life pattern.

In the United States, the family structure has undergone many recent changes, including such factors as separation, divorce, and living together without marriage. New trends toward single-person parenthood and nonrelated persons living in a single dwelling (such as a commune) are further changing the old understanding of the term "family."

Although the nuclear family is still the most common type of family unit, single-parent families, communal families, and other types of families are increasing in number. Every type of family has tasks that are very important in helping both children and adults to grow and develop to the highest possible level of wellness.

In every type of family situation, individuals affect one another in all common aspects of life: growing, maturing, aging, adjusting, trying to obtain the necessities of life, sharing joys and problems, perhaps bearing and rearing children, accepting death and the realities of life, and facing fear, frustration, and disappointment. People share their strength and affection and they depend on others for emotional, physical, mental, and social growth. In a family there is a high degree of closeness and communication, plus the sharing of common goals, outlooks, and culture.

RESPONSIBLE ADULTHOOD AND PARENTHOOD

The primary task of the family today is to prepare its members for the joys and sometimes the harsh realities of life. Most family tasks simply require having responsible persons who are prepared to communicate openly with each other and to make decisions together for the good of all family members. There is a growing awareness among sociologists, clergymen, family counselors, and many others that good communication and self-understanding before a new family is formed are the best preparation for marriage and family life. How well prepared a couple is for marriage and for the special tasks incurred by having children is often the difference between the wellness of all family members and such results as separation, divorce, and having children who are insecure and unprepared for the tasks of living.

Groups of people (of which the family is the primary example) need to try to discover the things that bind them together and to make plans for smooth functioning. Before deciding to establish a family, people might ask themselves certain questions:

- What do we argue about?

- How do we go about discussing and solving problems?
- Who will make the decisions and set the priorities in our family?
- How do we intend to divide responsibility?
- How easily and openly do we express our real feelings?
- How do we feel about having children?
- How do we plan to divide and spend our money after we form a family?
- What will be the role of religion in our family-to-be?
- How will we schedule activities?
- How much privacy does each partner need?
- How does each partner feel about the use of tobacco, drugs, and alcohol?
- How do we feel about pets?

Partners who are responsive to each other's needs and who have a sense of common purpose will usually have fewer problems in reaching agreements and in making decisions. Persons planning to form their own new family may find insight and practical tips through talking with older, more experienced families and also from talking with family counselors, health professionals, and clergymen. Any differences or conflicts, either before or after a family is formed, should never be left unresolved. In many cases, special guidelines are needed to reach a decision.

One suggested approach to seeking a common solution to problems might be as follows:

- Define the problem. Decide who is affected by the problem and in what way. What feelings are involved?
- Think of possible solutions.
- Decide which solution may be best.
- Try a solution and see if it works well for all concerned. If it does not work, try another one.

When differences of opinion are difficult to resolve, the following approaches may be helpful:

- Have one person make the decision and the other person agree to go along with it.
- Think of a compromise solution—one that allows each person to have some of his needs met, perhaps not quite in the way originally desired but for the long-range good of both.

- Keep in mind that in most differences of opinion, there usually is no entirely right or wrong way of doing something.

Communication occurs as one individual responds to another's facial expression, mannerisms, gestures, posture, and actions, as well as his words. When a person's words and actions seem to contradict each other, much discussion may be necessary in order to develop a clear understanding of his real feelings. Great satisfaction and new discoveries come to the person who can await the outcome of open and honest communication and decision-making without insisting that there is only one right way.

THE TASKS OF THE FAMILY

The tasks of a family are certain responsibilities that all families are expected to carry out, whether because of the authority of a religious body, the expectations of society, or the convictions of the family members themselves. The tasks rest on two basic ideas: (1) that the family unit is the primary source of the strength and encouragement from which children and adults develop to their highest potential and level of wellness and (2) that the family is the basic social unit. As the basic social unit, the family determines the wellness of society for years to come. The performance of the family tasks depends on the actions of adults who are responsive to each other, to the needs of growing children, and to the welfare of society as a whole.

Being able to provide shelter ("a roof over our heads"), food, clothing, and health care adequate for all family members is probably the most commonly thought-of task for couples beginning families of their own. Families who do not need to worry excessively about the necessities of life may be more free to concern themselves with other important aspects of growth and development for all family members.

Parents should be aware of the growth stages common to all children and of the parents' challenge to nurture each child's sense of basic trust, identity, initiative, industry, and self-esteem. (Such nurturing is referred to as carrying out "developmental tasks" in this chapter.) The above-mentioned qualities develop in a certain order during each stage of growth from infancy to young adulthood. Each individual grows and develops at his own rate but in a pattern similar for all people.

Each stage of life is important to the next. The sense of trust developed in the infant, who observes how quickly and well his parents respond to his needs, is basic to all future emotional, mental, and even physical and spiritual growth of the child. It will have a definite effect on his developing personality. The toddler gradually becomes aware of his own separate identity, and the preschool child develops a sense of initiative that enables him to put his best efforts into new learning and schoolwork. The child whose needs are recognized and whose growth is aided will be better prepared for the adolescent years, during which he reaches for independence and a stronger sense of identity and worth. All of these stages of growth are treated in more detail in chapters 5 and 6.

The developmental tasks are usually worked out within the family structure. Both children and parents have much to learn through experience about the value of their contributions to the growth of every family member. Time for communication and interaction with each family member must be allowed whether it is convenient or not. Young children need the attention they demand, even when they interrupt their parents' tasks or leisure. A child senses his parents' love by the quality of attention and guidance (discipline) that he receives. Respect and affection can never be taken for granted.

It is within the family that the individual develops his ability to show affection and his appreciation for the importance of loving and being loved. The give and take involved in meeting each other's needs and in the sharing of responsibility for work encourages each child to master both the mechanical and the social skills of daily living. Even when the child is at an early age, it is wise to foster his basic desire to be helpful and to do his share in meeting the needs of family members.

With the growth, development, and change of each family member, tasks and responsibilities will shift, both because of factors within the family and influences from outside the family. As each person develops his talents and masters skills, he will grow in self-esteem and become more ready to take part in family and individual decision making.

Although the needs of one family member often support the needs of another, the growth needs of all family members are not always in harmony with each other. One example of such a conflict is the adolescent struggling to free himself from the authority of the parents, who are seeking to guide and supervise the not-yet adult. It is important to realize that conflict as well as agreement can contribute to proper functioning of the family. Patterns of family interaction can be loving and stimulating or they can be sources of pain and confusion. It is also important to realize that problems do not arise from conflict itself but rather from the lack of adequate discussion to resolve differences.

Privacy and togetherness are other factors in family life. Each person needs some privacy and some respect for his privacy, whether or not these needs are achieved through separate bedrooms for each child. Privacy and the sharing of space also depend greatly upon the specific ages and personalities of family members. The concept of "togetherness" (doing things together in the family) includes not only family outings but also such rituals as the celebrating of Thanksgiving, religious holidays, and birthdays. These shared experiences foster the development of family loyalty and a shared philosophy of life. In its togetherness, the family teaches values, broadens its experience through proper use of leisure, and encourages sound mental health. Also, through "table talk," children are exposed to community, political, and other issues that will become more important to them as they grow older. In all these experiences, the child also learns a sense of priorities—the value of spending money wisely for needed and nutritious food rather than for candy and dangerous toys of questionable value and the values of love, harmony, and consideration for others rather than having one's own way at any cost.

CULTURE AND SOCIETY

In addition to carrying out the primary tasks aimed at each family member, individual growth and overall wellness in all areas, the family has the task of being the principal educator in every aspect of culture. The habits and traditions of any culture are often taken for granted by a family, unless the particular family stands out with a special ethnic or other identity because it is different from the community around it. A child's development is affected by the attitudes and experiences of many generations before him. Family traditions and ways of doing things—from habits of speech, favorite foods, religious customs, and folk tales and stories about ancestors to manners and values—bind the family in mind and spirit, create a specific and valuable learning environment for children, and give a child a sense of "roots" and a point of view in an often confusing age. The family not only imparts its own cultural background but also prepares its members for the expectations and values of society in general.

Both the family and society in general exert pressure on each individual to conform to expected ways of behaving within a particular cultural setting. Conflicting expectations from friends, parents, teachers, and other significant people are evident in the rewards and punishments that a child can anticipate for different forms of behavior. A child who has a cultural background or economic status (or both) that is considerably different from that of the community around him may be confused that his friends do things different from the ways in which his family do them. He may feel uneasy or rejected. How his parents cope with the realities of being different—racially, economically, culturally, and intellectually—will strongly influence the child's adjustment. If the parents convey pride in what they are and show the value in their way of life, the child will be able to sift out the essential values and avoid feelings of superiority or inferiority. His confidence in himself will also influence the way in which he is treated within the community.

In most communities, there are many organizations that play an important part in the social growth of families and their members. Groups such as the Girl Scouts and the Boy Scouts provide programs for youngsters and increase the awareness of the youngsters of the variety of cultural contributions and talents that make America great. Many communities also have organizations and even recreational facilities available for particular interest groups, such as the Jewish Family Service, the Christian Family Movement, the various religious, ethnic, and other associations. Most people have access to community resources and health professionals such as physicians, social workers, psychologists, family counselors, and health department services, and all can volunteer their services for the good of others through organizations such as the American Red Cross. These and many other programs and services can be helpful to families as they work to accomplish their individual and family tasks.

ACCEPTING CHANGE

In the family, as in any group, things never remain the same. New members arrive through birth, adoption, marriage, or invitation. Some members leave through death, separation, divorce, moving out to begin homes of their own, moving away to new jobs or schools, etc. Individuals in the family are constantly growing both physically and emotionally, and their needs, interests, and personalities change. Such constant change requires that family members be educated for change so that they may better accept new arrivals, growing and differing personalities, and separations and death. Such education is essential to sound mental health.

It is natural for the individual to have mixed feelings about his relationship to the family or, indeed, to any group. Although the warmth and closeness of any form of group living is very desirable, each individual also needs some privacy and the right to be who he is, to express himself as he chooses. Just as the toddler who is becoming aware of his own separate identity can make life difficult for those who love and care for him, every individual feels some conflict between his own needs and the values of group living.

When a new member enters the family, perhaps through birth or marriage, there are mixed feelings on both sides. For a young child, the welcoming of a new baby into the family can be very disturbing. Although the child may be proud to have a new brother or sister, he may also feel jealous and pushed aside. With the introduction of a new parent or children through remarriage, the newcomer may be worried about being liked and accepted. The existing family is also likely to miss the way things were before the new person came. Similar reactions occur when a new person or family moves into the neighborhood. People who recognize that such mixed feelings are normal can take special steps to help both the newcomer and those who are likely to have difficulty in accepting the changing situation. Families should take prompt action to welcome and get to know newcomers. Any delay may allow negative or fearful feelings to develop.

With death, divorce, separation, or any parting, people experience grief reactions and often require special support and comfort. When a family member leaves to start an independent life of his own, whether because of school, career, or marriage, the family's anticipation of a happy new life for the departing member is often mixed with fear and concern that things may not go well. When a family member or a friend dies, more emotions than simple grief may be involved. (For example, a child may be angry that a parent has deserted him.) When you are adjusting to any parting, it is important to communicate feelings honestly, to remember the past and the special relationship you have shared with the departing person, and to come to a gradual acceptance of the normal reaction of sadness and grief. Through such open communication, all family members gain new strength to make the best of the new situation. Then, too, not all separations are final. A couple whose children have grown and left home will see them again when they return to visit their "home base," and there will be a growing sense of the life cycle among all the generations.

During his life, an individual is usually a member of several social, work, leisure, and other interest groups as well as the family unit. It takes time to develop a good relationship with a new individual or group, and most relationships end after a period of time. Since American families today typically live in several different communities over a lifetime, most people will have to take steps to become part of a new social environment at some time during their lives. Relationships also begin and end because of changing interests. Becoming involved with a new group can be both an attractive and a frightening prospect, involving worries both that the individual many not really like the new people and that they may not like him. These feelings are often particularly traumatic for young children, who may need the support and encouragement of their parents in adjusting to a new situation.

The child who grows up in an affectionate and understanding family, where concern is shown for each individual's needs and personality, becomes the adult who is able to relate well to others and to make his own unique contribution to others. The broader his exposure through education and family outings, the more he will be able to enjoy and profit from new experiences. Through relations with friends, school and work associates, neighbors who come and go, distant relatives with whom he visits, he acquires a sense of the coming and going aspects of group life and the certainty of change. Eventually, he may choose to begin a family of his own.

SPECIAL PROBLEMS AND RESOURCES

Sometimes it seems that no previous age has challenged the family's role of providing a stable environment for individual growth and fulfillment as much as the present age. At the same time, more seems to be expected of the family than ever before. People who expect the family to function smoothly and perfectly along traditional lines in an era of rapid change and greater emphasis on seeking personal happiness and self-fulfillment are often shocked when they experience or hear about the growing frequency of divorce, child neglect and abuse, pregnancy occurring outside marriage, and emotional problems that arise when persons no longer know what to expect from life.

When the pace of life was slower, when religious beliefs and moral principles were unchanging, and when couples were expected to remain married for life, it may have been much easier to adjust to the realities of life. Now it is not uncommon for an adult to raise children without a partner or spouse, for a child to have to adjust to a "new" father or mother, for a person to hear that a priest has left the church and gotten married, or for someone to find his job eliminated by technological advances or his health seriously threatened by changes to the body that are brought on principally from anxiety or the environment.

People cope with the stresses brought by rapid change in a variety of ways. A child may fall behind in school; one person may withdraw while another may express his frustration in acts of violence; some persons will develop an ulcer, high blood pressure, or a drinking problem. The healthiest approach to stress is almost always to share one's problems in communication with others. In addition to the usually available ear of the clergyman or health professional, there are now a variety of community organizations and agencies that are able to help the individual cope with stress brought on by specific types of problems. These include the local public health department, family social service agencies, mental health centers or clinics, and various church and government agencies devoted to family counseling, such as Catholic Charities and Lutheran Child and Family Services. In addition, many self-help groups have sprung up, such as Parents Without Partners, special groups for widowed persons, and Alcoholics Anonymous.

Most communities have one or more of the above sources of help available. Every family should be aware of the types of resources available to help them and to help others who are troubled. Many of these resources can be found by inquiring and by checking the yellow pages of the telephone directory.

THE FAMILY'S ROLE IN SICKNESS AND HEALTH

The family has a special responsibility in caring for the health of its members. In the family, health decisions are made and personal care is undertaken. The family is the most frequent provider of health care and the channel through which most health education takes place. The family may prevent or may contribute to the health problems of its members. Although sometimes the family must learn to understand and accept a long-range health problem in one of its members, it can often do much to correct many poor health situations. The health of any one family member usually affects the level of wellness of all other members in some way.

The specific health tasks of the family might be described as follows:

- To maintain a home environment that fosters good health practices and sound personal development
- To prevent illness through immunizations, good nutrition, and other health habits
- To deal responsibly and effectively with all kinds of crises in the family
- To recognize interruptions of normal development such as illness or the failure of a child to thrive
- To make decisions about seeking health care: whether or not to see a physician, to check with a pharmacist or a nurse, or to "just wait and see"
- To maintain a relationship with the community and its health institutions and resources and to know the rights of the sick person to receive effective care
- To provide nursing care for family members with minor illnesses and injuries and for sick, disabled, or dependent members of the family, including special care for the very young

Serious illness can greatly disrupt family routine and even threaten family security. If a major illness or accident should require the hospitalization of a family member, there is a further threat of heavy medical expenses. Meeting such expenses can cause severe financial hardship, whether or not the family has health insurance. This is particularly true if the sick person is the family breadwinner.

The person acting as the home nurse in giving health care to a sick family member can help the family to function better if he is aware of the following factors:

- The seriousness of the illness
- The methods of planning and giving nursing care for short- or long-term periods of time

- The dependence of the family upon the ill person, and the ways in which the patient's responsibilities can be assumed by others
- Each family member's understanding of and response to the nature of the illness
- The needs of each family member that must be met

The home nurse can do much to lessen the family's fears and to make use of their willingness to be of assistance by demonstrating understanding of their feelings and paying attention to their needs as well as to the needs of the sick person.

Chapter 4

Preparation for Parenthood

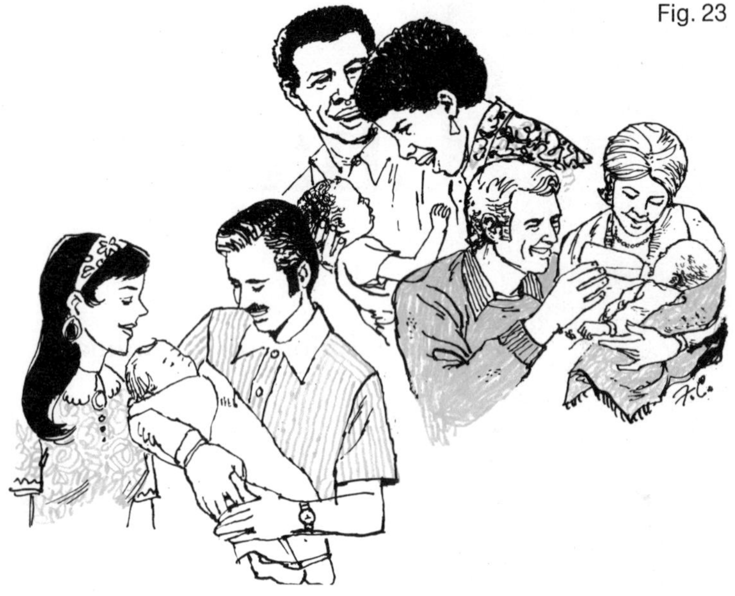

Fig. 23

The birth of a baby is a time of great excitement and the beginning of a new way of life. During the 9-month period before birth, a baby passes through many fascinating phases of development. The mother-to-be has much to think about and to do so that she can be sure of the healthy growth and safe delivery of her baby. Also, she must prepare for the effect that the baby will have on her own life and on the lives of her husband and any older children. Ideally, she has been preparing all her life for this important step, through good nutrition and health habits and through the building of healthy attitudes toward childbearing and the rearing of children.

Childbearing affects every body process. Changing the body's delicate balance to provide for the nutrition and growth of a developing baby is done most safely under the supervision of a health professional. Health care during pregnancy is preventive in nature. Everything possible is done to make sure, through testing, good diet, and sound health practices, that both mother and baby will always be in the best possible state of health.

The experiences of each mother through pregnancy and delivery are different. Some women may experience nausea, but many others will not. Some babies in the womb kick sooner or more vigorously than others. Although many women experience a long first labor and delivery, mothers having a second or third baby may breeze through the process relatively quickly—or the second or third experience may be as long or longer than the first.

Preparing for the birth of a new baby involves many aspects. In addition to getting a crib and diapers, many new parents-to-be will want to take advantage of courses being offered to prepare them for childbirth and infant care. Often a properly prepared father will have the chance to be present throughout labor and the delivery of his child. If properly prepared, he may actually help the mother (and thus the baby) in the process, and the experience may result in his developing an even stronger bond with both the mother and the baby.

Preparation for parenthood begins with thinking about the meaning of parenthood. Parenting includes giving love, attention, and guidance as well as providing food, shelter, and clothing. Particularly at the coming of the first baby, the mother and father need to plan together for the changes and adjustments that are going to take place in their lives, although the full impact of the differences will not be felt until after the baby has actually come. The expectant father should be involved throughout pregnancy, taking great interest in the progress of the growing fetus and sharing in the discomforts of pregnancy. He will acquire a strong sense of "our baby" through his active involvement.

Pregnancy is often accompanied by mixed feelings on the part of both parents-to-be. Along with joyful anticipation that there will be a child to love, guide, and share one's life with, there may be anxiety about the processes of pregnancy, delivery, and child care, about financial concerns, and about how the relationships with the family will change with the arrival of the new baby. Taking childbirth preparation courses will do much to prepare the family for what lies ahead and also will give them an opportunity to share feelings and experiences with other expectant parents.

BEGINNING THE PREGNANCY

Planning the Pregnancy

People have different ideas about the right time to have a baby. Personal values, social trends, religious beliefs, and desires in regard to planning for a certain length of time between children (child-spacing) influence decisions about having a baby.

The ideal time for pregnancy seems to be between the ages of 20 and 30, with about two or three years between the end of one pregnancy and the beginning of another. This approach results in fewer premature deliveries and increases the chance of having a healthy baby. Teenage mothers and those over 35 are more likely to experience complications during pregnancy.

Planning for child-spacing not only gives the mother time to recover from the physical and emotional strain of the last pregnancy but also helps to make sure that each child receives adequate care and affection during his period of greatest need, before another child is born. Some parents will want the previous child to be talking, toilet-trained, and able to manage some activities on his own in order to avoid the stress of caring for two very small children at the same time.

Some couples who have difficulty in conceiving now have more hope of becoming parents with the aid of new research and the help of obstetricians and gynecologists. It is often possible to determine whether the man or the woman has an unusual problem that prevents pregnancy and then to take steps to make pregnancy more likely.

Once a woman is pregnant, anxieties often occur about the timing, about finances, and about the way in which existing relationships will be affected, along with joy, pride, and loving anticipation. In the initial stages, the woman's mood changes, and early signs of pregnancy such as drowsiness and possible nausea make it difficult for her to sort out her emotions. It may take several months for her to adjust to the fact that a pregnancy has really begun.

Signs of Pregnancy

The most common sign of pregnancy is a missed menstrual period. In addition, the breasts may tingle or become sensitive. Some women will experience nausea, or "morning sickness," but this symptom is not as common as it was once thought to be. Excessive sleepiness is another sign of pregnancy.

After the second missed period, the existence of a pregnancy can be determined easily by a physical examination. It is possible to confirm a pregnancy sooner, however, through testing a sample of the woman's urine with a chemical. This test can indicate pregnancy only 12 days after the first missed menstrual period (about 26 days after conception). Several other forms of testing are also in use but are not always reliable. Early confirmation of pregnancy is particularly necessary for women who have a tendency toward miscarriage (delivery of the fetus before it has developed enough to live).

The sooner a woman knows she is pregnant, the sooner she can begin actions to protect the growing baby (fetus). Any female who suspects that she may be pregnant should avoid taking any medications without a doctor's approval. Research continues to show new links between medicines and diseases (such as German measles) that have a negative effect on the growing fetus. *A women who is pregnant or who may be pregnant should not receive any kind of vaccination under any circumstances, because there is a chance of risk to the fetus.* She should also not allow X-rays unless she is sure the fetus is protected.

The pregnant woman should choose the health professional carefully, especially if she prefers a particular method of childbirth. If she hopes to have her husband or a friend with her during labor and delivery, she should discuss these matters frankly with the health professional. Women should be able to participate in their delivery in the way in which they desire and are prepared.

HEALTH CARE DURING PREGNANCY

A woman who thinks she may be pregnant should seek health care within 2 or 3 weeks after the first menstrual period is missed. The objective of health care during pregnancy is to keep both mother and baby in the best possible physical condition throughout the pregnancy and to make sure of a safe delivery and speedy recovery. The mother-to-be will be examined regularly by the health professional, who will monitor her health and nutrition and the health and growth of the baby. The health professional will usually want to see the mother-to-be at least once a month until the sixth or seventh month, then more frequently during the last 2 months.

Health History

The medical history of the mother is very important, and that of the father too, in order to evaluate the general health of the mother and the prospects for a healthy baby. Special care may be needed if certain conditions are present (for example, diabetes, heart disease, tuberculosis, or extreme youth or advanced age). It is important for the health professional to know whether the pregnant woman has had, or is protected against, any communicable diseases that could affect her health or the health of the unborn baby. Any illness, accident, or condition that could affect the progress of the pregnancy or the delivery must be evaluated. Previous delivery by Caesarian section (baby removed surgically from the uterus), the blood Rh factor (see page 104), and previous complications are examples of elements that will have to be considered.

Physical Examination

On the first visit, the health professional may be able to confirm the pregnancy through physical examination by noting changes in the color of the vagina and cervix and noting softening of the cervix. He would also note the size of the uterus and examine the breasts for any abnormalities. He would make a routine check for cervical cancer (Pap smear) and gonorrhea. He may measure the internal dimensions of the pelvis to see if it is large enough for the baby to pass through. (X-rays are not usually taken in early pregnancy because of possible danger to the mother and fetus.) A sample of blood will be taken that will be used to determine—

- The blood type of the mother.
- The absence or presence of the Rh factor.
- The amount of time it takes the blood to clot. This information helps the health professional to prepare for the possibility of hemorrhage (excessive bleeding) during delivery.
- Hemoglobin content, which determines whether the mother has anemia.
- Whether the mother has syphilis, in which case treatment would be started.

Regular Visits

On follow-up visits, the health professional will usually check as follows:

- The urine is tested for sugar, albumin, and waste materials that show whether the kidneys are functioning properly and how well the mother is tolerating the increased strain of pregnancy.
- The blood pressure is monitored for any early signs of problems.
- The hemoglobin will be tested to detect anemia.
- The feet and legs will be observed for swelling and varicose veins.
- The growth of the fetus and uterus will be observed.
- The baby's heartbeat will be listened to.
- The mother's weight will be watched.

Any questions that the mother wishes to ask can be asked during the visit. If any complications arise, she should call the health professional.

Signs of Possible Complications

If a woman receives good care throughout pregnancy, she is less likely to develop any complications, although complications of pregnancy are rather rare. The health professional will want to be notified of any unusual discomforts. The following are possible danger signals and should *always* be reported promptly:

- Bleeding from the vagina, no matter how slight
- Sudden excessive weight gain
- Swelling or puffiness of face or hands
- Frequent headaches
- Sharp or continuous pain in the abdomen

- Severe or continuous vomiting
- Chills or fever, or both
- Dimness or blurring of vision, or flashes of light or spots before the eyes
- Sudden escape or dribbling of fluid from the vagina

Weight Gain in Pregnancy

In general, it is suggested that pregnant women should gain about 24 pounds (11 kilograms). A woman who is underweight at the time that pregnancy begins might be advised to gain 30 or more pounds (17 kilograms), while a woman who is definitely obese might be advised to gain only 22 pounds (10 kilograms).

Pregnancy is not the time to lose weight; however, chemical changes in the mother's body during weight loss can damage the baby's developing brain. The weight gain should be gradual: only 1.5–3 pounds (.07–1.4 kilograms) should be gained in the first 3 months, and about .5 to 1 pound (.02–.05 kilograms) per week after 3 months. The following information gives an idea of the general distribution of the weight just before delivery.

	Pounds	Kilograms
Baby	7.5	3.4
Placenta	1.4	.7
Amniotic fluid	2.2	1.0
Uterus	2.2	1.0
Breast growth	1.1	.5
Blood volume	3.3	1.5
Extracellular fluid	3.3	1.5
Maternal stores (fat and protein to support lactation)	3.0	1.5

NUTRITION AND HEALTH DURING PREGNANCY

The woman who puts effort into her diet, who follows good health practices in coping with the discomforts of pregnancy, and who perhaps attends classes that increase her understanding of pregnancy, childbirth, and infant care, can feel confident that she is doing her best for her child. The self-discipline she practices and the consideration she shows for her baby will carry over into her mothering. The woman who, with the father, prepares consciously for childbirth can expect to begin her labor with confidence and knowledge. Her positive outlook will benefit her whole family.

Nutrition

Good nutrition during pregnancy is based on the same principles as good nutrition at any time (discussed in chapter 2). There is a close relation between nutrition and the outcome of the pregnancy, the health of the mother and the baby, and the mother's ability to nurse the baby. The health professional who works with the mother throughout the pregnancy is the best person to advise on diet.

During pregnancy, there is need for a gradual increase in protein, vitamins, and minerals. During the last 3 months, the need for calories may also increase, since that is a period of rapid growth for the baby. However, some women become less active physically and do not require a higher calorie intake. Check with the health professional regarding diet during the last 3 months, because many health professionals guard the mother's weight gain very carefully during that period. The quality of the diet is most important. This means that foods containing essential nutrients should take precedence over high calorie, empty nutrient foods such as sodas, candies, cakes, pies, and many popular snack foods such as potato chips. Protein is important in keeping the mother's body healthy while it is undergoing changes. It is also important because it aids in the baby's growth.

GUIDE FOR RECOMMENDED FOOD DURING PREGNANCY AND LACTATION

Food	Pregnancy	Lactation
Milk (vitamin D fortified)	3–4 cups	6 cups
Meat, fish, poultry (liver once a week)	4 oz.	4 oz.
Eggs	3–4 per week	3–4 per week
Vegetables, including—		
Dark green	½ cup	½ cup
Other vegetables (one vegetable to be raw)	1 cup	1 cup
Fruits, including—		
Citrus	1 serving	1 serving
Other fruit	1 serving	1 serving
Cereal (whole grain, preferably)	1 serving	1 serving
Bread (whole grain, preferably)	5 slices	5 slices
Fats (polyunsaturated oil or margarine)	1 tbsp.	1 tbsp.
Sugars, sweets, cooking fats	Only to meet calorie needs	
Iodized salt	Daily	Daily

By following the food guide, you should be able to make sure that every calorie you eat carries nutrients with it. Foods that are high in calories but low in nutrients, such as popular snack foods, candy, and carbonated beverages, should be avoided. If weight gain is faster than is recommended, cutting down on fats in foods by substituting skim milk for whole milk, avoiding fried foods, and increasing exercise may be recommended.

It is very important that the expansion of blood and fluid volume that is normal in pregnancy be allowed to occur. Sodium (salt) intake should *not* be restricted during pregnancy. This recommendation is a change from recommendations of the past. Sodium not only allows normal fluid expansion to occur but is also needed in the development of tissues and bones of the baby. The pregnant woman should be allowed to salt her food to taste. Use of iodized salt is recommended because the baby needs iodine.

Vitamin or mineral pills cannot make a poor diet nutritionally adequate. A good diet based on the food guide will provide all the vitamins and minerals needed for the normal woman, with the possible exceptions of iron and folic acid for some women. Women who enter pregnancy with low body stores of iron may have iron supplements prescribed by the health professional to prevent anemia. Some women will also need to have folic acid prescribed to prevent anemia because of an increased need for this vitamin during the last trimester of pregnancy.

Some of the specific discomforts of pregnancy can be alleviated with special attention to the diet. For example:

- Having an adequate roughage intake of such foods as fruits, vegetables, whole-grain breads, cereals, and bran, and an increase in fluids, will do much to prevent problems with constipation.
- Increasing calcium intake may help in leg cramps.
- Avoiding greasy foods, highly seasoned foods, and foods high in sugar and starch will help to control heartburn.
- Getting enough iron in the diet will prevent anemia.

The woman who eats wisely during pregnancy knows she has done what she can to make sure of a healthy baby, to protect her own health, and perhaps even to make for an easier and less complicated delivery through maintenance of her own strength.

Good Health Practices

In general, pregnant women are encouraged to continue their usual activities. Work, most forms of exercise, tub baths, sexual intercourse, and travel are usually permissible without restriction until the last few months before the expected delivery. Any questions on these activities should be discussed with the health professional. Examples of good health practices that are especially important during pregnancy are as follows:

- Get ample rest. It is common to feel drowsy and fatigued during the early months of pregnancy.
- Continue sexual intercourse as long as both persons are comfortable, *unless* the health professional advises otherwise.
- Avoid douching, unless it is advised or approved by the health professional.
- Wear stable, supportive shoes, or at least avoid high heels or platform shoes.
- Take *NO* medication, not even vitamins or laxatives, without first checking with the health professional.
- Avoid alcohol. Alcohol reaches the fetus through the placenta. Frequent use of alcohol during pregnancy has been shown to cause serious health conditions in the baby, including low birth weight.
- Avoid smoking. Babies born to mothers who smoke are more likely to be born prematurely or to be of low birth weight if full term.
- Wash breasts and nipples to remove colostrum if present. (See the following section for information on breast care.)
- Do not wear constricting clothing (for example, tight pants, rolled or elasticized stockings) that cuts off circulation to the legs. Pantyhose (with cotton crotch) or a maternity garter belt may be useful.
- Continue exercise as usual. (Consult the health professional if there are any questions.) If you have no regular exercise, it would be good to add a 10-minute walk to your daily routine.
- Undertake exercises that are helpful in increasing comfort during pregnancy, strengthening muscles for delivery, and improving the physical condition of the body. (The health professional can demonstrate or explain these.)
- Do not have vaccinations.

Breast Care

Breasts will be examined for any abnormalities by the health professional. Lumps in the breast are not unusual during pregnancy, but only the health professional can determine whether they are of medical significance. The breasts should be kept clean. If the nipples are not washed daily, they may become encrusted with secretions (colostrum), and this condition may lead to cracking and unusual tenderness when the baby begins to nurse.

Wash the nipples with soap and warm water with a circling motion, and then move outward in a circular fashion until the entire breast has been washed. The health professional should recommend any special care. As the breasts become larger in preparation for nursing the baby, they become heavier, and extra support may be needed early in pregnancy. A larger brassiere will be needed, with wide, adjustable straps and cups large enough to support the breasts without undue pressure. The health professional will usually give advice regarding the type of brassiere to be worn.

Common Discomforts

Although pregnancy is a normal process, most women at some time or another during pregnancy experience some discomfort. This is usually due to the normal changes occurring in the body and is only temporary. Often, simple changes in the usual routine or in the diet, or simple exercise, will bring relief. Some of the more common discomforts and a few measures to bring relief are as follows:

- *Fatigue*—Drowsiness and fatigue are common during pregnancy. Plan for extra rest, particularly during the day. It is good to sit with your legs and feet elevated to decrease pooling of blood in the legs.
- *Frequent urination*—This may be caused by pressure from the growing uterus and is common in the first 3 months of pregnancy and again in the last 3 months. If nighttime urination is a problem, limit fluid intake after 6:00 p.m. or consult the health professional.
- *Morning sickness*—Nausea and vomiting may occur at any time of the day but are more common in the morning (if they occur at all). Keeping dry toast or crackers by the bed and eating them 5 to 10 minutes before getting up may be helpful.
- *Heartburn or indigestion*—Smaller, more frequent meals will often

help. Avoid greasy, fried foods and highly spiced foods and any other foods that are known to cause difficulty.

- *Constipation*—Avoid laxatives. Drink lots of water (1–2 quarts a day, or .946–1.9 liters), eat raw fruits and vegetables, or prunes. Exercise daily.
- *Backache*—Backache is caused by adjusting the posture to support the heavy abdomen. Do exercises to strengthen the lower back muscles, such as the "pelvic rock." Use a firm mattress or bed-board. Bend from the knees rather than at the back when stooping to pick up a heavy object. Try to maintain good posture.

  The pelvic rock is done either lying on your back or in a position on hands and knees. When lying on the back, bend the knees so that the feet are flat on the floor. Press the back against the floor, pulling in the abdomen and letting the buttocks lift slowly off the floor. Release the muscles and allow the small of the back to come off the floor.

  When on hands and knees, place the hands about 12 inches (4.8 centimeters) apart and the knees about 9 inches (3.6 centimeters) apart. Keep the knees in line with the hips. Let the back sag and raise the buttocks as high as possible. Take a deep breath. Then slowly raise the back, expel the breath, and, at the same time, squeeze the muscles of the buttocks and pelvic area and tighten the muscles of the upper legs. Repeat the pelvic rock exercises eight or ten times slowly and firmly.
- *Leg cramps*—Rub the feet and legs, then stretch the feet forward. Keep the feet elevated and warm when cramps occur. It may be wise to check with the health professional regarding calcium intake.
- *Vaginal secretions*—There is a normal increase in vaginal secretions during pregnancy. If, however, there is itching or a bad odor, there may be an infection present. The health professional should be notified so that treatment may be started. Synthetic pantyhose or pants may add to the problem; cotton-crotch garments may reduce the problem.
- *Hemorrhoids*—Straining at bowel movements when you are constipated is not advisable. Increase exercise and roughage intake to prevent or relieve constipation. Consult the health professional if the condition is severe.
- *Edema*—Edema is the excessive collection of fluids in body tissues. If this condition occurs in the legs, make an effort to spend greater

amounts of time sitting with your legs elevated and avoid standing still for long periods of time. If edema occurs in other parts of the body, consult the health professional and report the time of day it occurs and in which part of the body it occurs. Also, ask about the wearing of support stockings if the edema is in the legs or ankles.

- *Varicose veins*—Varicose veins may be caused by pressure of the growing uterus on the large blood vessels that carry blood to the legs. The symptoms are dull, aching pains, a sense of weight or heaviness, fatigue, sometimes itching, and the appearance of enlarged veins on the legs. Pregnancy may make already-existing varicose veins even more troublesome. Sometimes, women will develop varicose veins during the last few months of pregnancy, yet have no trouble with them after the pregnancy.

  Frequent rest periods, particularly with your feet raised on a chair or a stool while you are sitting, or on pillows when you are lying down, usually bring relief from discomfort. Avoid crossing your legs when sitting. Avoid wearing stockings with elastic bands or any clothing that restricts the free flow of blood from the legs. Avoid standing for long periods of time. If the health professional advises it, support stockings may be worn.
- *Difficulty in sleeping*—Sometimes late in pregnancy, you may have difficulty in sleeping. Such sleeplessness may be caused by the increased bulk of the body or by the tendency of the baby to kick while the mother is at rest. Pillows placed in the right spots may help you to find a comfortable position. A walk or a warm shower, or both, before going to bed may help.
- *Faintness or dizziness*—If this occurs while you are lying on your back, turning to rest on your side may stop or prevent the problem. Pressure of the uterus on a major blood vessel may cause the problem.

CHANGES IN THE BABY AND THE MOTHER

The normal period of pregnancy is about 9 months, or 280 days from the beginning of the last menstrual period. The 9 months are divided into three periods of 3 months each, known as trimesters. The word trimester is commonly used when various signs and developments that occur during pregnancy are referred to. General information about the growth of the fetus and changes in the mother is presented below.

First Trimester

Within 2 weeks after the egg (ovum) has been fertilized by the sperm in the Fallopian tube of the mother, it attaches itself to the lining of the uterus, and the mother will experience the first signs of pregnancy: a missed menstrual period and possible breast tenderness and tingling. By this time, the single egg has divided and redivided many times. Soon it will be developed enough to be called an embryo and will have its own protective covering (the sac) and fluids, and the umbilical cord and placenta through which it will receive oxygen and nourishment for the next 9 months.

By the end of the first month, the heart and brain have developed, the arms and legs are beginning to grow, and the sense organs are developing. The embryo is only ½ inch (1.3 centimeters) long. At this time, the mother begins to feel drowsy and may even feel nauseated.

By the end of the second month, the embryo begins to take on a human appearance, although its head is abnormally large. All its major body systems are developing, and its taste buds have formed. The growth of the uterus puts pressure on the mother's bladder, and she will have to urinate more often because of reduced space to hold urine. New hormones are circulating through her body, and her breasts become fuller and the nipples may darken. She may also notice a dark vertical line on her abdomen, called *linea nigra.*

At the end of the third month, the embryo (now called a fetus) is definitely recognizable as human. All its body systems are developed and have started to function together. Its fingernails and toenails are forming. The eyelids are formed but are still fused together. The fetus, which has been growing at a rate of about ¼ inch (.64 centimeters) a week, is now over 3 inches (7.6 centimeters) long and weighs about ½ ounce (14 grams).

Second Trimester

The second trimester is usually the most peaceful time of pregnancy, with the fewest problems. The mother begins to take on the "glow" of pregnancy, and with the first feelings of the baby kicking (called "quickening"), the mother begins to sense the fetus as an individual separate from herself. She may begin to reach full acceptance of her pregnancy. Nausea, if any, usually stops at about this time. The abdomen and breasts gradually grow larger, and stretch marks may appear. The mother may notice increased saliva and perspiration and may experience leg and foot cramps.

The fetus at 4 months is almost a fully formed human being, although it probably could not survive outside the womb at this point. Its major body systems are developed, its movements can be felt by the mother, its heartbeat can be heard by stethoscope, its posture is straighter, its facial features are better developed, its hands and feet have creases and fingerprints, and sexual differences can be seen. Tooth buds are present, and the bones are beginning to harden. The fetus is 6 inches (15.2 centimeters) long and weighs about one ounce (28.3 grams).

At the end of the fifth month, the fetus is covered with downy hair all over, and a white, cheeselike covering forms on the skin. The fetus is 8 inches (20.3 centimeters) long.

At the end of the sixth month, the baby's eyes can open, and eyelashes and eyebrows are formed. The skin is wrinkled. The heart and liver are enlarged. The fetus is 10–12 inches (25.4–30.5 centimeters) long and weighs about 1½ pounds (681 grams). If the baby were to be born prematurely at this point, it could, in some cases, live with medical help.

Third Trimester

The rapid growth of the baby during the third trimester causes a variety of discomforts to the mother. It may be difficult to maintain good posture, to sleep comfortably, or to move about as normal. The mother is likely to experience backaches, feel pressure in the lower abdomen, and have constipation, increased frequency of urination, indigestion and heartburn, and shortness of the breath as the growing baby crowds her internal organs. Aching legs and fatigue and restlessness and fretfulness while awaiting the delivery date are common experiences. The mother begins to think more about the coming labor and delivery. This is a good time to get things together for the hospital stay and for the baby. Late in this period, the head of the fetus settles into the pelvis (referred to as "dropping" or "lightening"), there is less pressure on the stomach, and breathing may be easier.

During the seventh month, the baby's brain increases in size and its complex functioning is more developed. The baby begins to move more freely in the womb. A sticky, greenish substance (called meconium) forms in the intestines. The fetus is 12 inches (30.5 centimeters) long and weighs 2–3 pounds (907–1361 grams). If born at this time, the baby would have a better chance to survive with proper medical care.

During the eighth and ninth months, the baby continues to grow rapidly, more fat forms under the skin, and the skin looks less wrinkled. The antibodies the baby needs for protection against disease in the first few months of life are being acquired. Head hair is present, and the skull hardens but its sections are not grown together. During birth, the sections of the skull will overlap to make the head smaller so that the baby can pass through the birth canal more easily. The fetus is 19–20 inches (48.3–50.8 centimeters) long and weighs 6–7 pounds (2,721–3,175 grams). All its systems are mature enough to maintain life outside the womb; however, the more growing that is done inside the womb, the better chance the baby has to begin a healthy life. A baby weighing less than 5½ pounds (2,494 grams) or born before the 38th week is referred to as premature.

PREPARING FOR THE NEW ARRIVAL

It is not necessary to spend a fortune for clothing and equipment for a new baby. Often, clothing for the baby is received as gifts. Some equipment may be borrowed. If this is not the first baby, there will be many items of used clothing and equipment on hand for the newcomer. When purchases are made, costs should be kept within the family budget. Some articles might be made at home better and more cheaply.

In addition to acquiring equipment and clothing, preparing for a new baby involves choosing a doctor or a source of health care for the baby. It also involves talking with any older brothers and sisters and planning measures to make all family members feel secure at a time when meeting the demands of a new baby will require a lot of time and attention. Another aspect of preparation may be childbirth or child-care courses. The expectant parents will also need to prepare for the hospital stay by gathering needed items.

Preparing Brothers and Sisters

Preparing for the baby's arrival is a family affair. When there are other children in the family, they too must be prepared for the arrival of a new baby. It is not wise to tell very young children about the expected birth more than a month or two in advance, since telling them before that makes the time seem like a very long wait. Older children, even with the most thoughtful preparation, are likely to have mixed feelings about the competition for the attention of parents that comes with a new baby. They may revert to more babyish ways of acting and may exhibit other unusual behavior as they seek to continue receiving attention from the parents. Patience and special efforts to give more, rather than less, loving care to the older chil-

Fig. 24

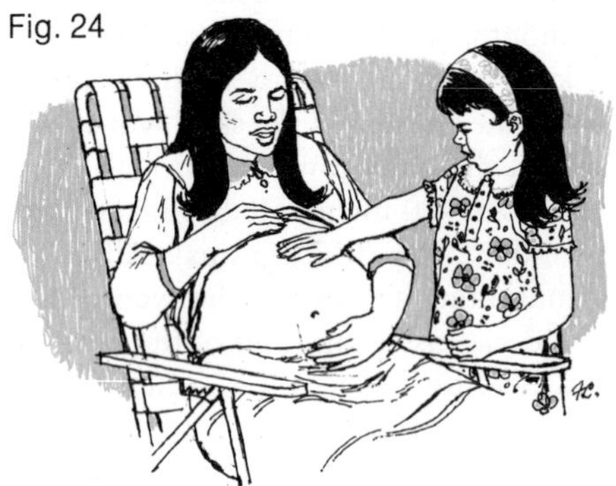

dren will avoid many of these problems. Even if the parents have less time to give, the quality of the time spent with each child is very

Fig. 25

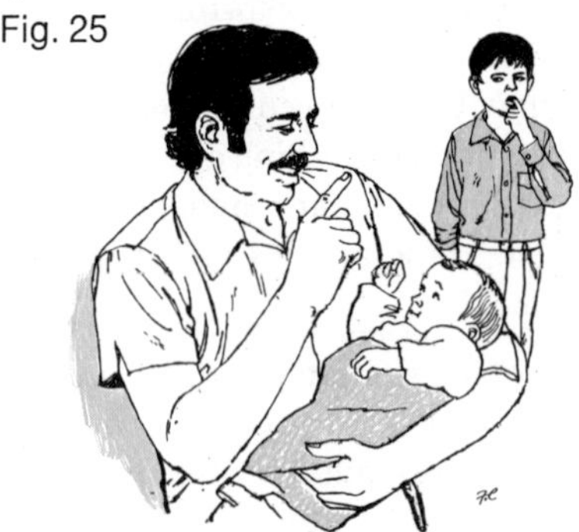

important. For instance, a mother might read to an older child while she nurses the baby or might enlist the help of the older brothers and sisters in caring for the baby. Fathers, especially, can be helpful during this period by giving more time to the older children.

Fig. 26

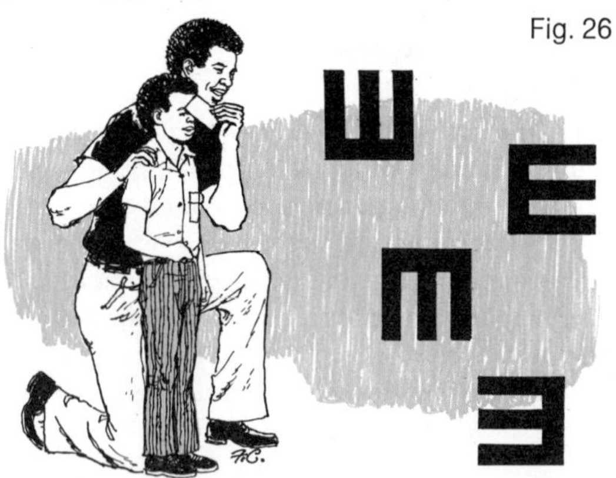

Choosing the Baby's Doctor

It is a good idea to choose the source of health care for the baby *before* his birth. The health professional or clinic can give advice as needed and will provide medical help if problems arise. It is customary for new babies to have monthly checkups and begin receiving immunizations within a month after birth. Many doctors or health clinics will answer questions over the telephone. Be sure to check to see whether this service is available or not.

The Baby's Bed

The baby does not need a bassinet but does feel more secure if his first bed is not as large as a crib. A box, dresser drawer, or large basket with towels for mattress and padding is quite adequate for several months. When acquiring a crib, look for the following features:

- Slats on crib sides no more than 2⅜ inches (5.8 centimeters) apart, so that the baby's head cannot slip through or become wedged.
- A latch for the sides that is not easily released, so that the baby cannot fall.
- High enough crib sides so that there is no danger of the baby's falling out. (When the baby is taller by one fourth than the rail, he is in danger of falling.)
- A firm mattress.
- A mattress that fits snugly in the crib so that the baby cannot become wedged in a crevice. (About an inch, 2.5 centimeters, can be allowed on one side when the mattress is pushed to the other side.)

It is not a good idea to use a pillow in the baby's bed. The following supplies are needed for the bed:

- A fitted plastic mattress cover or two or three flannelette-covered waterproof pads.
- Three or four crib sheets.
- One or two heavy blankets. (Four crib blankets can be made from one large blanket, usually at a considerable saving.)
- From two to four waterproof flannelette or quilted cotton pads about 18 inches square (45.7 centimeters) to place under the baby to protect the sheet (or the mother's lap) from wet diapers and drooling.

Diapers

Diapers are a necessity. Even if a diaper service or disposable diapers will be used, you should have at least a dozen cloth diapers on hand.

They are especially useful when burping the baby, to protect your clothing. Cost and convenience are the major considerations. Although diposable diapers are more expensive, they save much time in terms of laundering and are particularly convenient when traveling. The baby may use as many as 80–100 diapers a week. If cloth diapers are used, from three to four dozen will be needed. A diaper pail with a cover is needed to hold soiled diapers. Safety pins may be necessary, even though you may be using disposable diapers, which have self-sticking tapes.

The Baby's Clothing

Clothing should be lightweight, suitable to the climate and season of the year, loose enough to allow freedom of movement and ease in putting on or removing it, and nonirritating to the skin. Labels will provide information on the fiber content and the laundering procedures. You should select clothing that requires a minimum of care. It is a needless expense to buy very small clothing, because the baby will outgrow it quickly. The best buys are 12- and 24-month sizes. Many items of clothing may be received as gifts, and others may be borrowed or used. The following list should be modified or added to, according to the climate or season in which the infant is expected to be born. A basic supply of clothing includes—

- From four to six cotton-knit shirts
- Three or four cotton-knit nightgowns (perhaps with handy drawstrings or special cuffs to close over the baby's feet and hands to keep them warm) or kimonos
- Two sweaters and a cap
- From two to four pairs of waterproof pants
- Three or four cotton flannel receiving blankets to wrap the baby in
- A "blanket sleeper," or bunting, for cold-weather sleeping

Supplies for Bathing the Baby

The baby may be bathed in the kitchen sink, which should be cleaned and lined with a towel, or in a plastic or enamel basin, which may be set in the sink or on a table of suitable height. Other necessities include—

- Two soft towels.
- Two soft washcloths.
- Mild soap. (Shampoo is not necessary at first.)
- Scissors for cutting fingernails and toenails.

Preparation for Feeding the Baby

If the baby is going to be breast-fed, it is wise to start preparing the nipples during the last few months of pregnancy. Massaging them with lanolin for a few minutes several times a day is all that is necessary. Avoid soap on the nipples, since it will cause them to become dry.

Even if the baby is to be breast-fed, two or three bottles and nipples are necessary for feeding him boiled water and juice. Glass bottles are easier to clean and boil than plastic presterilized ones, although disposable plastic bottles are an alternative. If the baby is to be bottle-fed, the following items will be needed:

- From six to eight bottles
- Twelve or more nipples
- A pan for boiling the bottles during sterilization procedures
- A bottle brush to clean the bottles before boiling

Feeding and the preparing of feedings are discussed in detail in Chapter 5, "Infancy." The health professional with whom you have arranged to care for the baby will advise what kind of milk or formula to purchase. Even mothers who plan to breast-feed should have canned evaporated milk or a prepared formula powder or concentrate on hand in case feeding plans change.

Childbirth and Child-Care Education

There are many benefits from attending courses that prepare parents-to-be for labor and delivery and for child care. The more the parents know about what to expect in childbirth and how to care for their new baby, the more relaxed and confident they will be.

Topics usually covered in childbirth education classes include the normal processes of pregnancy, the growth of the baby, things to do for common discomforts, how to walk, sit, stand, and lie down comfortably as the abdomen grows larger, and what to expect during labor and delivery. Some programs teach special exercises that will help to make labor and delivery easier. Some exercises also help speed the recovery of the mother after childbirth. Breathing and relaxation techniques do much to reduce the fear, tension, and pain that may be associated with childbirth. Some courses involve the father as a coach in a planned approach to labor and delivery and provide opportunities to practice the techniques during class. Whichever type of course is chosen, there is an opportunity for the parents-to-be to freely discuss their feelings, fears, and hopes about pregnancy and childbirth, both with the instructors and with other expectant parents.

Courses that help new parents-to-be prepare to care for their new baby can be particularly valuable. The less anxious the parents are, the more they can relax and enjoy being parents. If both parents have the responsibility of caring for the baby, the father is less likely to feel neglected while the mother spends most of her time caring for the baby.

The time during pregnancy when parents may profit most from attending classes may vary with the emphasis of the classes. Mothers-to-be may be more comfortable if classes are attended during the second trimester. However, if the class is intended to prepare the parents for breathing and relaxation during labor, it may be advisable to take the course during the last 3 months of pregnancy. Some courses are aimed more at giving broad information that includes care of the newborn infant. Be sure to discuss the content of the classes with the health professional and with the group offering the class in order to determine the class preferred and the best time for parents to attend.

Demands for classes in prepared childbirth and child care are being met by a variety of sources. Some of these are the Childbirth Education Association, Parent-Child, Inc., Lamaze Childbirth Preparation, Family Life and Maternity Education (FLAME), and the Childhood-Parenthood Association. Courses may be offered by hospitals, health agencies, private health professionals, special-interest groups (including groups of parents), and adult education programs. The American Red Cross offers a course called Preparation for Parenthood, which includes broad information about pregnancy, labor, delivery, and caring for the newborn infant. Visiting Nurse Services offer courses in some communities. If information on special groups is not available in the community, you can obtain it from the International Childbirth Association, 1310 North 26th Street, Milwaukee, WI 53205, or check with your local Red Cross chapter.

Preparing for the Hospital Stay

If the baby is to be delivered in the hospital, the mother should have her bag packed fairly early in the third trimester, just in case she delivers earlier than expected. Some things to pack might include—

- Several nightgowns, robe, bed jacket, slippers
- Cosmetics and toilet articles
- Shower cap
- Sanitary belt
- Writing paper, envelopes, pen or pencil, stamps
- Basic clothes for the baby to wear home
- Book, magazines, deck of cards, knitting or embroidering—things to amuse the mother or to occupy her time
- Street clothes to wear home from the hospital

The father also should be prepared for this long-awaited event. He should—

- Keep enough gas in the car to reach the hospital
- Know the way to the hospital, where to park the car, which entrance is open day and night (a practice run may be a good idea if the area is unfamiliar), and where to take his wife in the hospital when she is in labor
- Have a taxi telephone number in a handy place and keep enough money on hand for the fare
- Have the telephone number for an ambulance, just in case
- Have a list with names and telephone numbers of the doctor, the hospital, the person who will care for the older children, if any, and those persons with whom the father will want to share the important news as soon as the baby is born
- Know where the insurance card or papers are
- Have change for telephone calls

LABOR AND DELIVERY

Labor is the work the uterus does to enable the baby to be born. During this process, which involves tightening (contracting) of the muscles of the uterus in a more or less regular pattern, the baby moves from the uterus through the birth canal (the vagina) into the outside world. During the first stage of labor, the contractions cause the gradual opening and thinning or shortening of the cervix (the "mouth" of the uterus). The second stage of labor refers to the time between the complete opening of the cervix and the actual birth of the baby. After the baby has been born, the placenta (afterbirth) is also delivered. This is called the third stage of labor.

Signs of Labor

The beginning of labor is usually indicated by discomfort caused by the contractions of the uterus. These contractions start in the lower back and radiate to the lower abdomen. Usually the contractions in the first stage of labor are mild and irregular at first, probably 20 minutes apart and lasting as little as 10 seconds. If this is the first baby, delivery is still a long way off, and there is plenty of time to get ready.

The uterus often begins practicing for labor during the last month or so before actual delivery, with mild, irregular contractions. It is sometimes difficult to determine when true labor has really started. True labor contractions are contractions that produce changes in the cervix that allow the baby to move out of the uterus. These contractions occur in a regular pattern, getting gradually closer together.

Sometime during early labor there is usually a vaginal discharge, either of mucus or of slightly bloody fluid. This is a sign that the cervix has begun to open (dilate) in preparation for the baby's birth. A sudden gushing or slow leaking of fluid from the vagina indicates that the membrane (bag of waters in which the baby is enclosed) has broken open (ruptured). Whether this fluid appears early or later in labor has no effect on the length or difficulty of the labor.

If the leaking or gushing of fluid or the discharge of bloody mucus occurs before labor has begun and before the baby is expected, the mother should go to bed, and the health professional should be contacted for instructions.

When Labor Begins

At the first indication that true labor has begun, the health professional should be notified. The mother-to-be will be advised when she should go to the hospital. If this is the first pregnancy, the mother should plan to leave for the hospital when the contractions are coming regularly with 5 to 10 minutes between contractions. With later pregnancies, she should plan to go when contractions are 10 to 15 minutes apart. Since at the beginning of labor the contractions are usually mild and infrequent, the mother usually has time to get things organized and to prepare for the trip to the hospital. She may drink fluids during this time but should not eat solid foods or drink milk. As the contractions become stronger, more regular, and more frequent, the mother may feel more comfortable if her back or abdomen is massaged and if she begins special breathing techniques that she may have learned in a childbirth preparation class.

At the Hospital

Upon arriving at the hospital, the mother is usually sent direct to the maternity section, and admission procedures are begun. The mother will be asked when labor started, how often the contractions are occurring, what food she has eaten in the last few hours, the date of her last menstrual period and the expected due date, how much weight she gained during pregnancy, how many previous pregnancies and miscarriages she has had, whether she has any allergies, and whether there are any unusual aspects to the pregnancy such as the Rh factor or special health problems that require medicine or a special diet. A general health history may be requested. She may also be asked whether the baby will be breast-fed or bottle-fed and whether the baby is to be circumcised if it is a boy. The hospital will also want to know who the baby's doctor will be.

A health professional will examine the woman to determine how far the cervix has opened and shortened. The vaginal area may be shaved or washed with a special solution to help keep the area free from germs during delivery. An enema may be given to empty the bowel, thus helping to avoid infection during delivery and giving more room for the passage of the baby. Blood pressure, temperature, pulse, and respiration will be taken, and a urine sample may be requested. The heart sounds of the fetus will also be checked.

When the routine preparation is completed, and if delivery is not expected immediately, the mother may be put in a labor room until labor has progressed further. Some hospitals and health professionals allow the father or a close friend to be with the mother in the labor room or the delivery room, or both. If the father can be present at the delivery of the baby, it is a great comfort and encouragement to the mother and helps to unite the mother and father as a family unit. In many hospitals, however, the father will be allowed in the delivery room only if he has been prepared through childbirth preparation classes. These classes provide the necessary information to reduce anxiety and to assist effectively in the birth process through teaching the mother special breathing and relaxing techniques.

The length of the first stage of labor varies and may last up to 14 or more hours. It is usually shorter for women who have had babies before. During this time, the mother will usually be allowed to sip water or suck on ice chips, and she may be given medicine to relieve discomfort. If the first stage of labor is longer than expected, she may be given other clear liquids. The contractions of the uterus should be timed, and the mother should be helped to breathe deeply and to relax as much as possible with each contraction.

The Delivery

During the second stage of labor (during which the baby is moving through the birth canal), the mother will feel more pressure in her pelvic area and will feel like trying to push the baby out ("bearing down"). She should not push, however, until the health professional indicates that she should do so. As the labor progresses, the contractions will be stronger and more effective in pushing the baby along.

As the baby moves down the birth canal, the top of his head will show during contractions. (Most babies are born headfirst.) At this time, the mother may be taken to the delivery room. (If the labor room is also equipped for delivery, changing rooms will not be necessary.) The delivery room has special equipment to care for the mother and baby in an environment as free from germs as possible.

The second stage of labor may last for a few minutes or for an hour or two. Medicine to relieve pain can be given as needed. Breathing in and out rapidly, with short, panting breaths is helpful both as a distraction to the mother and for better control while the baby is being delivered. The mother will be told when and how to push and how to breathe correctly to help in the delivery of the baby. If the doctor feels it is necessary, a cut (episiotomy) may be made in the vaginal muscle to provide more room for the passage of the baby and to prevent tearing. After delivery the skin is stitched back together to help it heal evenly.

The baby may be placed on the mother's abdomen while awaiting the third and final stage of labor, the delivery of the placenta (afterbirth). This usually occurs within minutes after the birth of the baby. The placenta will be examined to be sure that all of it has been expelled from the uterus.

After the umbilical cord is cut and while other health professionals will be watching the baby's breathing and other vital signs, the doctor will be checking carefully to make sure there is not too much bleeding from the mother's uterus. Sometimes medicine or an injection is given to help the uterus contract so that it becomes small and hard once again. The mother's lower abdomen will be massaged every few minutes to make sure the uterus does contract, since contraction is essential to control bleeding.

After the delivery, the mother usually feels very tired, but she feels a great happiness in seeing and holding her baby for the first time. Being able to touch the baby is very important to her and provides her first chance to form a close emotional attachment to her baby.

HOSPITAL CARE FOR THE NEWBORN

Immediately after the birth, hospital health professionals observe and test the baby for any undesirable health conditions and then begin any treatment that may be necessary. Then the baby is taken either to the hospital nursery or to the mother's room if she has chosen to have the baby share her room (a practice called "rooming in," see page 104).

Eye Drops

Immediately after delivery, a special liquid or antibiotic ointment is put into every baby's eyes to prevent blindness in case the mother has a gonorrheal infection.

PKU Testing

Hospitals routinely test newborn babies for the possible existence of phenylketonuria (PKU). This is a very rare condition that causes a nutritional deficiency and can lead to mental retardation if treatment is not begun right away. If this condition exists, part of the treatment is a special diet during the first few years of the child's life.

Jaundice

Hospital personnel will be watching for any sign of jaundice (a yellow coloring of the baby's skin and eyeballs) during the first few days after birth. Jaundice is not uncommon in newborn babies. A third or more of normal babies experience a mild form of this "normal" jaundice, and the condition will usually disappear in a week or so without treatment. "Normal" jaundice is caused by an oversupply of iron in the blood and liver. This excess of iron is actually helpful in preventing iron deficiency anemia later on.

Jaundice can, however, be a symptom of a disease or infection. Sometimes it is the result of the mother's and the baby's blood becoming mixed during pregnancy. Any jaundice that does develop must be checked carefully. Since the newborn baby's defenses against infection are not well developed, special care must be taken to prevent exposure to germs and to provide prompt treatment if an infection does develop.

The Rh Factor

If the mother has Rh negative blood and the father has Rh positive blood, special procedures may be necessary soon after the baby is born. This occurrence is relatively rare, since most people have Rh positive blood. However, if the situation does occur and if the baby has Rh negative blood, there is no complication.

If the baby has Rh positive blood, however, he must be observed carefully. If the blood of the baby and the blood of the mother have become mixed during pregnancy, antibodies against the baby's Rh positive blood will form in the mother's blood. If these antibodies get into the baby's blood, they may destroy some of his own blood cells, causing anemia and perhaps jaundice. If the baby is jaundiced at birth or soon after, or if there is any evidence of anemia, treatment may need to be started. Usually during the first pregnancy, not enough antibodies are produced to harm the child. Later babies, however, are very likely to be harmed if preventive techniques are not used after the birth of the first Rh positive baby.

After the birth of an Rh positive baby, the mother is usually given an injection of immune human globulin containing anti-Rh antibodies (Rhogram) within 72 hours after delivery. This injection stops the production of anti-Rh antibodies and prevents danger to the woman's future children. The injection must be repeated after each birth or miscarriage.

Rooming In

The practice of having the mother and baby share a room during their stay in the hospital is sometimes called rooming in or family-centered maternity care. Within hours after delivery, the baby is placed in a bassinet next to the mother's bed so that mother and baby can be cared for together in a relaxed atmosphere. Often the father is also allowed to hold and care for the baby.

Specially trained nurses show the mother how to care for the baby so that by the time mother and baby leave the hospital, the mother will be confident of her ability to care for the baby. She learns to bathe the baby, change the dressing on his navel, and feed and change him. She becomes familiar with the baby's personality and movements and with his every feature and wrinkle. Rooming in is thus the ideal learning situation for a first-time mother. Even experienced mothers will appreciate the opportunity for closeness and early acquaintance with their new son or daughter.

EMERGENCY DELIVERY

Occasionally there is an unavoidable delay in getting to the hospital, or the labor progresses much more quickly than expected or has started much earlier than expected. Only in such unusual cases is an untrained person required to assist in the delivery. Only a small fraction of all births present this kind of exceptional problem, but when such problems do occur, the important action is to assist the mother and baby during the birth process.

Supplies for Emergency Childbirth

It is a good idea to have equipment on hand that is necessary in the event that a baby must be delivered at home or in a car on the way to the hospital.

This equipment includes–

- Material to protect the bedding or the car upholstery–newspapers, clean towels, plastic bags, one or two folded sheets, or some other similar material
- Equipment for cutting the umbilical cord–a new razor blade (single-edged) in protective paper, or scissors and alcohol, and sterile cord ties or shoelaces that have been sterilized by placing them in a 350°F (176.7°C) oven in aluminum foil for 3 hours
- Sanitary napkins and a container of some sort for the afterbirth
- A blanket, diaper, and diaper pins for the baby

If the trip to the hospital is made during the night, take along a flashlight, a blanket, and a pillow.

Preparing for the Delivery

For a long automobile ride, have the mother wear a nightgown, slip, or robe but no other underclothing. If the bag of waters has broken, or if blood and mucus are draining from the birth canal, place a sanitary napkin or a clean folded towel between the mother's thighs.

The second stage of labor, during which the baby is being moved through the birth canal, is accompanied by strong contractions of the uterus, 5 minutes or less apart. During this time, the mother has a strong urge to push the baby through the birth canal. This stage may last a short time or for several hours. There is little that anyone else can do for the mother at this time except to reassure her, make her as comfortable as possible, and encourage her in any special breathing techniques that she has learned in preparation for childbirth.

When the labor contractions are approximately 2 minutes apart and the mother is straining and pushing with the contractions, the delivery will take place very soon, and the mother needs help immediately. She should be placed in a good position for delivery, and the assistant may inspect the birth canal to see how close the baby is to being delivered. There may still be time to get to the hospital, or there may be a complication that demands that special medical help be obtained. These are the procedures:

1. Remove any underclothing that will interfere with the delivery of the baby.
2. Have the woman lie on her back on the floor, bed, car seat, or any flat surface. If she is at home, she may lie across a bed with her feet resting on two straight chairs, with her thighs and abdomen covered with clean towels or sheets. If she is on the floor, her knees should be bent, with her feet flat on the floor and her thighs separated widely.
3. Place newspapers or clean cloths or towels under the woman's buttocks, if any such material is available.
4. Wash your hands if water is available.
5. In inspecting the opening of the birth canal (the woman's vagina), *do not* place your hands or fingers in the birth canal at any time because of the danger of infection.

Inspection of the Presenting Part

Inspect the opening of the woman's birth canal (vagina) to see whether the baby's head is visible at the time of contractions. (The head goes back up into the canal between contractions.) The back of the head is usually the presenting part. A wrinkled scalp and hair may be noted, although the head may still be enclosed in the bag of waters. If the woman has had previous pregnancies and the exposed area of the baby's head is approximately the size of a 50-cent piece, or larger, delivery will probably occur within a few minutes, during the next two or three contractions. If the woman is having her first child and the exposed area of the baby's head is smaller than a 50-cent piece, *proceed to the nearest hospital, if* it is not more than 20 minutes away. You probably will arrive in time. Meanwhile, encourage the woman not to bear down or strain with contractions but instead to breathe in and out rapidly with short, panting breaths.

Delivery of the Head

Fig. 27

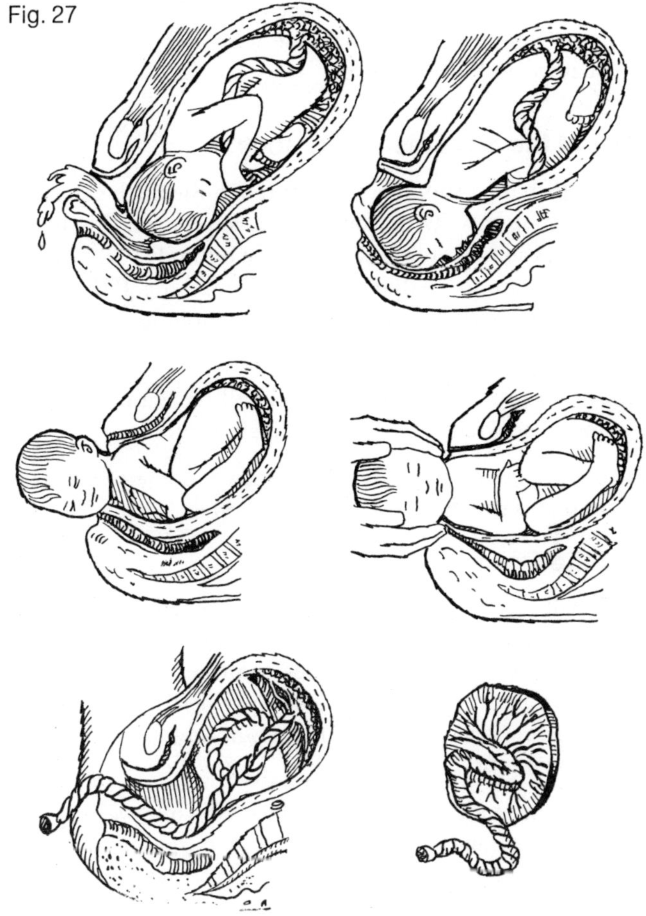

As the infant's head emerges, be prepared to guide and support it with your hands to prevent its becoming contaminated with blood, mucus, or fecal material. If the bag of waters breaks at this point, birth will probably take place rapidly.

When the head emerges, check it once to see whether the umbilical cord—which looks like a soft, thick, gelatinous, bluish-white rope—is wrapped around the infant's neck. If so, gently but quickly slip it over the baby's head with your forefinger between the baby's neck and the cord.

As the baby's head emerges, it turns naturally to one side. Do not turn it. Break the bag of waters immediately if it does not break as the head is delivered. Hold the head gently, and, as soon as possible, wipe out the infant's mouth and nose with clean cloth, gauze, or facial tissues to aid his breathing.

Delivery of the Shoulders and Body

As soon as the baby's shoulders start through the birth canal, lift the baby slightly upward with your hands, supporting his head and neck, to assist them to emerge. The rest of his body will be expelled. It is very important to see that the baby is breathing. If the baby does not breathe immediately, follow the instructions above under "Delivery of the Head."

The baby will probably be crying and will have a bluish color. As he cries more, he will become more pink in color.

Pat the baby's skin dry, then wrap the baby in something warm and place him on his side on the mother's abdomen.

Cutting the Cord

No harm will result if the infant is left attached to the afterbirth (placenta) by the umbilical cord until the mother can be taken to the hospital. This procedure is safer than cutting the cord with unclean instruments or using an improper cord tie. If the cord is strangling the baby as the head emerges, however, the cord *must* be cut as a lifesaving procedure.

If the decision is made to tie and cut the cord while waiting for contractions to resume to expel the placenta, wait until all pulsations of the cord have stopped—about 5 minutes. At home, use a new razor blade (single-edged, if possible) or take the time to boil scissors or soak them in rubbing alcohol (or after-shave lotion or other alcohol-based preparations) for 20 minutes. The scissors may be used while still wet. Sterile cord ties may be purchased or may be sterilized in advance by being wrapped in aluminum foil in an oven at 350°F (176.7°C) for 3 hours.

The umbilical cord *must not* be cut closer than 4 inches (10.2 centimeters) from the infant's naval. Using the sterile cord tie, make a square knot or two or three simple knots around the umbilical cord, tying one knot 4–6 inches (10.2–15.2 centimeters) from the baby and a second knot 8 inches (20.3 centimeters) from the baby. Cut between the knots. (The end of the umbilical cord attached to the baby dries out, shrivels up, and falls off within a week to 10 days.)

Expulsion of the Afterbirth and Care After Delivery

Shortly after the birth of the baby, the mother's contractions start again to help separate the afterbirth (placenta) from the wall of the womb (uterus). *Do not pull on the cord,* do not massage, and do not push hard on the mother's abdomen in an effort to hurry things along. Doing so could cause severe damage to the uterus, which may result in severe bleeding. As soon as the afterbirth comes out, however, place your fingers on the mother's lower abdomen and massage the top of the uterus gently but firmly for a few minutes like gently kneading dough. This massaging will cause the uterus to contract and form a hard ball the size of a grapefruit. This controls bleeding. Repeat every 5 minutes for at least the next hour to make the uterus stay hard. Also check for excessive vaginal bleeding until the mother is seen by a physician. Another way to cause the uterus to contract is to have the baby suck at the mother's breast. *Save the afterbirth and take it to the hospital with you.*

After an emergency delivery, gently cleanse the vaginal opening with a clean, moist towel—or place the mother on a bedpan if one is available and pour soapy water over the vaginal opening, from above toward the rectum, and rinse by pouring warm water over the entire area. Lay a sanitary napkin or other suitable clean cotton material across the vaginal opening.

Give the mother tea, coffee, or other sweetened nonalcoholic fluids and keep her warm. Do not attempt to cleanse the infant of the white, greasy protective coating covering its skin. Do not wash its eyes, ears, or nose. Check to be sure that its breathing is normal and that it is kept warm during transfer to the hospital.

If the afterbirth is not expelled within a reasonable length of time or if it is not completely expelled, there is danger of hemorrhage. Medical care should be sought without delay. *Do not pull on the afterbirth or on the cord.*

If there are tears in the birth canal, with serious bleeding, treat as for an open wound, by applying direct pressure to the bleeding area with a pad of sterile or clean cloth.

IMPORTANT POINTS TO REMEMBER

- Allow the delivery to proceed without interference until the baby's head has fully emerged.
- *Never* try to hold back the baby's head or tell the mother to cross her legs to delay delivery. Such actions may seriously injure the infant.
- *Never* place your hands or fingers into the birth canal at *any* time, because of the danger of infection.
- If the umbilical cord is wrapped around the baby's neck more than once, or if for some reason you cannot slip it over the baby's head, it must be cut *at once* to prevent strangulation. Squeeze the cut ends with gauze, cloth, or your fingers until ties can be applied.
- If any part of the baby other than its head is seen at the opening of the birth canal—for example, its buttocks (a breech birth), hand, or foot—the chances for a safe birth are much less, and you should *proceed at once to the nearest hospital. Do not pull on any part and do not attempt to deliver the infant yourself.*
- A rare but urgent crisis exists when, upon rupture of the bag of waters, the umbilical cord protrudes into the birth canal. The mother should be taken to the hospital *immediately* and meanwhile should stay in a knee-chest (jackknife) position to relieve pressure on the cord and to prevent shutting off the blood supply to the infant. (If the mother is in a situation where she cannot get to a hospital, as in a disaster, the knee-chest position is a temporary position, to be used until a physician can be found.)

Helping the Baby Breathe

The most important first aid procedure in emergency childbirth is assisting the infant to begin breathing. All babies have some fluid in their mouth and in the nose and throat passages that must be drained out. To drain the fluid out of the mouth and nasal passages, hold the baby for a few minutes by the feet, head downward, head and shoulders supported. Since the newborn baby is very often slippery, care must be taken in handling him. The following procedure is recommended:

1. Lay the baby along your arm, cup his head in your hand, and keep his head lower than his chest or legs.
2. Support the baby's head, face down, with the other hand, and let the baby's chest rest on your wrist and forearm, with your thumb and little finger part way around his neck (Fig. 28). If necessary, the baby's mouth can be held open with your index finger.

Fig. 28

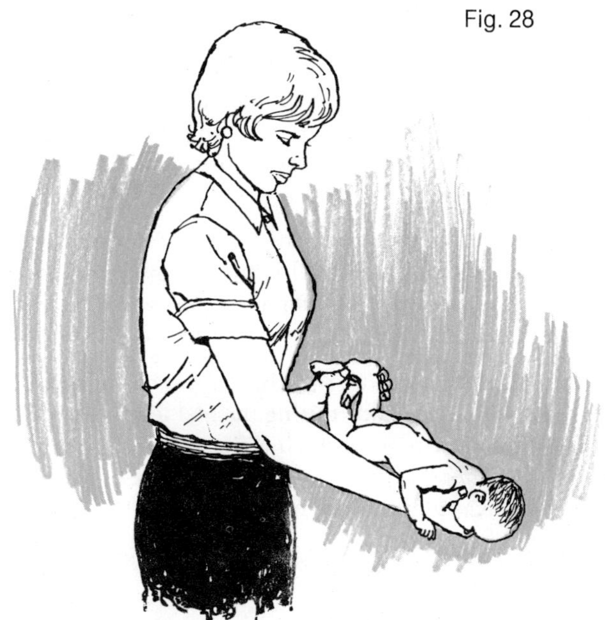

3. Handle the baby gently. Stroke along his neck from his chest toward his mouth in a milking motion and wipe his mouth again. Use no rough slapping or shaking.
4. If the baby does not cry and breathe, give him artificial respiration in gentle puffs through his mouth and nose, one puff every 5 seconds.
5. As soon as the baby is breathing well, wrap him loosely in a towel or receiving blanket to provide warmth. His skin color will change from blue to a rosy pink within 1 to 2 minutes after he begins to breathe and cry.

RECOVERY OF THE MOTHER

The new mother will be advised to rest, to conserve her energy, and to accept help with household routines. Following this advice is important at this time, when the mother's body is adjusting to no longer being pregnant. Having someone help with the housekeeping and meal preparation for the first week or two will help save the mother's energy while she is busy caring for the baby.

The new mother should expect to feel tired once the excitement of being home wears off. If she had an episiotomy (cutting of the vaginal muscle) during the delivery, she may also be experiencing discomfort from the stitches. This discomfort can be relieved by use of a heat lamp for 15-minute periods several times a day. Special hygiene measures will be necessary to prevent infection in the vaginal area, and these should be discussed with the health professional. The new mother may be advised to be off her feet for several hours a day and to avoid climbing stairs.

The new mother has the task of caring for the major portion of the new baby's needs and of helping all family members adjust to the newcomer. The baby may be fussy for a few days while he adjusts to his new environment.

The new mother should not be surprised if she has mixed feelings about the "joys of motherhood" during the first few weeks following childbirth. Many women go through a short period of depression, often referred to as "postpartum blues." The advice of a health professional may be helpful if this occurs.

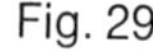

Fig. 29

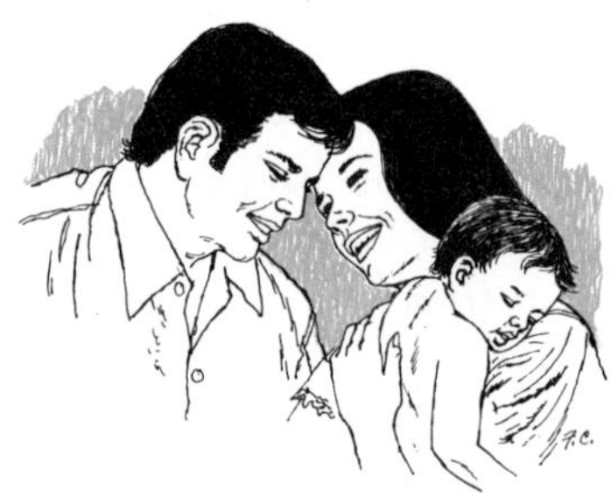

Chapter 5

Infancy

The physical well-being of the baby and his emotional growth and development are so interwoven that one cannot be isolated from the other. The physical needs of a young baby are really quite simple: food, sleep, warmth, cleanliness, protection from infection, and a lot of tender, loving care. To parents with their first baby, everything is new and different. Feelings of uncertainty are common, but the parents will soon learn that their own common sense is an excellent guide.

Each child is different, both in his personality and in the way he grows and matures. The baby's personality will affect his reactions to his environment from the moment of birth. Each baby has his own routine. Each will perform some activities better than others. The most valuable thing a parent can give to the child is love and encouragement as he learns to master his environment.

Fitting the care of a newborn baby into the family routine involves a trial-and-error period while the baby is setting his own schedule of eating and sleeping. Some newborn babies have a way of turning night into day or may prefer to be awake during the evening hours. Parents should expect irregular patterns during the first few months of the baby's life. Gradually they can fit the baby's needs to their own requirements and schedule.

Health supervision during childhood is important. During infancy, the baby should be under the continuing care of a health professional or a health clinic. Regular health supervision makes it possible for the child's growth and development to be evaluated and gives the parents the opportunity to ask questions about any matter that concerns them. Regular supervision will also insure that the child has the immunizations recommended at his age.

THE NEWBORN BABY

Many people say that all newborn babies look alike. Perhaps they do, but each baby is an individual and is totally unlike any other human being. In general, babies vary from about 18–21 inches (45.7–53.3 centimeters) in length and from 5½–8 pounds (2.5–3.6 kilograms) in weight. Boys are usually a little longer and heavier at birth than girls. Some babies appear to have no hair at all, while others may have long or thick hair. Hair that is dark at birth may become lighter, even blond, as the baby grows older, or it may stay dark and become kinky or straighter or curlier.

Appearance

The most striking physical characteristics of the newborn baby are the relatively large head, receding jaw, small chest, and large abdomen. The baby's head may be somewhat out of shape from being squeezed through the birth canal, and his body may be covered with a cheesy, white substance called vernix caseosa. His skin may be wrinkled or red. His back, arms, and legs, and occasionally even face, may be covered with a fine, downy hair, which will eventually disappear. There may be bruises or blotches present, most of which will disappear within several days. Some babies may have slate-blue pigmented areas on the back or buttocks. These are called Mongolian spots and tend to disappear within the first year of life. It takes a few months for the newborn infant to become the round, rosy baby that most people picture when they think of babies.

Changes as the Infant Grows

The growth of a baby is orderly: one stage of development follows another in a certain system. At birth the baby cannot hold up his head, but as his muscles become stronger and his nervous system develops, he will support the head. The baby develops coordination in his hands before he learns to control his feet. This head-to-foot development is the result of the maturing of nerve and muscle control from the brain. The baby will learn to turn over, then sit up, perhaps crawl, then stand alone, and, finally, walk. A child will be able to perform complex hand activities long before he learns to dance or skate. These steps show what is meant by orderly development.

The baby's head and face change rapidly in the first few months of life. Before birth, the head grew rapidly to allow for growth of the brain and the nerve centers, both of which control development. During the birth process, parts of the skull overlapped so that the baby's head could pass through the birth canal more easily. The sections of the skull do not grow together permanently for some time after birth, and there are two soft spots (called fontanels) in the newborn baby—one above the brow (usually closed between 12 and 18 months) and the other close to the crown in the back of the head (usually closed by the end of the second month). The head continues to increase in size until the child is 4 or 5 years old. By that time, the skull has reached about 90 percent of its total growth.

The newborn's face appears small because of the relatively large brow. The lower jaw is smaller than the upper jawbone and will grow at a faster rate to accommodate the first teeth. The first and second sets of teeth are already well developed in the jaw and are waiting to come through the gums. Occasionally, a baby is born with one or two teeth, but usually the first teeth will come in at about 6 or 7 months. These are usually the two lower front teeth (central incisors, or cutting teeth). The mouth and lips are well developed at birth because they are essential to eating (getting) food. Changes will occur in the face until about the teens but occur fastest in the first few months of life.

The height eventually achieved by the person depends on heredity, sex, and how the bones grow. The newborn baby's bones are soft and will become harder as their mineral content, chiefly calcium, increases. Bone growth is influenced by the supply of minerals and the utilization of them by the body. Studies show that children who have not had proper nutrients during their infancy and childhood are shorter than those who have had balanced diets. The studies also show that young adults of today are taller than their parents or grandparents were as young adults, a situation that is a direct result of improved nutrition during the last half century. The bony structure of the body will eventually increase to about 20 times the original size of the newborn.

The newborn's large abdomen is caused in part by the enlargement of the liver, which has been storing up iron. Also, the abdominal muscles are not yet strong enough to compress the intestines, which distend with food and gas. This potbellied appearance will disappear as the child begins to stand and walk, as the abdominal wall tightens and muscle strength increases.

Characteristics of the Newborn Baby

Much has been written about the shock to the baby as he is being born. He has come from a sheltered environment in the uterus, where he floated in warm liquid, to a world that is very different. His sensory perceptions vary in their acuteness. He is extremely sensitive to heat and cold and reacts sharply to loud noises. He can taste and smell. He is especially sensitive to being touched: he enjoys being touched and fondled but is quick to sense tension and insecurity in his handling. Although he is aware of light, darkness, and moving objects, he cannot see very well at first. He will not be able to focus his eyes on an object until his nerves and muscles are more developed.

The newborn baby has a number of natural abilities that are important in sustaining his life. He controls the amount of air he breathes, he can yawn to get needed oxygen, and he sneezes or coughs to get rid of excess mucus. He blinks his eyes to avoid bright lights. When he is cold, he shivers to stimulate circulation. He cries to indicate distress and discomfort.

It is instinctive for the newborn baby to nurse. When his cheek is touched, he will turn his head in search of the breast and will begin to "root" (try to find the nipple and get it into his mouth). The baby sucks both because he is hungry and because he loves to suck. If he does not get enough opportunity to suck at the breast or bottle, he will suck his fists, fingers, or clothing.

Babies seem to have a built-in clock that tells them when to eat. How the baby takes the feeding is often an indication of his personality. Some babies can hardly wait to eat and will suck vigorously until satisfied. Some do not appear interested and may dawdle. Some scream and squirm so impatiently that it is difficult for them to get food at all.

Each child has his own rate of growth and development and cannot be compared with another child. One baby may walk at 9 or 10 months, while another may not walk until he is a year old or more. Some babies' teeth come in unusually early. Some babies sit, crawl, or talk sooner than others. These characteristics do not mean that one child is more advanced or more intelligent than others.

THE PREMATURE BABY

The premature, or immature, baby is one who is born before his organs are able to function well outside the womb (uterus). The normal gestation period (period from conception to birth) is about 9 months, or 280 days. The nearer to the end of the gestation period that the baby remains within the uterus, the better is his chance for survival and for freedom from handicaps. Sometimes even a full-term baby, particularly a small baby, may not be fully ready to live outside the uterus without special help.

The diagnosis of prematurity is based on the baby's birth weight and on the number of months of development before birth. There are different levels of development, and each premature infant will vary in weight, amount of fatty tissue under the skin, ability to suck, vigor of movement, and efficiency of breathing. The premature infant's digestive system and ability to control his own body temperature are not fully developed, and special measures are necessary to insure his survival.

Modern medical and scientific advances have done much to conserve the lives of both immature and premature infants. The premature baby has his best chance for survival in a hospital, where there are special facilities for taking care of him, where his environment can be controlled, and where trained personnel can care for him. The first few days of the premature baby's life are important, and every day that he lives increases his chances for survival. If the baby is not born in the hospital, he should have immediate medical attention. Some hospitals and health departments, particularly those in large cities and university teaching hospitals, have special provisions for transporting premature babies from home to hospital.

If the premature baby is born without the doctor present, the following care is necessary:

- Avoid unnecessary handling.
- Keep the baby warm by wrapping him loosely in a soft flannel or wool receiving blanket, with his face exposed so that he can breathe.
- Improvise an incubator, using one of the methods described below.

  Place well-wrapped hot-water bags around the baby outside the blanket, taking every precaution to avoid burning his sensitive skin. Refill the hot-water bags frequently so that an even temperature is maintained.

  Place a padded cardboard carton inside a larger carton and put hot-water bags (or heated bricks or stones, or glass bottles filled with hot water) between the sides of the two boxes (Fig. 30). The radiating heat will warm the baby.

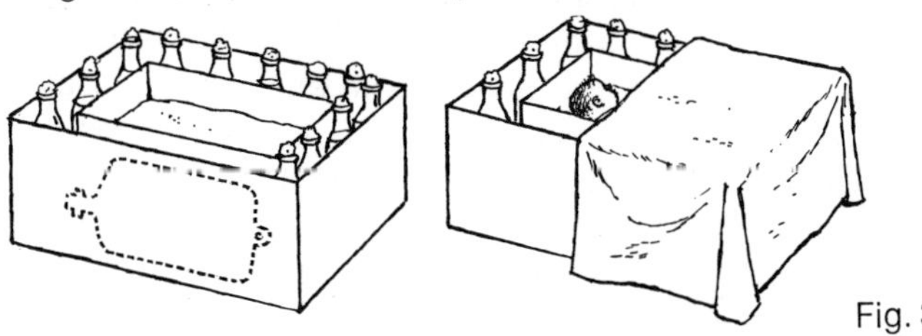

Fig. 30

- Arrange the baby in his incubator so that his head is lower than his feet.
- Place a diaper or a soft pad under the baby's buttocks so that the diaper can be changed with a minimum of handling.
- Do not give the baby food or water for 6 to 8 hours or until the doctor gives definite instructions for his care and feeding.

Like all babies, the premature infant needs tender, loving care and attention. Parents are often afraid to handle the baby at first because he is so little. While the baby is in the hospital, the mother should visit him often, holding him and doing whatever the hospital will allow according to his condition. By the time the baby is ready to leave the hospital, usually when he has reached the weight of 5 pounds (2.3 kilograms), mother and baby will not be strangers.

As the premature baby begins to gain weight, he begins to catch up in other ways. Usually there is no difference in the pattern of his growth and development except that the growth stages may come somewhat later than those of the full-term baby. The premature baby is therefore often slower in beginning to sit, stand, and walk. By the time he is 2½, however, he will usually be doing all the normal activities for his age.

FEEDING

Initially the baby's diet consists of milk, either from the breast or from a bottle. Years ago, all mothers breast-fed their babies because it was the only way to feed them. Breast-feeding is certainly an easier and less costly way to feed a baby, and it gives great satisfaction to both mother and baby. The mother who does not think she has enough milk for her baby at first should not give up too easily. The more the baby sucks at the breast, the more milk will be produced. Bottle feeding, however, is a safe alternative. Either way, the mother can cuddle and fondle the baby, talking softly to him to add to his sense of comfort. More important than the method chosen is the attitude of the mother toward feeding her baby. If he is held during his feeding and is loved and cherished, he will gain the security, confidence, and trust that every infant needs, no matter whether his food comes to him in a bottle or from the breast. Feeding time is a relaxing time for the mother also. She may want to lie down with the baby or use a pillow to support both her arm and the baby for more comfort during the feedings.

Fig. 31

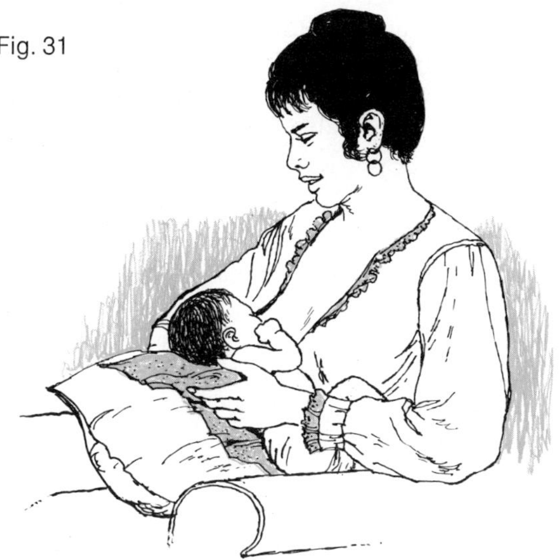

The newborn baby usually loses weight during the first few days after birth, while he is adjusting to the outside world. Within a week or 10 days, he usually is back up to his birth weight or past it. He usually doubles his birth weight by the time he is 4 to 6 months old and triples it by the age of 8 to 12 months. It is not healthy for a baby to be fat, although some cultures think fat babies are beautiful. Studies show that overweight babies will often be overweight as adults, with tendencies to heart problems. Solid foods, therefore, should not be started too early, usually not before the baby is 5 months old.

What To Feed

The mother who is breast-feeding does not need to worry about her baby's diet as long as she eats properly herself and allows the baby to nurse when he is hungry. The mother should drink extra fluids and eat a balanced diet. Milk products are an especially good source for the extra protein she needs while she is nursing. Until he is 6 months old, the nursing baby will usually not need any iron or vitamin supplements.

The type of formula for use by a baby will usually be determined by the health professional. Formulas usually consist of some combination of milk and water. The amount of dilution depends upon the age of the baby and the type of formula used. Although directions for preparing the formula are usually given on the can or jar, it is best to confirm them with the health professional. The health professional will also advise when to use a formula containing vitamins and iron, which are available both as liquid concentrate and powder.

Babies and children will vary with regard to how hungry they are from one feeding to the next. In general, the small baby will drink 2–3 ounces of formula (56.7–85.1 grams) for every pound he weighs. An 8-pound (3.6-kilogram) baby will take 16–24 ounces (453.6–680.4 grams). The baby should not be forced to eat if he is not hungry. If the baby consumes more than 25–30 ounces (739.3–887.2 milliliters) of formula a day, other foods can be added to satisfy his hunger. Prepared baby cereals are good sources of nutrients and can be given from a spoon.

When To Feed

Until the baby is several weeks old, he cannot take enough food into his small stomach to last very long; therefore, frequent feeding will be necessary during this early period. By the time he is a month old, the bottle-fed baby usually can wait 3 hours between feedings. By the time he is 3 months old, he will have a more regular schedule and may want to be fed about every 4 hours during the day. Parents should recognize that every baby has his own feeding schedule. If they need to adjust the schedule for a special reason, they might wake the baby a little early or let him stay hungry just a bit longer than usual.

Breast-Feeding

The nursing mother should pay special attention to her own diet and should remember that the more the baby nurses, the more milk the mother's breasts will produce. If she has any problems or questions about nursing, she might talk with other women who have breast-fed or might contact the local chapter of the La Leche League (see Appendix for address of national headquarters). The following tips should be helpful to the nursing mother:

- Keep the nipples clean by washing them with clear, warm water, but do not wash them with soap, since soap may cause cracking of the nipples.
- Allow the baby to find the nipple himself. Touch the breast to the

baby's cheek, and he will turn to find the nipple. (Such seeking is called rooting.)

- Be sure that the baby takes the entire nipple (the dark part, or "areola") into his mouth. This helps to prevent sore nipples.
- When you are starting to nurse for the first time, it may be necessary for you to limit the amount of sucking time to avoid nipple soreness.
- Shorter and more frequent nursings will help to avoid soreness caused by a hungry baby's nursing too vigorously. The average feeding time is about 10 minutes on each breast, although some babies will want to nurse longer.
- To remove the breast from the baby's mouth, gently insert your finger at the corner of the mouth until the suction is broken, then pull the breast away slowly.

Breast-fed babies need more frequent nursing than bottle-fed babies during the first few months, because breast milk is digested very quickly. The baby may want to nurse every 1½ to 2 hours for a few weeks. As the baby's stomach capacity increases, he will be able to go longer between feedings. Most babies get 4/5 of the available milk from the breast within the first 5 minutes of nursing. The longer the baby nurses, the more the milk supply will increase.

During the first few weeks, it is common for milk to leak from the breasts between feedings. Gauze or cloth pads can be placed in the nursing bra to absorb the milk and protect the clothing. The nipples should be exposed to air occasionally to prevent cracking or soreness. The nursing bra should provide good support but should not be too tight.

Burping

A baby swallows some air when sucking either the breast or the bottle, even if good feeding techniques are maintained. Burping (or "bubbling") the baby will allow him to expel this air; otherwise, the trapped air may cause gas to form in his intestines and make him uncomfortable, or it may cause him to spit up milk when he burps without help.

You can burp the baby either over your shoulder or with him sitting on your lap. Always be sure that the baby's mouth and nose are not blocked.

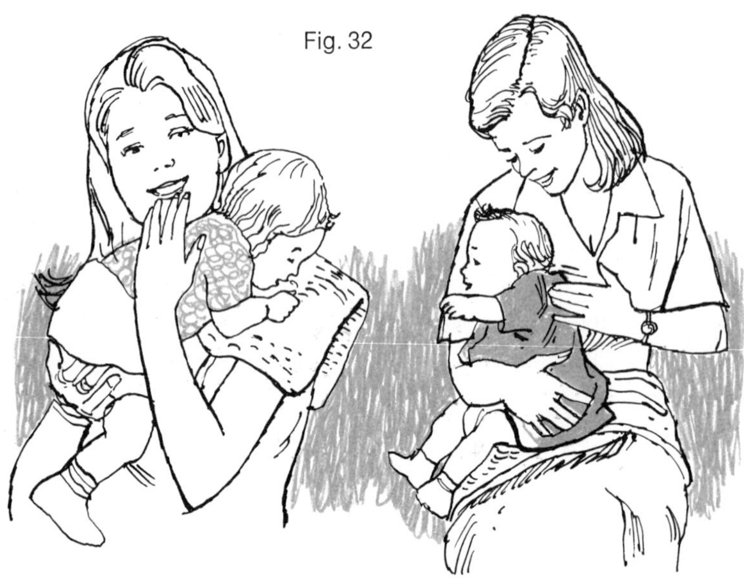
Fig. 32

Shoulder Method

- Place a clean towel or diaper over one of your shoulders.
- Pick up the baby and hold him with his head on the protected shoulder.
- Be sure the baby's head is turned to the side so that he can breathe.
- Gently rub or pat his back to help him release the swallowed air.

Sitting Method

- Place a protective covering on your lap.
- Support the baby by putting your arm across his chest and holding his far shoulder with your hand. His chin will be supported by your arm.
- Bring the baby to a sitting position, letting him lean forward for support.
- Gently rub the baby's back to help him release the swallowed air.

If the baby is asleep at the end of the feeding, it may not be necessary to wake him. Lay him down on his side or on his stomach.

Preparing the Formula

Formulas can be prepared from liquid concentrates or powders or may be obtained ready to use. The health professional's directions should be followed.

Whether or not the bottles, water, and milk must be sterilized depends on the water supply, the age of the baby, and the judgment of the health professional. If the water supply is pure and the health professional has not advised sterilization, milk and water may be mixed in proper proportions in a clean bottle and given immediately to the baby. If the quality of the water supply is questionable, or if the baby is experiencing diarrhea, sterilization is advised. Certainly no harm is done by sterilization. If the mother sterilizes properly, she is confident that the baby is not being exposed unnecessarily to infection. Sterilization is usually no longer necessary by the time the baby is 6 months old.

If the formula is being given by bottle, if there are enough bottles for one day, and if there is refrigeration available, the terminal sterilization technique is a convenient procedure. It is as follows:

- Wash the bottles, nipples, and nipple covers thoroughly with soap and water, using a bottle brush inside the bottles, then rinse them.
- Mix the formula and pour it into the bottles.
- Cap the bottles with clean nipples and nipple covers.
- Place the bottles in a pan and add water halfway up the side of the pan.
- Cover the pan and bring the water to a boil.
- Boil for 20 minutes.
- When bottles are cool, place them under refrigeration.

Once the formula has been mixed, it must be properly refrigerated. Unused milk should be covered and put in the refrigerator. The baby should never be fed with the formula in a bottle or from an open can that has been standing at room temperature for more than 30 to 40 minutes. Although many people warm a refrigerated formula, it is not really necessary to do so.

If there is no refrigerator, powdered milk should be used and made up bottle by bottle as needed. It can be mixed with water from the tap and put in a bottle. If the water is not pure, the terminal sterilization method should be used.

Introducing Solid Food

The baby usually does not need the extra nutrients in solid foods until he is 5 or 6 months old. When solid foods are introduced, they should be started slowly, and the baby should be observed for signs of allergy. A couple of spoonfuls once or twice a day (usually in the morning or at noon) is a good way to start; then if there is any allergic reaction (rash or vomiting), it will be likely to occur before night.

Fig. 33

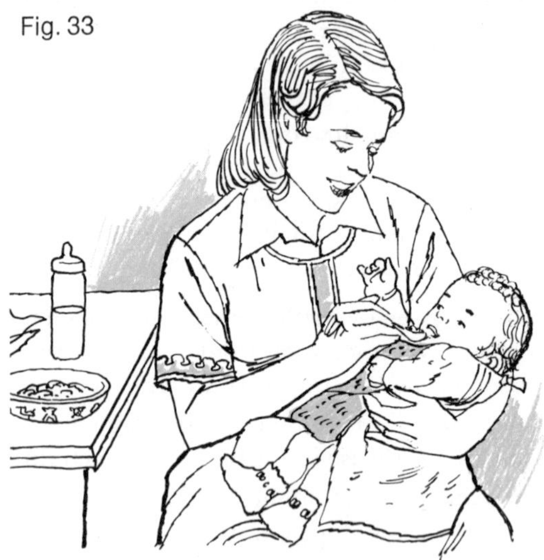

Only one food should be used for at least 3 to 4 days before a new food is added. This method will not only allow time to observe the baby for allergy but will also help the baby get used to the taste. Foods that cause allergy in some infants are orange juice, egg white, green beans, green, leafy vegetables, and wheat cereals. If the allergic reactions persist or are severe, the health professional should be called.

The solid food may be started with cereal enriched with iron, then vegetables, then fruit, and, finally, meat foods for protein. The food should not be heaped on the spoon. If baby foods are being purchased, only the plain ones should be bought, not mixtures. There is more nutrition for less money in the plain foods than in the mixed dinners or desserts.

Some parents prefer to make their own baby food. The food should simply be cooked well and put through a strainer or blender (for a small baby) or mashed well (for a baby 6 months or older). Quantities of prepared foods can be frozen in ice cube trays and then removed and placed in bags to be thawed when needed. The tray should be covered while the food is being frozen. Vegetables and fruits should be kept in separate bags. One or two cubes will make a meal for a 6-month-old baby. Many adult foods are quite adequate as "junior foods": applesauce, mashed potatoes, ground meat, mashed banana, and so on. When the baby is getting foods that are prepared for the entire family, there should be no chunks or strings in the food that the baby can choke on. (Particular care should be taken with raisins, peanuts, string beans, and celery.) The baby gradually gets used to the different tastes and textures.

Do not add butter or fat, sugar, or salt to any baby foods. The baby needs each calorie to be well packed with nutrients. Babies get plenty of sodium (salt from milk and other foods) and should not be given extra salt because of possibly increasing the risk of their developing hypertension.

After the baby is 6 months old, a nutritious diet for him consists of several servings of food during each 2-day period from each of the four basic food groups:

Milk, cheese, cottage cheese, butter, margarine

Fruits and vegetables (at least one green, leafy type)

Meat, fish, poultry, eggs, dried beans, peanut butter

Bread, crackers, cereal, rice, spaghetti

The child should be allowed to have food preferences within the limits of these kinds of foods.

Babies will soon begin to take an interest in feeding themselves. Although a baby of 6 months will still be using the breast or bottle, he can be helped to drink from a cup. He can also be helped to use a spoon himself. If the mother stands behind him to guide his actions, he will learn more quickly. He may also eat pieces of cracker, bread, cheese, and meat with his fingers. This is not only good for the baby's nutrition but also will entertain him. The mother should be prepared for the fact that mealtime will be a messy time. Although feeding himself will take longer for the baby, he will become relatively independent sooner than if the mother continues to feed him.

Weaning

The first step toward weaning the baby (decreasing his dependency on breast or bottle) is to offer him milk from a cup. Drinking from a cup should begin at 5 to 6 months of age, when the child is eager to explore and may not be interested in nursing or drinking from a bottle any longer. Juices and water, as well as milk, should be offered by cup.

Weaning is begun by stopping one feeding from breast or bottle at a time. The first week, the feeding that seems least important to the baby is stopped. The second week, another feeding is eliminated, and so on. Generally, the evening bottle is the last to go. The bottle that helps the baby to relax before sleeping may still be used at age 2 or so. Some mothers will be concerned that the child is not getting enough nourishment, but by age 9 to 12 months, 12–16 ounces (354.9–473.2 milliliters) is sufficient each day.

Weaning is a gradual process in most instances. Mothers who have enjoyed their child's dependence on them for breast or bottle feeding may want to postpone weaning. It is a difficult time for them. Since breast or bottle feeding has been a time of closeness, mothers may want to give extra cuddling to replace the holding that was a part of the former feeding method. The responses of the baby should guide the weaning process. The health professional should be consulted if there are any questions.

COMMUNICATION AND TRUST

From the moment of birth, the baby is learning about the world—and, most important of all, learning about human contact. The attention a baby receives during his first year will give him a basic sense of trust that is essential as he grows older and learns more grownup behavior. The baby whose needs are taken care of quickly and lovingly will feel good about himself and about his environment.

Crying

When a baby cries, he is communicating his discomfort or dissatisfaction. He may need to be burped, to have a soiled diaper changed, to be fed, fondled, or played with, or to have clothing added or removed so that he will not be too hot or too cold—or he may just be lonely. Some babies will have a fussy period during the evening no matter what has been done to make them comfortable.

It is the parents' responsibility to discover the cause of a baby's crying and to do what they can to make the baby comfortable. If the baby's needs have been met, it may be safe to ignore the crying if it doesn't last too long, but no child should be left to cry for long periods of time. It may be that the baby is lonely. Often he will be satisfied just to be in the room where his parents are. Also, some babies rest better and feel more secure when they are snugly wrapped in a blanket.

It is important that parents avoid always trying to quiet a baby by feeding him. Obesity in later life may develop because, from infancy, the person has learned to try to fulfill emotional needs by eating.

Some fussiness by babies can be prevented by careful planning:

- Before beginning to feed, change, or bathe the baby, have all the necessary equipment organized and ready for easy use.
- During diaper changing, give the baby something to attract his attention or to play with.
- Have a flexible routine for various activities so that the baby knows what to expect and can anticipate events.

Talking to the Baby

Fig. 34

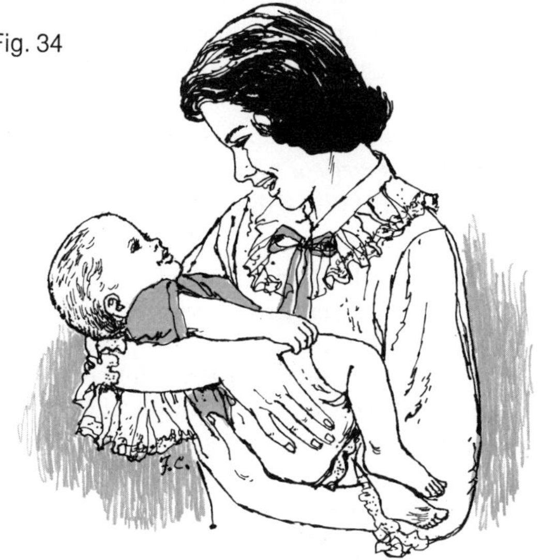

The baby learns to communicate with his parents in new ways when he is talked to. Parents can encourage this learning by making certain responses to the baby:

- Smile at the baby when he smiles and when he is looking at your eyes.
- Talk to the baby about what he is doing, hearing, feeling, and seeing, and when he is eating.

- Set aside some time each day for you and the baby to "talk" to each other. You might even read to the baby. The room should be quiet (no radio or TV). The direct contact helps the baby relate directly to you as his caretaker. He also gets the feeling that he is someone special.
- Respond to the baby's noises by repeating his sounds and by saying the words for objects that he may be looking at.
- When the baby begins to use words, reward him by talking back promptly, looking at him, and listening attentively.

Activities for the Baby

Providing the baby with activities will help him to learn about the world, the objects in it, and his ability to control such objects. This can be done by—

- Moving the baby about in the infant seat, playpen, or walker so that he can see the world from different angles.
- Allowing the baby to explore his home freely in a safe area.
- Playing games involving searching (peek-a-boo, hiding a toy under a pillow, etc.) and allowing the baby to find objects. (This fosters security.)
- Providing toys of varying shapes, sizes, and colors that can be looked at, held, squeezed, or pulled.
- Providing toys that do something special, such as make noise, when the baby touches them.
- Providing toys that allow exploration of relative sizes or shapes—toys that can be stacked, or nesting toys that can be put inside one another.

Any object that is safe and that the baby enjoys is a good toy. Many household items are good toys, and simple toys can be made at almost no cost. If the baby loses interest in some toys, he will be excited to see them again if they are put away for a while and given back to him a month or so later.

HINTS FOR BABY CARE

Handling the Young Baby

Careful handling of the small baby is essential both to insure the child's safety and to give a sense of security. Any sudden motion that may frighten the baby should be avoided. Support should be given to the heaviest parts of the baby's body: head, back, and buttocks. The procedures below are recommended.

Picking Up the Baby

- With the baby on his back, grasp his feet at the ankles, placing a finger between his ankles for security and comfort, and lift his buttocks slightly.
- Slip your other hand under the baby's buttocks and up along his back. With fingers spread, support his head and shoulders.
- Shift the hand that is holding the baby's ankles to his buttocks, supporting them in the palm of the hand, and raise the baby gently into your arms.

Using the Football Hold (Holding the Baby With One Arm)

- Pick up the baby, supporting his head, back, and buttocks with both hands.
- Holding the baby in both arms, gently move him to one side of your body so that his hip rests on your hip and your arm and hand support his back and head. Clasp him securely with your elbow.

This position will free your other hand and arm and is very useful when washing the baby's hair.

Care of Skin, Hair, and Nails

A daily bath is not necessary, although the baby should probably be bathed every other day. Bathing also provides a play time for the baby. When he is bathed—

- The water should feel comfortable and should always be tested first on the parent's wrist or elbow. It should be neither hot nor cold.
- Plain water should be used to wash the baby's face.
- The baby's body should be rinsed thoroughly.
- The baby should be dried carefully, especially in the cracks and creases of the body.

Cotton-tipped sticks should not be used to clean the navel, nose, ears, or any other place; a soft washcloth is sufficient.

Skin rashes on a baby may be caused by harsh detergents and some fabric softeners, by inadequate rinsing of clothing, bedding, or diapers, or by too infrequent changing of diapers. If a rash occurs, exposing the irritated area to the air is often helpful.

Cut the baby's toenails and fingernails while he is asleep, so that he will not get excited and jerk away.

The baby's hair may be washed weekly, or more often. If "cradle cap" (a greasy crust or scale formation on the scalp) occurs, apply baby oil or a bland ointment at night and shampoo in the morning. Repeat the procedure until the crust is removed.

Diapering

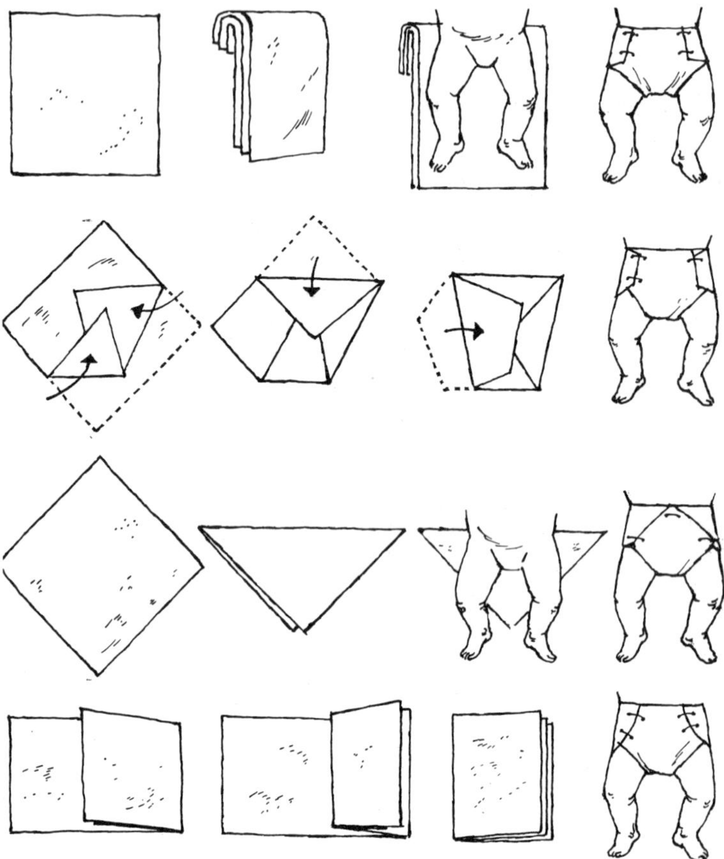

Fig. 35

After removing the wet or soiled diaper, cleanse the baby's bottom with a damp cloth to remove the irritating urine or stool. Then put on a clean diaper. Place the thickest layer of the diaper at the baby's back for a girl and in front for a boy. When pinning the diaper, place your fingers between the diaper and the baby to help guide the pin away from the baby. A diaper that is properly snug will allow two fingers to fit between the diaper and the baby at the waist and legs.

Bathing the Baby

A daily bath is not necessary, although the baby should probably be bathed every other day. After the cord has dropped off and the umbilicus (or navel) has healed, the baby can be given a tub bath. This will usually occur in the first 2 weeks. Baths are given to keep the baby clean, but the process gives the baby and the parents a very good chance to get acquainted. The baby usually enjoys being bathed and as he grows it can be a time for play, a time for mimicking sounds made by the parents, and a time for making other growth responses to the parents' laughter and cuddling. The bath should be given in a room that is warm and free from drafts, so that the baby will not get chilled. The baby may be bathed in a bathinette, in a baby bathtub, in the washbasin, or in the kitchen sink if it is cleaned well both before and after the bath. Bathing the baby in the family bathtub allows him more freedom to kick and splash than does a bathinette or a baby bathtub. NEVER LEAVE THE BABY ALONE in a tub, on the bathinette, or on a table. ALWAYS keep one hand on the baby.

Equipment

Bathinette, tub, basin, or sink
Bath water of proper temperature, about 100° Fahrenheit (38° centigrade)
Bath pad covered with a clean towel
Newspaper for soiled clothing
Bath towel and washcloth, clean clothing
Bath tray containing soap, oil or lotion, powder or cornstarch, cotton balls, safety pins, waste disposal bag

Procedure

1. Make sure the room and all equipment are ready before the baby is undressed or removed from his crib.
2. Wash your hands thoroughly and put on a coverall apron before handling the baby.
3. Lift the baby out of the crib, providing support to his back and his head, and place him on the bath pad.
4. Remove all clothing except the baby's shirt and his diaper, both of which are needed for warmth.
5. Clean the baby's nostrils with a small piece of cotton twisted into a wick and moistened with clean water. Use a separate wick for each nostril. If commercial cotton applicators are used to clean the nose, remove the stick to avoid injuring the nose.

6. Test the temperature of the water. It should be comfortably warm, about 100° Fahrenheit (38° centigrade) when tested on the inside of your wrist.
7. Palm the washcloth to prevent dragging and dripping. Wash the baby's eyes from the ear toward the nose. Wash his face without soap. Use a firm, gentle stroke, supporting his head with one hand. Dry his face.
8. Wash the baby's neck, washing only the outer part of his ear and behind it. Give particular attention to the folds of skin in which moisture, lint, and dust may collect. Rinse and dry.
9. Use the football hold to hold the baby so that his head is over the bath basin.
10. Soap and wash the head with a gentle rotary motion, using your hand or a washcloth. Rinse and dry.
11. Remove the baby's diaper. If it is soiled, cleanse his buttocks with oil, lotion, or water-moistened cotton balls.
12. Remove the baby's shirt.
13. Place the soiled clothing on a newspaper or other protective material.
14. Wet and soap the baby's hands.
15. Beginning at the baby's chest and arms and using firm, gentle, continuous strokes, soap his entire body.
16. Using the body-arm hold, pick up the baby and slowly slide him feetfirst into the water to avoid frightening him. Maintain a firm grasp on the far arm and shoulder.
17. Rinse the front of his body.
18. Reach across his chest and grasp his far arm and shoulder. Lean him forward against your wrist and rinse his back.
19. Remove the baby from the tub. Carefully dry him, especially in all the folds of skin and between his fingers and his toes.
20. Wash the baby's genitals, using cotton moistened with water or oil. If the baby is a girl, separate the labia and cleanse downward once on each side. If the baby is a boy, gently push back the foreskin (if he is not circumcised) and wipe with moistened cotton. Do not use force.
21. Apply a small amount of powder, baby oil, or lotion to the baby's buttocks to prevent skin irritation. Avoid using excessive amounts.
22. Put a clean diaper on the baby.

23. Put a shirt on the baby. Open the neck of the shirt wide so that the baby can see through as it is placed over his head. Slip his fingers through the wrist end of the sleeve, grasp his hand, holding all his fingers to prevent injury to them, and draw his arm through the sleeve. A gown may be put on in the same way.
24. Wrap the baby loosely in a blanket so that he can move freely and without restraint:

    Arrange a blanket so that it lies diamond-shaped on the bed or table.

    Place the baby so that his head is toward the top point of the blanket.

    Turn one pointed side loosely across the baby. Cover his feet by folding the bottom point upward and then bring the other point across the baby.
25. Put the baby in his crib or in a safe place.
26. Clean and dry the bath equipment and put it away.

Sleep

Most newborn infants sleep about 20 hours a day. For the first few months, their sleeping schedule may be quite unpredictable. It is good if the baby can have a sleeping area of his own, but if a room of his own is not available, his crib could be rolled into a hallway at night.

The baby will make noises as he breathes and may breathe irregularly. If he is uncomfortable, his cry will be strong enough to wake the parents.

Baby Carriers, High Chairs, and Car Seats

Many mothers find a reclining seat handy for their small babies. The seat props the baby so that he can see the world around him and is especially useful in the home. A baby carrier should be sturdy and able to resist tipping, and it must have a harness to keep the baby in place.

As the baby grows older, a high chair is desirable. Again, sturdiness, stability, and a safety belt are important. A high chair that has an adjustable footrest and is easy to clean is more satisfactory.

A baby or small child held in the arms of an adult is not safe from injury in an automobile accident. The child should always be securely fastened into a car seat while riding in a car. For infants, a rear-facing device that holds the baby in a half-reclining position is recommended. The device is fixed to the seat by using the car seat belt. When the baby can sit, a conventional child's car seat, perhaps with a protective shield, can be used. The car seat should be carefully checked to be sure that it gives superior protection. The Consumer's Union is a good source of information on such devices.

Babysitters

All parents need some time for themselves away from the baby. However, any child under 5 years old should never be left alone. The babysitter should be chosen carefully and should be someone known and trusted. It is good to use only one or two regular babysitters and to observe the babysitter to be sure that the person knows how to handle, feed, diaper, and comfort the child. The babysitter should know—

- Where the parents plan to be and when they are going to return.
- What and when to feed the baby and any special instructions for his care
- The name and telephone number of a responsible friend or family member in case the parents cannot be reached
- The telephone numbers of the baby's doctor, the fire department, and the police

Mothers who breast-feed can leave their babies too. The baby should be breast-fed shortly before leaving. If a feeding will be necessary while the mother is gone, the baby could be given a bottle of formula or of milk that the mother has expressed (squeezed) from her breasts in advance. The mother should be sure to acquaint the baby with the use of the bottle before leaving him with a sitter.

The baby or young child may be unhappy when he sees that the mother is about to leave him. The time of leaving is made easier if—

- The mother does not leave as soon as the babysitter arrives but gives the baby time to adjust to the babysitter while the mother is still there.
- The child is left with a favorite toy.
- The mother tells the child she is leaving, kisses him, and tells him she will be back at the time of a specific event in his day (not at 4 o'clock but after his nap). The child will soon learn to trust in the fact that she will return.

(Most chapters of the American Red Cross offer a Mother's Aide course to prepare babysitters.)

Fig. 36

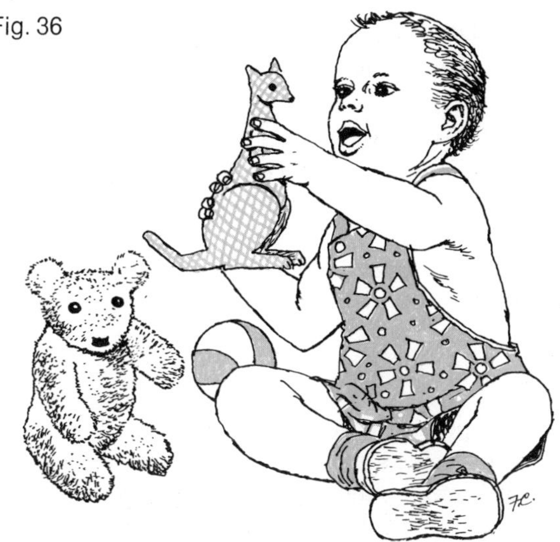

HEALTH CARE

Many patterns for healthful living are established in the infant and young child by good nutrition, routines for eating and sleeping, and opportunities for socializing and play. In addition, the child should be under the care of a health professional for regular checkups, immunizations, and care during illness. Parents should know the signs of illness and seek medical attention as necessary. They will also need to know basic home treatments and home nursing procedures.

The Health Professional

Babies and children should be taken to a health professional or a clinic for regular checkups. The scheduling of these checkups will be made according to the child's needs and the health professional's judgment. Usually, babies are given checkups at 1, 2, 3, 6, 9, and 12 months of age. After that, yearly checkups are advisable. The health professional will insure that immunizations are received at the appropriate age and will be available if the child becomes ill.

If the child becomes ill, the health professional should be consulted immediately. Some symptoms that should be observed and reported are—

- Vomiting or weakness, or both, that lasts more than one day.

- Frequent watery, loose bowel movements. (The presence of mucus or blood in the bowel movement should also be reported.)
- Difficulty in breathing, which may or may not be accompanied by turning blue (cyanosis).
- Fever over 101°F (or 38°C) when temperature is taken rectally, especially when accompanied by restlessness, crying, flushed face, and irritability. (If the temperature is taken under the armpit, the health professional should be notified if it is over 98.6°F, or 37°C.) Correct procedures for taking a child's temperature are given in chapter 18.

Immunizations

It is extremely important that the child receive all immunizations (shots or drops of vaccine into the mouth) that are recommended by the health professional. These immunizations provide protection against various communicable diseases of childhood and adulthood that can lead to serious complications and even death. Infants have a natural immunity during the first few months of life but they soon lose it. Infants should be protected against diphtheria, whooping cough, tetanus, polio, and measles during their early months. Booster doses of some immunizing agents are given at specified times according to the advice of the health professional. Many health professionals also advise routine protection against other diseases such as mumps, scarlet fever, and typhoid fever.

Every community in the country has an interest in insuring that precautions are taken against the spread of communicable diseases. There is a period of time following an immunization before it actually becomes effective, and booster doses are often needed to continue the protection. Most states require that recommended immunizations be current before a child is allowed to start school. When a health emergency occurs, immunizing materials may not be available, or there may be no authorized person to administer them. Immunizations must be given as a preventive measure, since immunization after exposure is often too late. It cannot be overemphasized that precautionary measures against diseases are available in every community and should be taken advantage of.

The immunization schedule that follows is based on current practice and recommendations.

Childhood Immunization Schedule

(Prepared by U.S. Department of Health, Education, and Welfare; Public Health Service; Center for Disease Control.)

At This Age:	Your Child Should Have Received:
2 months old	1 DTP immunization 1 polio immunization
4 months old	2 DTP immunizations 2 polio immunizations
6 months old	3 DTP immunizations 2 polio immunizations[1]
15 months old	3 DTP immunizations 2 polio immunizations[1] 1 measles immunization[2] 1 rubella immunization[2] 1 mumps immunization[2]
18 months and older	4 DTP immunizations 3 polio immunizations[1] (If your child has not already received measles, rubella, and mumps immunizations, they are needed.)
4 to 6 years, before starting to school	A DTP booster (the 5th immunization) A polio booster (the 4th immunization)[1] (If your child has not already received measles, rubella, and mumps immunizations, they are needed.)
Thereafter	Tetanus-diphtheria (Td) booster should be given every 10 years or following a dirty wound if a booster has not been given in the preceding 5 years.

[1]Some doctors give one additional dose when the child is 6 months old.
[2]Only one shot is needed. Some doctors combine these vaccines in a single injection (MMR).

Home Treatment

Home treatment for the sick child includes keeping the child comfortable and giving him foods and medicines that will aid in his recovery. The health professional's advice should be followed carefully, particularly during illnesses such as croup.

The sick child will be more comfortable if he can continue to engage in his usual activities if he feels like doing so. If he has a fever, he will be more comfortable with fewer clothes and covers. A baby or child who is ill needs more fluids than usual. Water and juices are the best choice. The health professional should be consulted for guidelines on the use of aspirin. Children's dosages of medicine will be smaller than adult dosages and may vary according to the weight of the child. All precautions listed in chapter 19 should be followed.

Medicines may be given to babies by mouth with a medicine dropper. The procedure works well if the medicine is placed on the baby's tongue. Care must be taken, however, so that the child does not choke, spit out, or cough up the medicine. A small paper cup or cupcake paper is also easy to use because it can be squeezed between the mother's fingers to direct the medicine into the baby's mouth, as with a funnel. The mother might also pinch the baby's mouth open from the cheek sides and drop the medicine into his mouth. His cheeks should be held until the medicine has been swallowed.

Giving medicine is made easier when the medicine has a pleasant flavor, and many children's medicines do taste good. Medicines should not be mixed with food or put into the baby's formula. All of the formula might not be taken. Also, this practice might cause the baby to refuse the usual formula. A cracker, water, juice, or milk might be offered after the medicine has been swallowed. The parents should check with the health professional about what to use.

Croup

One serious threat that often ocurs in children under the age of 6 is croup, which can be recognized by difficult breathing and a peculiar barking cough. The attack usually occurs at night, with the child awakening from sleep with a croupy cough that gradually gets worse and may be accompanied by his turning blue (cyanosis). The child becomes frightened with the increasing severity of the symptoms. His symptoms will be eased if he is allowed to sit up in bed and if the parents reassure him that he is not going to choke.

The parents should try to stay as calm as possible and should call the health professional immediately. They should report the child's breathing, coloring, and emotional state to the health professional, and it may be recommended that the child be taken to an emergency facility for treatment.

Croup is caused by muscle spasms of the larynx, which cause breathing obstruction. Caring for the child with croup involves measures that will help him to breathe without difficulty. The most effective treatment is to place the child in a high-humidity environment, either by placing him in a steamy bathroom or by the use of a humidifier. This will help to reduce the spasms and will help to liquefy secretions. Attacks may occur during the day also but usually involve a croupy cough without the child's turning blue.

Chapter 6

Childhood

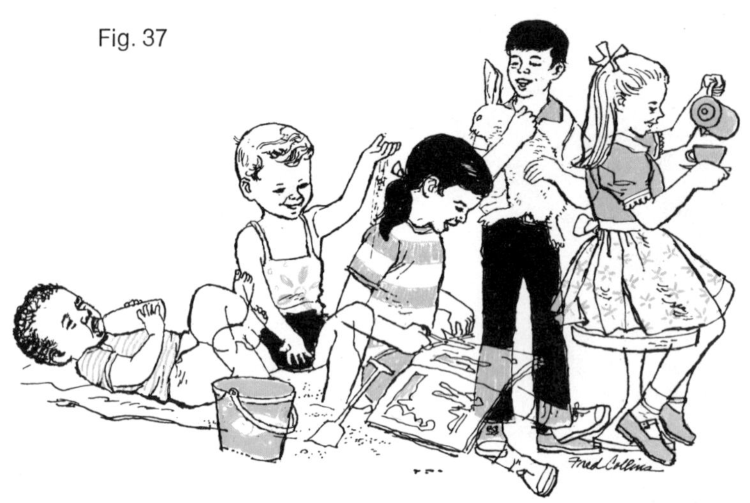

Fig. 37

In this chapter, childhood refers to the time of life from 1 year of age to about 10 to 12 years of age, when adolescence begins. During this period, personality is unfolding and important patterns of behavior are being established by the child. The child develops skills, attitudes, and health habits that affect the rest of his life. So that the stages of growth and development and the needs of the child that cause the greatest concern to parents can be considered, childhood will be discussed here in three stages: the toddler (1 to 3 years), the preschool child (3 to 6 years), and the school-age child (6 to 12 years).

Physical growth includes many things—among them, changes in general body growth, head circumference, diameter of the thorax (that part of the body between the neck and the diaphragm), abdominal and pelvic measurement, and weight and height.

Development refers to progressive increase in skills and capacity of functions. *Growth* refers to an increase in physical size of the whole body or any of its parts and can be measured in inches or centimeters and in pounds or kilograms.

Every child is an individual who differs in terms of the rate of growth from other children. He grows and develops physically, mentally, socially, emotionally, sexually, and spiritually at different rates, although the result is a progressive development of the whole individual child.

There are factors in growth and development that have to be considered when learning about how a child grows. These factors are—

Race
Nationality
Sex
Heredity
Environment—prenatal and postnatal
Socioeconomic status of the family
Nutrition
Illness and injury
Exercise

THE TODDLER

By his first birthday, the baby has learned to trust (or mistrust) by observing how well and quickly his parents meet his basic needs. The

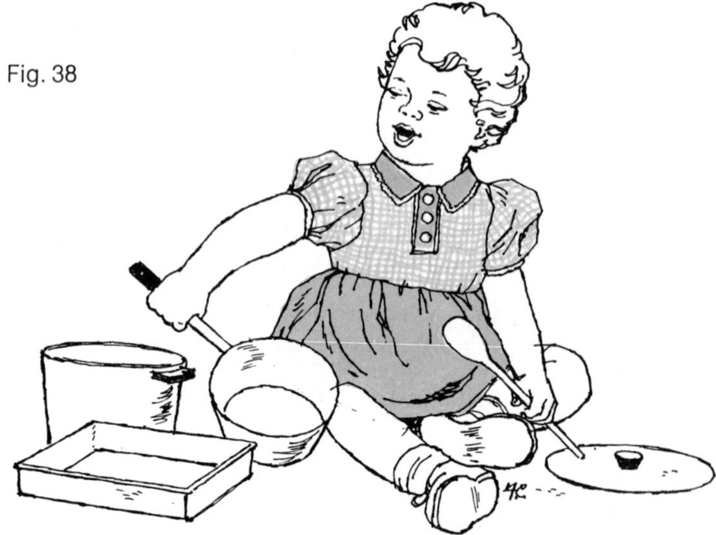

Fig. 38

toddler is becoming aware of himself as an individual. If he is respected as an individual, he tends to want to do what he feels is right.

Physical Growth and Development

The child's physical growth spurts during the first year. His weight, which doubles at 4–6 months, now triples. The child who earlier was just starting to crawl all over the place and into everything can now pull himself up and stand alone. At first he is unstable, but then he learns to hold onto something, to take a step, then two, and finally to walk stiffly, sometimes backward, falling down now and then. He picks himself up easily if he falls. He runs up walks and driveways, jumps and hops with both feet, and goes everywhere, in and out, upstairs and downstairs. He cannot sit still. He uses his power of locomotion to increase his ability to estimate distance and depth. He gains much enjoyment and surprise from various activities that stimulate his senses and use his muscles.

Children, however, are individuals, and there are differences in their growth and development. They walk at different ages, and not all of them develop the same skills at the same time. The average child usually walks by 12-15 months, but it is not unusual for a normal, healthy child to walk as late as 22 months.

At approximately age 2 or 3, the child learns to move with more sureness and safety, as he continues to explore his surroundings with interest. Activities in exploring and investigating are indications of the child's desire for independence. Other activities, such as climbing stairs, exploring, and learning about the world, may steadily unfold; as the child grows, he begins to sense that he now can control certain aspects of his environment. He pokes into everything he can get his hands on, shakes tables or objects, and tears magazines. His grasping ability and control of fingers and thumbs are well developed, and he can open containers with screw lids, build blocks into towers, turn doorknobs, and use crayons to color a book. His neuromuscular coordination has increased to the point where he can also put on simple items of his clothing, can climb stairs without crawling, and can kick or throw a large ball.

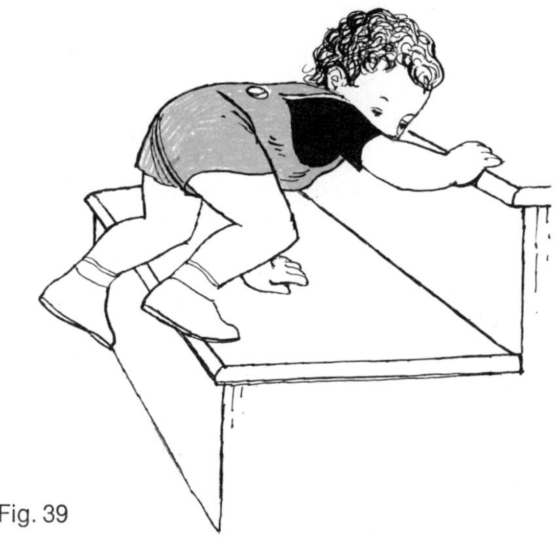

Fig. 39

At this period, the child's growth rate slows down, as reflected by the fact that between 1 and 4 years of age, he will gain only 4–6 pounds (1.8–2.7 kilograms) in weight and increase 2–3 inches (5–7 centimeters) in height per year. A 3-pound (1.36-kilogram) gain may be healthy and normal for some children, while a 6-pound (2.7-kilogram) gain is healthy and normal for others. Boys may begin to have a leaner, bony look, and girls may develop a feminine roundness. All other physical and motor skills also continue to improve, although at a slower rate, and are affected by practice and the child's maturation process.

Speech Development

The baby hears much that he does not understand, but this very lack of understanding is a challenge to learning. The child understands words long before he is able to say them. He knows his name and the meaning of the word "no." When he is about a year old, he begins to imitate the sounds that have meaning to him. The happy, outgoing child usually talks earlier than the quiet, less active one. If the mother is tense and silent when caring for the baby, he is often slower in learning to speak.

People tend to use single words and short sentences with the young child so that he can more easily understand. Nouns such as *mama, daddy, bottle, ball,* and *dog* are learned first, along with a few action words such as *bye-bye, up, out,* and *wait.* Nearly all children mispronounce words when they begin to talk but improve gradually. Usually, by the end of the second year, the child will know about a hundred words.

You must speak simply and clearly with the toddler to be sure that he understands, especially when he is in an unusual or frightening situation such as a visit to a dentist or a clinic. Rather than telling a crying, kicking child to behave, you should speak calmly and give simple explanations.

Eating

A growing child has a good appetite and has developed a well-defined preference for certain foods. He may drink his milk from a bottle or a cup. Learning to eat can be a messy business. Although most toddlers are able to feed themselves with a spoon, they still spill a lot. A child may become restless, noisy, and messy about his meals. He may take a bite and hurl the next spoonful into the air. He may also eat with his fingers and smear food on his chair and clothes. He may yell. He may bang his utensils. Whether the child eats with the family or not will depend upon his behavior when he eats with people around him and how tolerant his family is about his feeding behavior.

The parents should be understanding and tolerant of the child's behavior. Some suggestions are as follows:

- Allow the child to feed himself as much as he wants to but give help when he seems tired or appears to need some help.

- Ignore the child's table manners. He will outgrow his being messy as soon as he develops the skill of handling his utensils properly.
- Serve the child's meals regularly and in small amounts.
- Provide rest for the child before and after meals, especially when he has had active play and exercise.
- Make mealtimes learning times, to introduce and master ideas and skills that might present difficulties at other times.
- Never use food as a reward. ("If you eat your spinach, you can have ice cream.")
- Never withdraw food as a punishment. ("If you don't eat your spinach, you can't have ice cream.")

Sleep

Getting the child to sleep at suitable times and in suitable places will be easier if the right conditions are provided. If possible, the child should have a quiet room of his own, where he can sleep undisturbed. The small size of a bassinet gives the very young baby a sense of security. His next bed should be a crib that he can use until he is 3 or 4 years old. The mattress should be firm to provide body support and promote proper sleeping posture; firm foam rubber is ideal. The mattress should have a waterproof covering (not a plastic bag) to keep it clean and free from odor. (Plastic bags may cause death by suffocation.)

During the second year, the child's sleep pattern changes. Usually, the morning nap is eliminated and the afternoon nap becomes longer. There is a stage when one nap is not enough and two naps are not required; then the child can be put to bed earlier in the evening.

The 2-year-old often resists going to sleep, perhaps because he does not want to be separated from his mother. He finds many excuses to bring his parents back into the room, such as asking to go to the toilet or to have a drink of water. After the child has had his wants satisfied, he should be left alone. Although he may cry at first, giving in to his demands will encourage him to continue resisting bedtime.

Toilet Training

During the first year, the baby wets and soils his diapers with little awareness. He may grunt, strain, or pull at his diaper when a bowel movement is coming. Until the child understands the relation between a bowel movement and the use of the toilet, it is a waste of time and emotionally disturbing to both the child and the parents to try to train him. The child is usually about 2 years old before his nervous system and muscles are sufficiently developed for toilet training.

In training the child, parents should use a term such as "BM," which will be clear in meaning both to the child and to most adults. If the child will be using the regular toilet, he may need a special child's seat at first, and steps so that he can use the toilet without adult help. Some children, however, are afraid of a regular toilet. A potty chair is very valuable in the toilet training process and gives the child much more independence.

Bowel training is usually started first. Bladder control is more difficult for the child and usually takes longer. First steps in bladder control might include helping the child to be aware that he is wet, then that he is wetting, and, finally, that he is about to wet. This procedure will help him understand the relationship between the process of wetting and the result: wet pants. He may then want to take the steps necessary for the most comfortable result: dry pants. Children vary so much in their personalities and development that what works with one child may not work with another. Some children even train themselves late in the second year, sometimes in just a few days. Once the child understands the process, he can be taken to the toilet or the potty at intervals or be reminded to go by himself.

The child's desire for approval and his wish to imitate his parents or older brothers or sisters are important factors in toilet training. The toddler will, of course, have accidents and at times will refuse to go to the toilet. It usually takes longer to learn to remain dry at night. Children usually do not wet the bed on purpose and should not be punished for doing so. In general, parents should try to be understanding and to avoid shaming the child. The important things are the child's state of readiness and the parents' attitude of encouragement and approval.

Developing Good Habits

It is important to help children learn habits of cleanliness while young. The child should be taught to wipe himself after a bowel movement. Girls should be taught to wipe from front to back to avoid bladder infections. The toddler must be taught not to play with urine or stool. The child should be helped to wash his hands after going to the toilet. A small step to help him reach the sink will encourage him to wash his hands by himself.

Safety

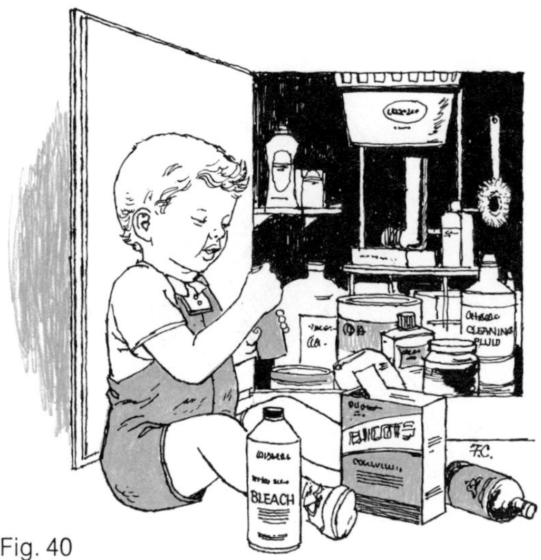

Fig. 40

The toddler is an explorer. He tries to touch and taste everything within reach (Fig. 40). His parents should understand that this is the way he learns and develops his skills. Within the limits of safety, the child should be allowed to inspect and become familiar with everything around him so that his natural curiosity is satisfied. Every room in the home, however, should be examined carefully for safety, and hazardous objects should be removed or put where the child cannot get at them. Doing this is called child-proofing the home.

The baby's furniture should always be in safe condition. Crib bars should not be more than 2⅜ inches (6 centimeters) apart, and the mattress should fit snugly in the crib, to avoid enabling the baby to get his head wedged in an unsafe position. Never use thin plastic bags to waterproof the mattress. The locks that hold the crib side in position should be in working order. The high chair should have a broad base that prevents it from tipping over. The tray catch should be secure, and a safety belt should be used. Never use a stroller without fastening the safety belt. If there are stairs, gates should be used at the top and the bottom to prevent falls once the baby becomes interested in climbing (Fig. 41).

The kitchen poses special safety hazards for toddlers. Many children enjoy playing with pots and other items from kitchen cupboards.

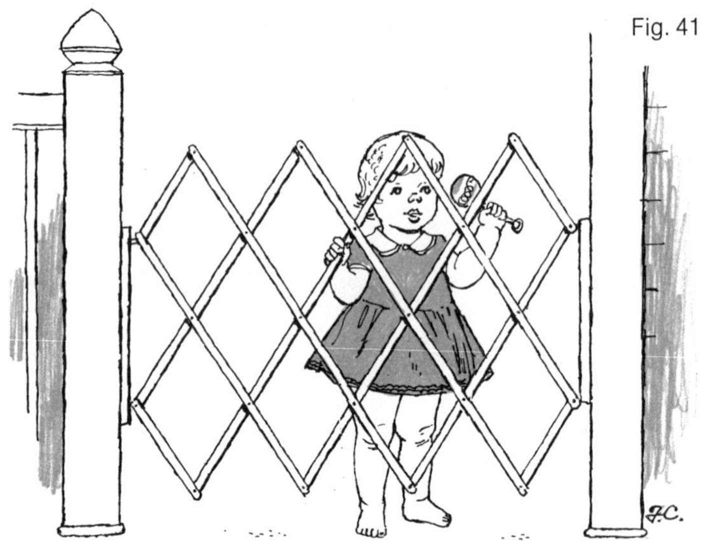

Fig. 41

Since the toddler usually wants to be with or near his parents, it would be wise to keep him in a playpen in or within sight of the kitchen during meal preparation. If the child is not kept in a playpen, there is also a danger that someone may trip over him. Be sure to observe the following precautions:

- Keep pot handles turned toward the back of the stove so that a child cannot reach them and an adult will not accidentally bump them, perhaps causing a dangerous spill.
- Do not let the child play near the stove when the oven is hot or when there is any danger of grease spattering or pots boiling over.
- Do not store within a child's reach any soaps, detergents, cleaning substances, insect poisons, drugs, knives, or matches. All of these are potentially fatal.

Electrical appliances and cords fascinate the young child but can be the source of serious shocks and burns. Although the child should be taught not to play with any electrical equipment, parents should never take unnecessary chances. Electrical cords should be as inaccessible as possible to avoid serious mouth injury if the child should bite into them. Unused electrical outlets should be covered with adhesive or safety plugs so that a child cannot stick anything into them. Light bulbs should be kept in all lamp sockets. Adults should avoid any unsafe practices in the handling of electrical appliances, since a child is very likely to imitate such practices.

All medicines and poisonous substances should be stored in a locked cabinet, if possible, out of reach and out of sight. These items should be stored in their original containers to avoid any confusion. A child should not be allowed to play with empty containers that once held harmful substances.

Suffocation hazards include allowing the child to play with thin plastic bags and storing unused refrigerators that have not been padlocked or have not had the door removed. A refrigerator or icebox is an airtight box, and a child cannot be expected to know the danger of such a hiding place.

Teething

From the time a child is 5 or 6 months old until he is 2 or 3 years old, new teeth will be breaking through the gums periodically. Teething can cause much discomfort to the child and may be accompanied by drooling, swollen gums, nausea, vomiting, diarrhea, a runny nose, and, occasionally, even a slight fever. The pain can often be eased by chewing on teething crackers, rubber toys, or something cold. If the child is too uncomfortable, a health professional will be able to make further suggestions.

Teeth usually appear in a predictable order, although variations do occur. The two lower front teeth are usually the first to appear, then the two upper front teeth. The first molars appear about the time a child is a year old. The total set of baby teeth includes eight front teeth (incisors), four "canine," or "eye," teeth, and eight molars, and is usually complete by age 3.

Thumb-sucking

The child who sucks his thumb is often a source of special concern to the parents. Parents need not worry about the child's mouth being deformed if the habit does not continue into older childhood. The cause of the thumb-sucking is the more important issue. It may simply be a sign that the child did not have enough sucking pleasure during infancy; however, it is often an outlet for the child's feelings of insecurity. The best course of action is to attempt to correct the cause, which may mean providing more consistent discipline, more regularity in the child's schedule, or more affection. Pressuring the child to give up the habit will only increase his unhappiness. The busier and happier a child becomes, the less he will need to turn to thumb-sucking for comfort.

Temper Tantrums

The active toddler or preschool child will sometimes have experiences that he really cannot handle well and will not be able to find behavior to meet his needs at the moment. He may express his frustration by crying or in violent bodily activity. His actions are usually aimless, but they may be directed toward hurting himself, for example, by banging his head against a wall or the floor. During a temper tantrum, the child loses all sense of reality; he may not hear or react to anything said to him. The child should be restrained only as a last resort to keep him from hurting himself or others or from breaking objects around him. Calmness and patience on the part of the adult are important during a temper tantrum.

Consistency by adults in applying rules of behavior does a great deal to prevent temper tantrums. Rules and procedures should not be modified as a result of this type of behavior; to do so only confuses the child and may give him reason to repeat the behavior.

If a child has frequent temper tantrums or if they continue after he begins school, parents may want to consult a health professional. Child guidance clinics, which exist in many communities, can give valuable advice in helping the child to form healthy behavior patterns.

Discipline

Loving parents have always wished to guide their children toward good habits, sound values, and socially appropriate behavior. This teaching process is referred to as discipline. The best means to achieve these results are, of course, the good example of the parents and expressions of approval when the child does well. The child who does not receive such expressions of parental concern rightly feels unloved and often seeks attention through disobeying whatever guidelines may exist.

Punishment is often the adult's first response to undesirable behavior on the part of the child. Although punishment is useful in emphasizing which behavior is not acceptable, it is not always effective. Some children persist in negative behavior despite repeated spankings, scoldings, or other methods of correction. It may be that the child would prefer being punished and at least having the adult's total attention, rather than being ignored while obeying rules and receiving no special recognition. The parent who is getting nowhere with a child should seriously consider giving the child more praise when he does well and calling much less attention to the undesired behavior.

Punishment should be thought through carefully by the parent to be sure it will bring the desired results. Punishment that consists merely of angry words or striking out at the child, with no particular regard for the child's self-respect or potential for improvement, may be useless or even harmful in the long run. A corrective course of action tailored toward improving the specific undesired behavior might include both some form of restriction to indicate that the behavior will not be tolerated in the future and a special task designed to set the child on the right track.

THE PRESCHOOL CHILD

Growth and Development

Physically, the preschool child has a full set of baby teeth, consisting of ten upper and ten lower teeth. He weighs about 30–35 pounds (13.6–15.9 kilograms) and is approximately 30–36 inches (76.2–91.4 centimeters) tall. He has reached about half of his adult size and, as stated earlier, his physical development slows down.

The child has better muscular coordination, and his motor skills are more refined. He can dress and undress himself completely and can button his shirt and even pull zippers up and down on his coat. At 3½ years, however, there is a great change in his behavior. His smooth motor functions are replaced by clumsy actions. He falls easily. He may stutter. He may feel tense and insecure, may be jittery and whiny, and may suck his thumb more.

At age 4, the child's feelings of uncertainty and insecurity start to change again. The child gains back his brash self-confidence. At this stage, he is often described as "out of bounds in almost every direction." He becomes bossy, belligerent, and rambunctious. He breaks things. He swears, swaggers, and boasts. He laughs and he gets very angry. He may engage in physical fighting, hitting, kicking, and biting in the process. At age 5, he begins to regroup his abilities. He shows more control of his skills. The frustrating 4-year-old is again transformed into an "angel" of 5, who has mastered the developmental tasks expected of him (Fig. 42).

The preschool child has begun to develop a sense of himself as an individual. His main task now is to learn more about his surroundings and about other people. His constant questioning may annoy others. He may feel threatened by changes in his surroundings. He needs to be able to cope with major changes such as moving to a new

Fig. 42

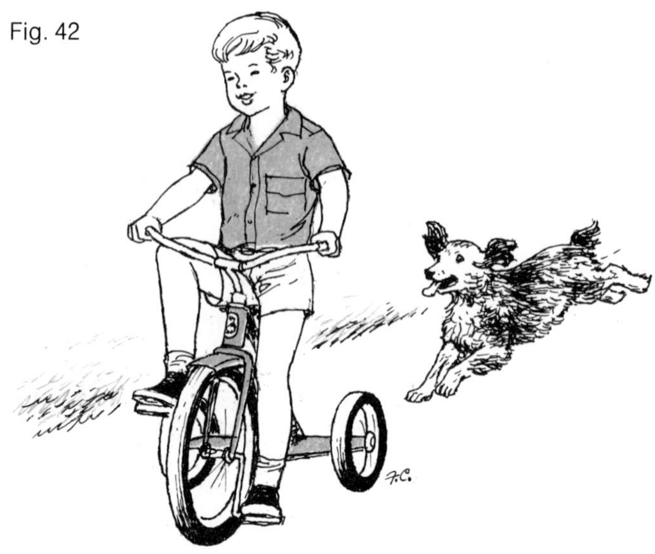

home or the birth of a brother or sister. He has a rich imagination and is also very active physically, almost to the point of violence. This is a period when the child begins to take initiative and will be doing more things than ever before. Critical or discouraging comments from adults could lead him to doubt himself, while guidance, praise, and a warm and loving attitude on the part of the parents help him toward self-confidence and avoidance of bad feelings about himself.

The preschool child begins to use longer and more complex sentences, and his vocabulary grows rapidly: he may learn as many as 600 new words a year. Parents who wish to discourage the use of slang or "bad words" should avoid paying attention to them, since they have little meaning to the child. Punishment serves only to emphasize the importance of the words to adults.

Play

Play has been called "the business of children." It has three basic aspects:

It provides outlets for the child's feelings and imagination.

It develops the child's physical skills.

Through play with others, the child learns cooperation.

As early as age 2, the child has a rich imagination. A corner becomes a playhouse; a piece of cloth becomes a cape; a box or chair becomes a car, train, or airplane. The child is very happy in his fantasies. This tendency to make believe should be encouraged, since it widens the child's understanding, enables him to express his feelings, and encourage creative skills. The child also imitates adults or characters he has learned about from fairytales, records, television, or books. He may play at being a fireman or a super-hero or may protect his stuffed toys as a parent would protect children. The child should have toys such as modeling clay, watercolor or finger paints, building blocks, or other materials to express his imagination and creativity.

The preschool child's physical skills are also developed through play. As he climbs, hammers, swings, or pedals about, he repeats each act until he masters it. Useful toys for this age group include slides, swings, balls, wagons, tricycles, toy tools, and climbing equipment.

The preschool child progresses from playing alone to simple, cooperative play with other children if playmates are available. A child between 3 and 6 is often ready for a play group or a nursery school.

Sleep

The preschooler is often so active that he does not know when he needs rest or sleep. The 3-year-old's sleep may be disturbed by dreams, and he often cannot tell whether they are real. A nap during the day often helps a child to sleep more restfully at night. By the time the child is 5, he rarely needs a daytime nap. Having a room of his own that is cheerfully decorated promotes sleep and provides a quiet place for the child to play or think.

Sexual Awareness

The attitudes that the preschooler forms about his body are more important than any factual information he may be given. The parents should not be alarmed to find the child playing with his genitalia and enjoying it. The parents should avoid any comments or scolding, which may lead the child to feel guilty or to feel that any part of his body is "bad." The wise parent, however, will help the child to find other activities that give enjoyment.

Teaching the Child

Teaching sensory and intellectual stimulation is very important for a preschool-age child. At this age, the child's reasoning and conceptual powers are more developed. He asks questions in a never-ending search for information. He can tell time and can count to at least 50. He can recognize the alphabet and in most instances can read or write his name. As his vocabulary expands, he can communicate better with his parents and friends. He reads, watches TV, and observes people to get more knowledge of the world around him. He loves stories of adventure and imagination and searches endlessly for the real hero. He enjoys his family, school, and life in general.

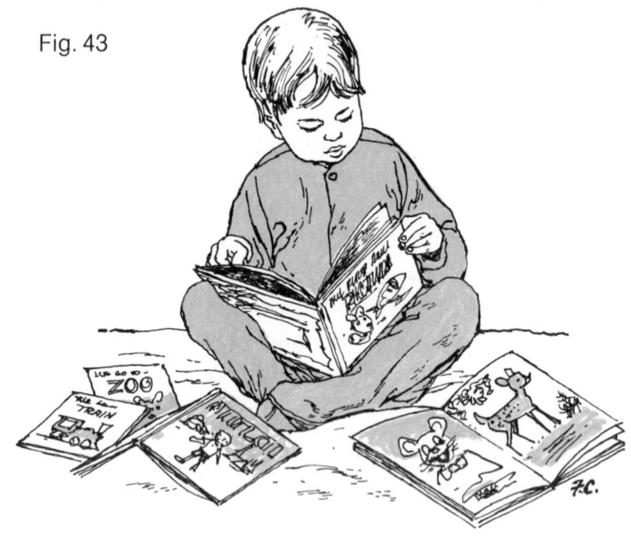

Fig. 43

New words, new ideas, and new information can be taught in many ways to a child. The use of food is one method of introducing first-hand experience in many aspects of life. Simple arithmetic can be taught in terms of the use of money to buy foods, the use of recipe measurements, and the timing of cooking. Beginning knowledge of science can be derived from the kind of foods that make us grow and their effects on how we feel, look, and behave. Concepts of "soil," "climate," "geography," and "transportation" can be taught by explaining the role of the family in obtaining foods and the factors that make food available. Appreciation of art can be taught through the colors, shapes, forms, and textures of food. Games are another method of teaching the child simple mathematics. Dice can be used to teach him to count; also the numbers of stoplights at a traffic crossing, keys, buttons, oranges, etc.

Games can also be used to identify and locate symbols. Learning to read can open doors to a great deal of information and enjoyment for the child. Reading stories to the child can help him develop his imagination.

The following are suggestions when teaching a child:

- Consider the readiness of the child when presenting a learning task or a concept.
- Children have short attention spans. Keep games short and they will continue to enjoy them.
- Avoid pressuring the child. Drop a game or activity immediately if a child indicates lack of interest in it.
- Make learning a fun experience for the child.

THE SCHOOL-AGE CHILD

Growth

The school-age child is full of enthusiasm and adventure. He is in constant motion. He takes more responsibility for himself than the preschool child, but he generally does better at the start of his task than at the end. He can run around the playground with speed and dexterity and is skillful in the use of his hands in activities such as cutting and pasting and stringing beads. He can use simple tools such as scissors, hammers, and other equipment.

Going to school is the most important event in the life of the school-age child. He is interested in everything, wants to learn, and is eager to please the teacher. Increasingly, he shows independence.

As the child grows older (between ages of 6 and 21) he begins to lose his baby teeth, and they are replaced by permanent teeth. A slow, steady growth continues. The child then gains about 5–7 pounds (2.3 to 3.2 kilograms) a year and grows about 2½ inches (6.4 centimeters) a year until puberty, when his growth spurts.

Development

The years between 6 and 12 are fairly calm years, during which the child enjoys purposeful activities and becomes a more responsible person. Many children show artistic talent or inventiveness or become very involved in hobbies or sports. If the parents show encouragement and approval of the child's activities and projects, the child develops good feelings about his own worth.

The school-age child is learning to conform to social norms and to play fairly. The parents serve as models to the child in relation to the rules of society. If the parents frequently break rules, it is difficult to teach children to obey the same rules.

The values of other children his own age become increasingly important to the child. Parents should not try to be "buddies" to their child but should encourage the child's confidence in them as parents. Although the child still depends on the parents for love and companionship, he may begin to reject hugging, kissing, and other signs of affection.

The closer the child comes to adolescence, the more he will start to waiver between conformity and rebellion against adults and between dependence and independence. Preadolescence is a time of growth. It is through the confusion that accompanies this growth that the child matures. Maintaining good communication—really listening to the child and answering his questions honestly and promptly—will lay a firm foundation for dealing with the problems of the adolescent years.

Developing Good Habits

The child often rebels against adult standards of cleanliness and dress during the school years. At the same time, he may be learning more about the importance of good health and safety habits at school. It is wise to encourage and utilize these health and safety measures in the home. If the parents have any questions, they can check with the teachers regarding the intent (or content) or other sources for information. The parents should avoid discouraging the child's initiative in these areas.

Privacy and Independence

The relationship of mutual respect that parents establish with their children in early childhood is the foundation for later years. Privacy is based on that respect. Rules for privacy should be established, and neither parents nor child should violate the other's rights except in a real emergency. The child should be encouraged in his efforts toward financial independence through the performance of small jobs after school and during vacations. The parents might choose to pay the child for the performance of some household chores or might give him a regular allowance.

Sexual Awareness

One aspect of sexual awareness is identification of the child with the parent of the same sex. Children perceive quickly whether both parents do the same things each day or that only one goes to work while the other prepares meals and cares for the home. The child should realize that there may be room for free choice in such matters. In America there is an increasing tendency for women to work and for men to assume more responsibility for daily home activities. Tradition, economic circumstances, and personal characteristics often determine how families will organize their lives. Different cultures vary in their attitudes toward the role of each sex.

In matters of sexual awareness and education, there should be an attitude of openness and mutual trust between parents and child. Mothers and fathers should explain menstruation and nocturnal emissions (wet dreams) to their sons and daughters several years before such events are likely to begin. Children should be told where babies come from in a clear, straightforward fashion by either parent, and the parents should be available to answer further questions as they arise. Straightforward, correct answers should be given. For example, a boy who is aware of the menstrual cycle can avoid embarrassment by knowing the reason when a girl says she cannot go swimming with him.

Attitudes toward the body and toward sexual relationships are among the most important values that parents can convey to their children. This learning begins early, with the parents' response to the child's exploration of his genital area. It continues through the imparting of information about anatomy, reproduction, and the related body processes. Throughout the learning, the parents will be conveying to the child through their behavior and casual comments, as well as during specific discussion, their attitudes about the responsibility each person assumes in any sexual relationship, for both himself and his partner.

Chapter 7

Adolescence

The adolescent years are a time of rapid physical, sexual, and emotional growth and a time of reaching for responsibility and independence. Through his "growing pains," the teenager comes to a sense of his own identity, the feeling of "who I am." He will shift back and forth between dependence and independence and will experience wide swings of mood. The growth and changes come so rapidly that the adolescent is often awkward and uncomfortable with his "new" body and new emotions. The challenges of adjusting to schooling, being like his friends, channeling his abundant energy, experiencing strange new physical sensations, breaking away from his parents, and learning to relate to the opposite sex may put him in a constant state of confusion at a time when he wishes to appear confident and mature.

The adolescent who has been properly prepared for the changes he is now experiencing will find that the teen years can be a constructive and satisfying time, especially if he has certain goals clearly in mind:

- To arrive at a sense of identity
- To become independent
- To achieve emotional maturity
- To strive for social and intellectual growth
- To establish good relations with the opposite sex
- To develop a definite outlook on life (for example, spiritual, philosophical)
- To develop his interests through the proper use of leisure time

Parents must remember that their child is preparing for adulthood, that drawing upon his talents and interests, he must integrate new growth and biological drives into an identity he can live with. He is preparing to get along on his own.

PHYSICAL GROWTH AND CHANGES

Although each adolescent matures physically at his own rate and pattern, the general trend is for the girls to develop about 2 years before the boys. During this time lag, both girls and boys are self-conscious as the girls begin to tower over the boys. The average age for the development of the girls' bodies is from 11 to 13, although some begin to change as early as 8 or 9. Boys begin to change sometime between the ages of 10 and 15.

The first obvious change is often the growth spurt. All at once, clothing does not fit. Girls' breasts begin to grow, and their hips become wider. Boys' legs grow longer first, then their trunks grow, and a few months later their shoulders and chest will broaden. Adolescents who seem to shoot up overnight often find their new height awkward and embarrassing.

Adolescence is often thought of as the awkward age, because body changes occur so rapidly during these years that many boys and girls feel unfamiliar with their own bodies and find it difficult to handle them gracefully. The conflicts and confusion of adolescence also contribute to this feeling of awkwardness. It is easier to take any clumsiness in stride if one thinks of adolescence as a time of increasing physical strength and activity, more energy, and improving coordination. Adolescence is the fastest growth period experienced since infancy and early childhood. The actual height attained is influenced not only by family and racial heredity but also may be influenced by quality of nutrition, state of health, and even climate and altitude.

Teenagers develop an almost constant appetite in connection with their rapid growth and increased activity. They will often be seen raiding the refrigerator. Many teenagers do not take time to eat

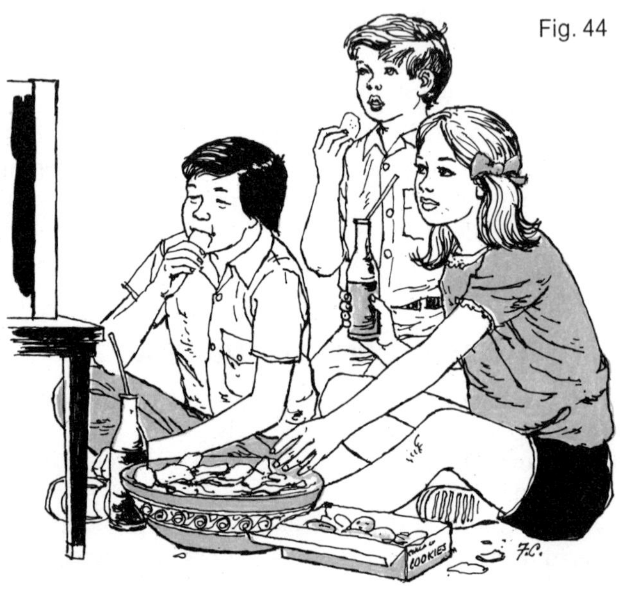

Fig. 44

properly; they grab for candy bars and soft drinks that contain calories with very little nutrients or none at all. As with people at all stages of life, the best diet for teenagers is food from the four basic food groups (see page 35). Such a diet will not only help them to maintain their energy and avoid unwanted weight but also will contribute to clear skin and shining hair. Fresh fruits and vegetables should be easily available, so that adolescents will be encouraged to choose foods that are good for them for snacks.

Hormone changes cause the sweat glands to develop in adolescence. This condition often leads to increased perspiration and acne (eruptions of the skin caused by infection and inflammation of the sweat glands). Several steps can be taken to minimize this problem:

- Keep the skin and hair clean.
- Expose the skin to sunlight.
- Eat a balanced diet.
- Avoid chocolate, nuts, and foods with a high fat content.
- Do not squeeze the pimples, since scarring may result.
- Consult a health professional if acne continues or increases.

Adolescents will suddenly find it necessary to use deodorants and antiperspirants as adults do to control perspiration.

The voices of both girls and boys become deeper as the voice box (larynx) grows. This process is gradual and is more obvious in boys. A boy may be embarrassed to find his voice "cracking" in the middle of a sentence as his deep, adult voice reverts briefly to the high-pitched tones of childhood.

One physical change that is not readily noticed is that most adolescents have all their permanent teeth (28) except the wisdom teeth by the time they are 13. The second molars usually erupt at the beginning of adolescence; their appearance is a sure sign that puberty (sexual growth) is close. The third molars, or wisdom teeth, may erupt in later adolescence or early adulthood.

SEXUAL DEVELOPMENT

About the time of the growth spurt, girls begin to develop breasts and both boys and girls begin to grow pubic hair. About 2 years later, underarm hair begins to grow, facial hair appears on boys, and girls begin to menstruate. As with physical growth, boys will generally mature sexually about 2 years behind the girls' schedule.

Adolescents who begin to develop early may either be pleased or embarrassed. The first girl in a group to develop breasts may try to hide them or otherwise deny their existence, especially to boys who might tease her. On the other hand, she may be the envy of her girlfriends, who can hardly wait for their own figures to develop. Boys who develop early are usually more proud than embarrassed.

Girls

A girl's breasts begin to develop between the ages of 8 and 13. The first sign is the breast bud, which is a swelling just under the nipple. Occasionally one side will develop before the other. At the time the breast buds are forming, a girl's hips begin to widen. It usually takes 2 years after the breasts begin to develop before the reproductive organs begin their functioning. With the onset of ovulation (production of eggs) and menstruation (periodic bleeding from the vagina), the girl is capable of conceiving a child. Menstrual periods are often irregular in the beginning but usually occur from 26 to 35 days apart.

Girls begin to experiment with makeup, dieting, and clothes during this period. They are often very much influenced by what their groups of friends are doing. Mothers are wise to encourage their daughters in the direction that will heighten natural good looks and self-confidence. It is unwise for the teenage girl to diet unless she is under the supervision of a health professional, because there is a real danger of malnutrition at a time when her body has a greater need for food than ever before.

Boys

The first sign of sexual maturation in boys is usually an increase in the size of the testes and scrotum, sometime between the ages of 10 and 15. About a year later, the penis gets longer. The moustache and beard are among the last changes to appear.

When boys are between 12 and 14 years old, they experience involuntary ejaculations (release of semen, the thick liquid that carries the male reproductive cells). This usually occurs at night and is referred to as a "nocturnal emission," or "wet dream." These ejaculations are often accompanied by sexually exciting dreams. If the parents have prepared the boy for this occurrence and explained that ejaculations are a normal, healthy sign of approaching manhood, the adolescent boy will realize there is no need to feel guilty.

The Role of the Parents

Wise parents will have prepared their sons and daughters for adolescent growth and change several years in advance of their expected occurrence, perhaps when the parents are also explaining the reproductive processes. It is not fair to the developing adolescent to experience a first menstrual period or nocturnal emission with no idea of what is happening. Throughout the teenage years, both parents should be easily approachable in regard to questions about sex and many other subjects of great importance to the developing young man or woman. Although schools may offer courses in sex education, it is the parents' responsibility to provide the guiding framework that helps adolescents to understand their bodies and to build a healthy attitude toward sex.

EMOTIONAL CHANGES

As the adolescent searches for identity, values, purpose, and an idea of his own destiny, he experiences much frustration, many mood changes, and mixed feelings about whether to forge ahead into adulthood or cling to the security of childhood. When he tries to do something on his own, he often feels the restrictions of parents, school demands, and rules in general. New problems are always arising before he is finished coping with the old ones. The adolescent may often feel embarrassed or frustrated for reasons he doesn't fully understand. He and his parents should realize that these emotions are common to adolescence and are only temporary.

Sense of Identity

Adolescents are trying to develop their own identities. They struggle with questions that adults have already answered: "Who am I?" "Why am I here?" "What will I become?" Their bodies are maturing sexually and they are beginning to take an interest in the opposite sex. They lack confidence, knowledge, and experience. They can't decide how much the standard rules should determine their behavior, and the ideas of their peers suddenly seem more important than any pat answers that adults can give. Every new experience becomes a testing ground for the adolescent's values.

Adolescents may not want to be like their parents. They may not really agree with their peers' values, but they do not have enough confidence to choose a way of their own. They may develop a personality that brings them the most social approval, yet may feel they are not really being themselves. Their real feelings, likes, and dislikes may become submerged as they work out an image of opposition to adult values and of conformity to their peers.

Independence Versus Dependence

Adolescents waver between independence and dependence: the need to be their own boss, to be self-sufficient in work, play, and friendships versus their human need to rely on others. Adults have already worked out the answers to this tension in their lives, while adolescents are breaking away from the total dependence of childhood in search of self-reliance. In one and the same action an adolescent may be sending two messages: "Don't tell me what to do" and "I'm scared. Please take care of me." The task of a maturing adolescent is often frightening and even overwhelming.

Moods

The mood swings of adolescents are often caused by hormonal changes that are totally beyond their control. Because they do not understand what is happening to them, adolescents often overreact. A normally even-tempered child can become an unpredictable adolescent, with moods ranging from being loving and delightful to angry and sulky. Adolescents may alternate between great activity and laziness, between complete acceptance of the values they have been taught and an attitude of questioning and scorn. They frequently show resentment of authority and advice. It may be harder to concentrate, and there may be an increased tendency to daydream. Both the parents and the adolescent are often uncertain about what is really going on.

Crushes

One common phase of adolescent emotional growth is the crush—the sudden infatuation with and ardent admiration of usually an older person. The boy's or girl's crush may be directed toward a person of either sex. The adolescent can hate as intensely as he can love—it is all part of the struggle to define his feelings, identity, and social role. Parents can help in these often fleeting crush situations by respecting the adolescent's feelings and noting the good qualities of the admired person. If handled in this way, the crush can be very helpful to the adolescent in developing his values.

SOCIAL CHANGES

Peer Pressure

Teenagers have a strong need to be accepted by their friends. They do not want to feel or appear different. They do not want to be taller or shorter, fatter or thinner, more or less intelligent, richer or poorer than their friends; they like to dress alike, talk alike, and do the same things. They are not yet self-confident enough to be different as individuals. This pressure to conform to the values of others of the same age and interests is called peer pressure.

As a group, teenagers try to be different both from the children they have been and from the adults around them. They experiment within the security of their own group. Since peer pressure is difficult to resist, disciplining the teenager who occasionally becomes involved in irresponsible behavior requires special understanding.

If the parents disapprove of the behavior of the adolescent's friends, the parents should confine their comments to objections to specific actions. Instead of saying, "Your friends are careless and disrespectful," a parent might say, "I was very upset when I found that your friends burned the coffee table with their cigarettes" or "I worry about your friend's driving because he peels rubber whenever his car leaves the driveway." The adolescent will appreciate the reasonable approach and the genuine concern of the parent.

Dating

Interest in friends of the opposite sex usually begins in the preadolescent to early teen years. Group activities with boys and girls are often the first social contacts. Girls of 13 to 14 often go through a "boy-crazy" period, while boys do not show a similar interest in girls until they are 16 or 17. Because they mature earlier, girls usually begin to date earlier. Boys often do not feel self-confident enough to ask a girl for a date and often feel they cannot afford it anyway.

Dating is a time of learning, sorting out conflicting emotions, and developing respect for sexual differences. Parents should be available for guidance and for answering questions. If an adolescent should become involved in steady dating before he was up to the emotional demands and responsibilities, the wise parent might encourage him to devote more time to his hobbies and other interests, to participate in family and social activities, and to widen his range of social contact, perhaps through dating more than one person, so that he would have the opportunity to mature emotionally and sexually in less demanding situations.

Parenting

Children who have good feelings about themselves and who know what to expect during the teen years are those who are best prepared for adolescence. From earliest childhood the parents have guided the child to trust, to take the initiative, to arrive at self-esteem through individual activities, and to practice sound health habits. The challenge to guide the adolescent as he integrates physical, sexual, and emotional growth, emerging biological drives, and new social demands calls for special sensitivity on the part of the parents.

While still unsure of his own identity, the adolescent begins to try to take control of his own life. The power struggles of early childhood become more clearly defined in terms of independence versus dependence. The adolescent balances time spent away from home with his peers against the demands of the family; late hours and junk foods against the schedules and habits of the family; an outside job against home responsibilities. He experiments with new styles of dressing and popular hairstyles.

The familiar reaction of the adolescent is often, "Everyone else gets to do it, why can't I?" Realistic limits should be set and consistently enforced. Although it is good that the adolescent is trying to take responsibility for his own life, parents cannot suddenly throw their own judgment to the winds. The teenager must be dealt with as a maturing individual, and the parents' values and reasoning should be discussed openly. The teenager still needs guidance, since he is often unsure of himself, no matter how confident he may appear.

One sound approach in matters of conflict is to work out a compromise around specific rules. There should be no changing of rules; otherwise distrust and resentment are fostered. The wise parent will continue to keep abreast of the adolescent's behavior in addition to simply enforcing a compromise when it becomes necessary.

Some common matters of conflict are—

- Intensive dating versus adequate opportunity for the adolescent to mature emotionally and socially
- The time at which an adolescent should return from a date or activity
- Rules of behavior dictated by the parents

- The use of time: schoolwork, leisure, outside job, etc.
- The teenager's attitude toward discipline and moral guidelines
- The teenager's manner of spending money
- Life-styles, clothing, friends, social life, and activities outside the home
- The adolescent's share of housework or other home responsibilities
- An attitude of respect or disrespect toward parents or other adults

Some guidelines for parents toward resolution of these conflicts are as follows:

- Encourage the adolescent to be as independent as possible.
- Learn to stand aside and let the adolescent make mistakes, and help him to profit from his mistakes. (Protection from experience does not educate; it only prolongs childishness.)
- Accept the adolescent's friends even though his choice of friends may be unwise. Encourage him to bring his friends to the house. Danger arises when an uncompromising parent forces the adolescent to meet his friends elsewhere.
- Be aware of the influence of your behavior and values (both good and bad) on your children.
- If home life is interesting and stimulating, the adolescent will enjoy spending a good portion of his leisure time in the home.

Like most people, the adolescent wants and needs to be treated with the respect accorded a free person and an individual capable of reason. The preceding matters of conflict and the guidelines toward resolving them are merely starting points; from there, the adult and the adolescent must evaluate the nature of their particular conflict and seek a compromise that is genuine, meaningful, and fair.

The key to successful communication and compromise between parent and adolescent is talking *with* rather than *to* the young person. If parents listen carefully and do not command, threaten, or criticize the adolescent, he will have feelings of acceptance, trust, self-confidence, and self-esteem, and a sense of being loved. The adolescent will then be more likely to talk with his parents about anything. The parents can then present their point of view as *one* approach to a problem, encouraging the adolescent to express his own point of view.

DEVELOPMENT OF A HEALTHY OUTLOOK

Adolescence is generally a healthy period of life. The real challenge is the development of a healthy outlook on life and good feelings that come from knowing that parents, teachers, and others value the adolescent as a person and respect his qualities and abilities. Adults should help the adolescent to affirm his values, to cope with stress, to become socially involved, to develop his physical and emotional abilities, to experience self-esteem and confidence, to develop intellectually, and to use his natural talents. The causes of many statistics such as those concerning teenage drug abuse, deaths in automobile accidents, suicides, and delinquency are mainly the social and psychological conditions under which young people are growing up.

Like most adults, teenagers are both realistic and idealistic. They are interested in the arts and in proving themselves intellectually. Their capacities for sustained work, concentration, and serving others are almost unlimited. The strong idealism of the adolescent is perhaps the greatest of his gifts. It is the wise parent or adult who fosters this idealism and helps the adolescent to channel his personality, abilities, and energy into a whole pattern of positive identity.

Fig. 45

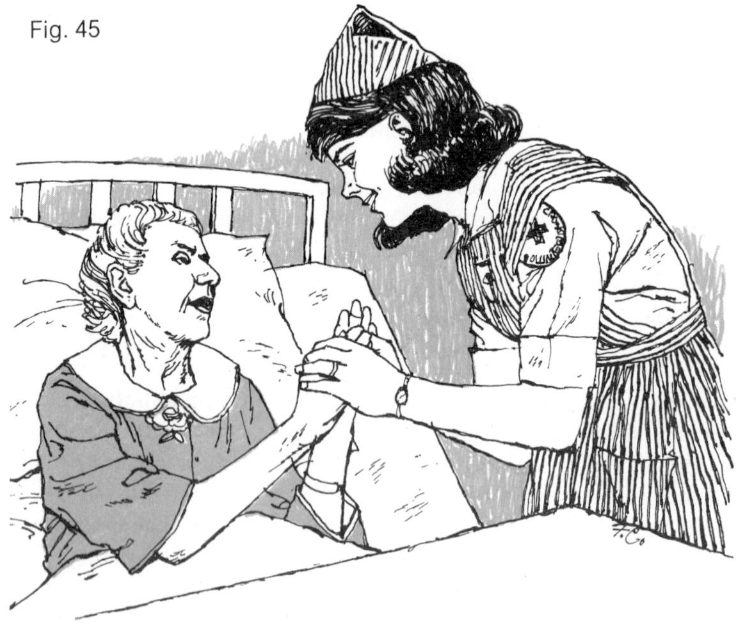

Chapter 8

The Adult Years

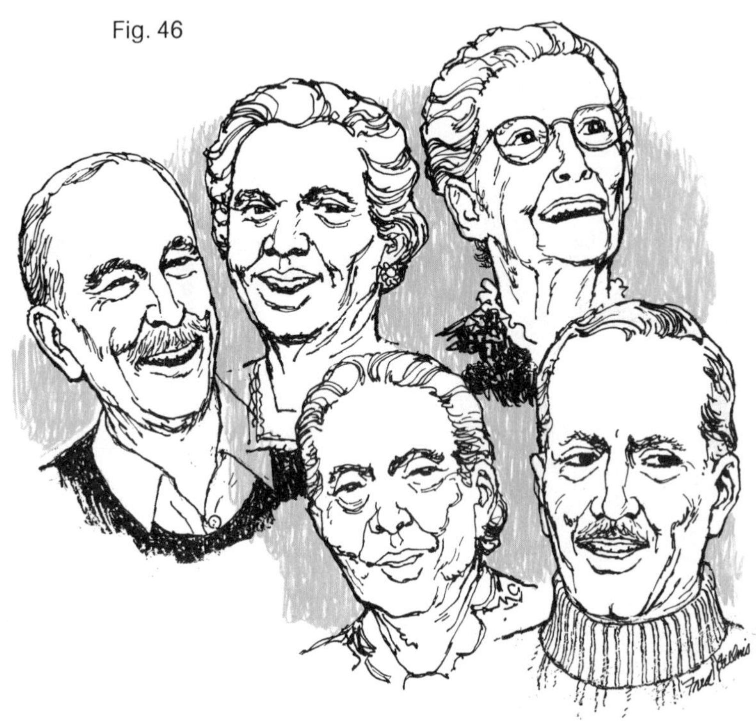

Fig. 46

Although the adult years span the ages from 20 to 70 and older, there is obviously quite a difference between a 20-year-old adult and an adult who is approaching 70. Physical and psychological changes occur, society changes, and a person's fund of experience grows considerably during the continuous process called aging. No two persons age at the same rate or in the same way. Life-styles, health habits, physical and emotional stress, and heredity influence a person's health as he grows older. While some people may become weaker, more frequently ill, or less able to tolerate change, others maintain their physical and intellectual abilities, resist disease easily, and may enjoy life more than ever.

The developmental stages and activities of infants, children, and adolescents can all be viewed as preparations for adulthood. At every stage, the individual masters tasks and concepts that enable him to get along successfully in the world. Impulses and energies are channeled into work, homemaking, and social skills. A sense of identity and personal strength is developed, as well as the ability to initiate and maintain close human relationships. Skill develops through the processes of deciding priorities, managing money, meeting the reasonable expectations of family, friends, and society, and maintaining the self-discipline to attain goals. Old age is not a unique condition in life that begins with a certain birthday or with retirement, any more than "growing up" is a condition that occurs overnight. We are all growing older, regardless of our age.

This chapter deals with common events and physical and psychological changes that take place in most individuals during early, middle, and later adult years. Commonly experienced effects of aging are described, and suggestions are given for a program of practical preparations to contribute to peace of mind in the event of unexpected illness, accident, or death.

EARLY ADULT YEARS

The early adult years are a physically active time when a person's education, training, and experience are channeled into some meaningful and rewarding pattern of activity that includes work, homemaking, and deepening personal relationships. A philosophy of life and a sense of personal strength and identity are formed, and many people become more aware of their need for companionship and the sharing of confidences and affection.

Marriage is one particularly rewarding way of life that young adults often choose for greater fulfillment. Successfully married persons are described as those who can give and receive affection, cry in each other's presence and not be ashamed, and quarrel badly and know it is not the end. The skills necessary to maintain such a relationship do not come naturally: they require effort. Young people now have available many opportunities to learn about and prepare for the special challenges of married life.

A few questions that should be considered before marriage are listed below.

- How confident are both partners that their marriage will be successful?
- How willing is each to please the other?
- How easy is serious conversation?
- How is conflict handled? Do conflicts result in better understanding of each other?
- What responsibility does each partner expect the other to assume?
- How self-sufficient or dependent is the proposed mate?
- What are his or her best friends like?
- Does the relationship survive loss of glamour, such as when one partner is ill?
- How is the physical health of the potential marriage partner?
- How are decisions made? (When two people agree on everything, only one person is thinking.)
- How much does each one value material things, money, intellectual pursuits, and togetherness?
- How willing is each to accept little annoyances?

Other factors that may influence the success of a marriage are religion, race, financial status, age, the changing roles of men and women, and individual life-styles. Similarity in these factors does much to strengthen the marriage by reducing potential areas of conflict. Although strong differences in any of these factors do not by any means rule out the possibility of success in marriage, they do require extra effort and adjustment if a harmonious relationship is to result. The degree of maturity at the time of marriage also affects the relationship; teenage marriages are especially prone to difficulty, and the partners may benefit from professional counseling.

Young married couples usually start by establishing a home base and insuring financial stability through rewarding jobs. Together they work toward better communication, shared decision-making, and mutually satisfying sexual relations. Together they determine how money will be spent, what types of relationships they wish to have with relatives, friends, and associates, and when to start a family of their own. Through serious discussion and shared decisions, they develop a philosophy of life and their identity as a couple.

The decision to have the first child brings additional adjustments. Often housing arrangements have to be altered, and the couple must decide whether one partner will temporarily forego a career to be home with the child. The couple's relationship will be affected, and their association with relatives and friends will also change.

Most young adults enjoy good health during this period when physical strength and endurance and emotional flexibility are needed to meet the needs of the family and to adjust to the demands of the community. Through positive attitudes and good habits of nutrition, exercise, and personal hygiene, they may continue to enjoy good health for many years.

MIDDLE AGE

By the middle adult years (40–60), a person's children may be on their own or may be finishing their schooling, the person's career is usually well established, and it is possible for the individual to pursue his own interests anew. It is a time of increasing self-awareness, of letting go of involvement in the decisions of one's children, and of planning for the future. For many, the middle and later adult years are a time of fulfillment, deepening insight, and a greater interest in social acitivity. There is a sense of achievement in one's work, and time for developing a more satisfying relationship with one's spouse.

Often, however, stress arises from competition at work, the sudden quiet at home with the children gone, changes in body image, loss of parents, spouse, or friends, and concern for the future. These situations often call for altering priorities, reevaluating abilities, and reviewing values. Sound practices of mental health and of leisure are very important to people who may have difficulty with these new concerns.

Most persons at middle age are healthy. They may feel some decrease in energy but they adjust to it and continue to grow in interests, activities, and inner resources. If, however, they have a chronic illness they must be careful about adhering to the prescribed treatment. Everyone should continue the basic good health practices discussed in chapter 2.

Menopause

Menopause is the process by which, as a result of hormonal changes, a woman stops menstruating and loses the ability to bear children. This process occurs in women anywhere from the mid-forties to the late fifties. Although some women may mourn the loss of the ability to bear children, many women feel a sense of relief. Any woman who does not want a pregnancy at this time should continue family planning measures until 6 months after her last menstrual period, as ovulation and menstruation stop gradually over a period of time. Although menopause marks the end of the ability to bear children, it does not, of course, mean the end of sexual activities.

Although many women experience no symptoms at all during menopause, others may occasionally experience "hot flashes" (a feeling of warmth and flushing of the face, neck, and upper body) and emotional swings. A heavier menstrual flow, or "flooding," is *not* a usual sign of menopause. Excessive bleeding or bleeding between periods, regardless of the time of life, should always be checked by a physician.

Male "Midlife Crisis"

There is increasing talk of a "male menopause." Although there are differences of opinion among experts, it does appear that during the forties and fifties many men undergo certain physical and emotional changes that are comparable to the female menopause. Since these changes do not affect the man's ability to father children, the term "midlife crisis" is more appropriate. Since the man's sexual performance may be affected, this is a time for straight, intimate talk between man and wife. Symptoms appear to be influenced by work-related problems, and men often review their strengths and weaknesses at this time. Many begin to feel that they have, after all, not achieved much, and they begin to fear that they may have missed opportunities and that there is now little time left. It is helpful if men realize that the midlife crisis is temporary in nature.

Studies indicate that regular sexual expression by men and women can continue until they are in their 70's and 80's. All persons continue to have sexual needs. A sense of loss of sexual vigor and of a youthful body can be minimized by warm, supportive expressions of love between partners.

Planning for the later adult years should begin during the middle years. Long before a person retires, he should—

- Develop interests, activities, and social involvements to be pursued after retirement
- Evaluate his financial resources and compare them with anticipated expenses and desired activities (travel, moving to a new living situation, the need for special medical care, etc.)
- Consider the suitability of his current living accommodations (climate, the nearness of church, shopping facilities, and friends and relatives) and the difficulties and expense of maintaining a large home
- If a move is desirable, consider his preference in regard to living with his family or a friend, in a retirement community, or in a mixed-age neighborhood

Any changes in regard to living arrangements or financial investment should be made only after inspection and careful evaluation of desirable features and limitations.

LATER ADULT YEARS

The major difference between old people and young people is how long they have lived. Most individuals proceed confidently into old age, maintaining their health, alertness, and interest to the end of their life. A happy and healthy old age can more likely be achieved if a person starts early in life to bring it about. Healthful living during the first 40 years of life is a priceless contribution to the second 40.

Although each person adjusts to change in individual ways, the ability to meet change and stress in a calm manner is evidence of adaptability and sound mental health. Those who are prepared can meet the complex problems of today's living with wisdom and flexibility. Many older adults choose life-styles quite different from those they have pursued in the past.

Although some older adults choose to withdraw gradually from active involvement in the community, many others seek to take advantage of leisure to try new things. What is important is the pleasure and meaning each person takes from his various activities.

Human contact and warmth are required by human beings at all stages of life, and the older person is no exception. Having spent the earlier years accumulating experience and wisdom and enjoying social life, the older adult now needs as much contact as ever with family and community. As a retired professional or technical expert, the older adult can both gain personal satisfaction and make great contributions to others by sharing knowledge in areas such as income tax preparation, community planning and development, legal matters, or perhaps by raising funds for community projects. An older adult may also choose to utilize talents by participating in volunteer activities through churches, schools, and organizations such as the American Red Cross. A person might serve as a teaching assistant, a "foster grandparent," a storyteller or reader, or a "friendly visitor," or might even assist in the "Meals on Wheels" program. Many older persons will enjoy the recreational and service activities found in government-supported senior citizen programs.

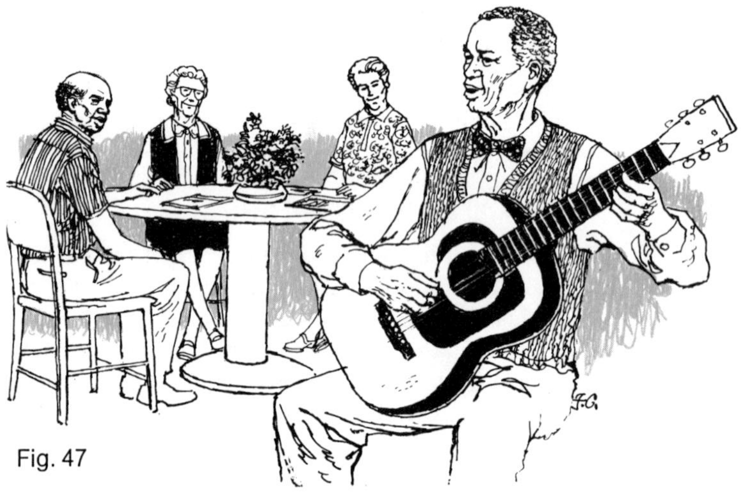

Fig. 47

Many cities, counties, and states have an "Office on Aging" or "Commission on Aging," which provides information on recreation programs, service opportunities, eating programs (see chapter 2), counseling, housing, legal matters, pensions, insurance, tax matters, and health programs. Booklets that give information on different types of programs for older Americans are available from the Administration on Aging, U.S. Department of Health, Education, and Welfare, Washington, D C 20201. If the programs referred to do not already exist in the community, persons are needed to get them started. Booklets are available free of charge that suggest ideas on employment and volunteer opportunities for older people, planning for the future, telephone information services, and other projects and programs.

Other resources include organizations for retired persons. Some of these organizations offer special benefits such as economical mail order drug service and health, life, and auto insurance designed especially for older people. Special services provided by these organizations include membership in local chapters or units, participation in programs and courses, and access to publications designed for older persons. The best known of these organizations are the American Association of Retired Persons and the National Retired Teachers Association (see the Appendix for addresses).

Older persons should not overlook the possibility of continuing their education. Many colleges and universities provide both leisure-oriented and academic courses of special interest to the elderly, often at reduced prices. Education is a lifelong process, and many retired persons obtain college degrees.

Adjusting to Physical Changes

Naturally, there are changes that take place in the human body as it ages. Graying hair, wrinkled skin, and bowed shoulders are common outward signs of aging that occur at different times in different people. Aging also greatly decreases body efficiency. The results are loss of strength and decreased resistance to disease; a decreased need for calories, which threatens to increase weight if dietary habits are not changed; poor circulation, which may cause hands and feet to feel cold or to swell; reduced sensitivity to temperature extremes; and poorer vision and hearing.

Adjusting to the physical changes brought on by aging may include taking the following measures:

- Exercising moderately to maintain muscle and joint function and to aid good circulation of the blood; avoiding constricting clothing on legs; elevating legs to decrease swelling and help blood circulation; maintaining good posture to aid breathing.
- Decreasing calorie intake to minimize weight gain, but being sure that the diet includes adequate supplies of essential nutrients.
- Seeking routine health care, including dental care, and checking of vision.

- Taking medicines as directed; if necessary, making notes to insure taking them as scheduled.
- Taking measures for extra warmth when appropriate. (Cold hands and feet can be helped by warm slippers, afghans, and warmer floors.)
- Allowing more time for routine activities, since reflexes and body movement may be slower; avoiding rushing; and moving carefully in situations where accidents are possible.
- Writing down appointments and engagements if a tendency toward forgetfulness is noticed.
- Evaluating daily tasks and routines for changes that could be made to conserve energy for more enjoyable personal and social activities.

Fig. 48

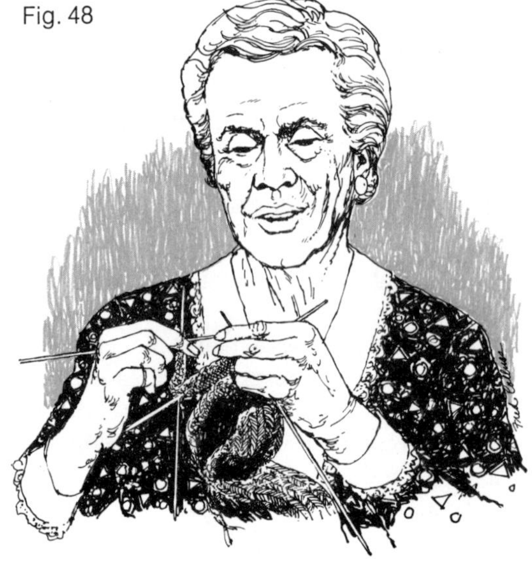

- Modifying the living environment to reduce the likelihood of accidents and to insure brighter and more even distribution of light. (Some modifications are nonskid rugs and floors, handrails on steps, hand grips in the bathroom, and rearrangement of furniture and other items in the home to permit safer movement.)

Because it is helpful to know the common physical changes that occur during aging and what steps can be taken to adjust to them, a description of the aging process follows.

The Aging Process

POSSIBLE BODY CHANGES	EFFECTS	SUGGESTIONS
Bone, Muscle, and Cell Structure		
Chemistry of the bones changes as calcium shifts from bones to tissues.	Bones become more brittle and are more easily broken.	Eat foods rich in calcium, such as milk and milk products and green, leafy vegetables.
Joints deteriorate.	Joints stiffen and are harder to move.	Use care at all times when walking; wear broad-heeled, medium-height shoes; avoid walking on snow, ice, or wet sidewalks, or be cautious.
Ligaments, tendons, and cartilage lose water and stiffen.		Use safety precautions in the home, such as hand grips on bathtubs, nonskid floors and rugs, and handrails. Rooms should be well lighted and uncluttered to prevent tripping and falls.
Muscles become weaker.	Strength decreases; body movement and other body functions become slower.	Carry out activities that include the normal range of motion. Allow more time for activities.
Tissues in the backbone shrink.	Height decreases and posture changes. Back, neck, hips, and knees may become bent.	

The Aging Process (continued)

POSSIBLE BODY CHANGES	EFFECTS	SUGGESTIONS
Worn-out body cells are replaced more slowly.	Wounds heal more slowly. Recovery from illness takes longer.	Prevent infection by carefully cleaning wounds. Seek early medical attention for wounds that do not heal. Eat a balanced diet. Avoid exposure to infectious disease. (Avoid crowds.)
Tooth enamel is not replaced.	Teeth tend to deteriorate.	Eat a balanced diet. Eat easy-to-chew foods. Brush and floss after meals.
Gums may shrink.	Gum infection is more likely, and teeth may be lost.	Care for dentures and gums to avoid infection. Obtain regular dental care.
Breathing and Blood Circulation		
Lungs become less elastic. The rib cage changes, and chest muscles become weaker.	Less air can be inhaled and exhaled. It becomes more difficult to breathe deeply. There may be shortness of breath.	Avoid smoking. Avoid exertion that may cause shortness of breath. Maintain good posture.

The Aging Process (continued)

POSSIBLE BODY CHANGES	EFFECTS	SUGGESTIONS
Less oxygen circulates in the bloodstream.	Resulting weakness may limit body movement and activities.	Do breathing exercises.
Blood vessels become narrower and less elastic.	The heart must work harder to supply blood to internal organs and to hands and feet.	Wear support hose. Elevate the feet when sitting.
Blood vessels of the brain may become clogged.	Blood pressure increases. The flow of blood is slower. Following exercise, the pulse rate does not return to normal as quickly. Poor circulation of blood may cause hands and feet to feel cold.	Have your blood pressure checked regularly. Engage in moderate exercise. Keep active to promote good circulation. Wear clothes appropriate for preventing loss of body heat. Keep home and floors comfortably warm.
Nervous System		
Brain cells are decreased, and blood vessels in the brain may become clogged.	Reflexes are slower. Learning process is slowed, and there may be reluctance to accept new ideas.	Allow more time for activities. Allow more time for learning. Engage in new or favorite activities.

The Aging Process (continued)

POSSIBLE BODY CHANGES	EFFECTS	SUGGESTIONS
	Loss of memory may result, and there may be occasional mental confusion.	Write things down to compensate for memory loss.
	The voice may change, and pronunciation may become less clear.	
	Heat, cold, and other touch sensations are not felt as readily.	Be cautious in using hot water bottles and electric heating pads. Test hot fluids before drinking and test bath water before bathing. Wear adequate clothing for warmth.
	Sleep patterns may change: it may be harder to fall asleep or to sleep for very long; napping may become more frequent.	If you want a longer period of sleep at night, reduce the number of daytime naps and increase activity, but do not become too tired.

The Aging Process (continued)

POSSIBLE BODY CHANGES	EFFECTS	SUGGESTIONS
Digestion and Elimination		
Tissues that absorb food function less efficiently.	Nutrients may be poorly absorbed. Poor iron absorption may result in anemia. Poor vitamin B absorption may cause fissuring of the mouth. There may be weight loss.	Consider the use of diet supplements. Eat foods rich in iron and vitamin B. Eat frequent, smaller meals. Obtain medical care. Have blood checked.
There is a reduction of digestive juices.	The stomach may be more easily upset.	Limit highly seasoned and other hard-to-digest foods.
Structural changes in the kidneys and prostate gland (in men) increase frequency of urination.	There may be a greatly increased frequency of urination, especially at night.	Limit fluids in the evening. Urinate immediately before sleep.
Intestinal muscles become weaker.	Constipation may result.	Increase fluid intake. Increase roughage in the diet, if it is tolerated.

The Aging Process (continued)

POSSIBLE BODY CHANGES	EFFECTS	SUGGESTIONS
	Hemorrhoids may result from straining with bowel movements.	Don't lift heavy objects. Put cold, wet packs onto rectal area. Seek medical care if hemorrhoids are severe.
Sight, Hearing, Smell, and Taste Changes may occur in the lens, blood vessels, and fluid in the eye.	Vision may be impaired or blurred. Eyes may become dry and irritated because of reduced tear production. Eyes become more sensitive to glare of lights. Cataracts and glaucoma may develop. Activities may be limited.	Have eye examinations annually or oftener if necessary. Wear glasses if needed. Provide adequate lighting for close work or reading. Rest eyes frequently. Eat a balanced diet. Avoid night driving. Take steps to adjust to changes. Use care when walking; avoid clutter in living areas. Take any measures necessary to prevent accidents.

The Aging Process (continued)

POSSIBLE BODY CHANGES	EFFECTS	SUGGESTIONS
Hearing may be reduced in one or both ears. Deafness for high tones occurs first.	Reduced ability to communicate may threaten to limit social relationships and enjoyment of activities. There is an increased possibility of accidents.	Have your hearing evaluated; if it is recommended, use a hearing aid. Ask others to face you when speaking and to speak slowly, distinctly, and in lower tones.
Sense of smell becomes less keen.	Odors are more difficult to detect.	Beware of potential dangers such as harmful gases.
The number of taste buds decreases, and taste becomes less keen.	Loss of appetite due to decreased enjoyment of food may occur.	Serve foods attractively; serve hot foods hot and cold foods cold.
Skin, Hair, and Sweat Glands		
Blood vessels under the skin break easily. Cell and tissue replacement is impaired.	Bruising is more likely. Growths and brown and yellow spots may occur. Fingernails and toenails develop ridges and become thicker.	Avoid bumping into objects and other accidents by putting things in their proper places.

The Aging Process (continued)

POSSIBLE BODY CHANGES	EFFECTS	SUGGESTIONS
Skin loses its elasticity.	The skin becomes thinner, drier, tougher, and wrinkled.	Avoid daily baths if the skin is excessively dry. Dry the skin well after bathing. Avoid overexposure to the sun. Use lotions and moisturizing creams as necessary.
Less fat is stored under the skin.	Lack of insulation from fat decreases the ability to regulate body temperature. Lack of cushioning from fat makes pressure sores more likely.	Dress warmly when necessary.
There is a decrease in sweat gland action.	Perspiration is reduced.	
Decreased gland activity affects hair and skin.	Hair becomes gray or white, and becomes drier. Skin color becomes paler.	

The Aging Process (continued)

POSSIBLE BODY CHANGES	EFFECTS	SUGGESTIONS
Hair follicles die.	In men, there may be a progressive loss or thinning of the hair; in women, the hair thins.	Consider the use of wigs and hairpieces if hair loss is excessive. Obtain a medical checkup if hair loss comes too suddenly.
Sex Functioning and Hormones		
Females' sex organs stop functioning, and menstrual periods stop.	Some women may experience hot flashes, headaches, sweating, loss of appetite, nervousness, depression, listlessness, or crying spells.	Obtain medical advice.
Hormone output is decreased.	Women may grow facial hair.	Remove hair by electrolysis, creams, or shaving.
There is less lubrication in the vagina.	Sexual relations may be uncomfortable.	Use a lubricant during sexual relations.
In later years, males' sex organs do not function as well.	There may be some decrease in sexual activity.	

BEING PREPARED

It is the rare person who escapes all sickness or who never has an accident requiring medical attention. Although a conscientious program directed toward positive health and the prevention of accidents does much to enhance the quality of life, either sickness, injury, or death can come to anyone at any time. It is wise to have a well-thought-out plan to meet these crises with a calm outlook. Much anxiety at times of crisis can be removed by having a regular doctor or clinic to turn to, by knowing that medical and other expenses will be met whether or not there is a large bank account, and by knowing that one's family will be provided for if an accident or illness should result in death.

Choice of a Personal Physician or Dentist

Most people prefer a doctor or dentist who not only is competent but also has a pleasant disposition, listens attentively, and answers questions patiently. If a person does not have a personal physician when a health problem arises, it is often difficult to decide what type of health professional to contact. If a person has a personal physician in whom he has confidence and with whom he feels comfortable, there is much less hesitation about seeking prompt medical attention as the need arises. The personal physician will know which kind of specialist to call upon if any conditions are present that demand further attention. (See chapter 2 for more information about choosing health professionals.)

Be sure to inquire whether the prospective doctor accepts payment from the available health insurance plan. A time of crisis is not the time to learn that the doctor does not accept insurance payments as full payment for special services.

Low-cost or free clinics are available in some communities, but some will not handle medical emergencies. People living on reduced incomes may want to take advantage of these clinics, at least for routine health care. Less active people will want to choose a doctor or clinic that is near their home or otherwise conveniently accessible.

Health and Life Insurance

Health and life insurance plans are often available at lower rates through a person's place of work; this is called group insurance. The amount and kind of coverage vary considerably. If the coverage is low or unavailable, health and life insurance might be taken out through a private insurance company. It is wise to apply for this coverage before reaching the age of 30, since most insurance companies will charge substantially higher premiums if any health problems are detected during the required physical examination.

Health and life insurance plans should be carefully studied so that one is familiar with the amount and kind of coverage offered. Many health plans will not pay some kinds of expenses unless they exceed a certain figure (called the deductible); some may not pay at all under certain conditions. Many insurance plans refuse coverage for dental work, eyeglasses, maternity care, and optional surgery. Some life insurance plans have special provisions for disabling injuries and loss of income. The contract should be carefully studied before it is signed. The coverage should be worth the monthly premiums.

Medicare is available to older or disabled persons. If coverage is not complete and medical expenses are expected to be high, it may be wise to supplement the coverage from a private insurance plan. Again, the additional coverage should be worth the premiums paid.

Preparation of a Will

Many people avoid preparing a will until serious illness or old age is upon them, with little thought as to what would become of a spouse or children if the individual were to die in a totally unpredictable manner such as in a car accident or from a heart attack. There is definite peace of mind in knowing that in case of death, property will be distributed according to one's wishes and in the manner most appropriate to the needs of the family. Provisions can be made in the will for the care of small children so that their fate will not depend upon the decision of a court if both parents should die. In the absence of a will, the state follows its own laws for the distribution of property.

Young people would be wise to consider the making of a will part of their transition to adulthood; married couples in particular should be prepared for the unexpected. If the will is carefully drawn up the first time, it is relatively simple to update. It should be updated when family or financial circumstances change, and if the person moves to another state.

A will is a legal document. It should be drawn up by a lawyer who is familiar with the laws of the particular state and who knows how to protect the person's interests. Homemade wills are upheld only if they conform to state law. An oral statement of one's last wishes may be valid if properly witnessed. State laws require at least two witnesses. The witnesses, however, cannot be persons who are to benefit from the will. The laws about what constitutes a valid will are quite rigid, and it is worth the legal fee to have a will prepared properly. Although the main purpose of a will is to give legally binding instructions, just as important are the purposes of giving peace of mind and sparing grieving relatives the burden of decision-making.

Chapter 9

Threats to Health and Life

There are many threats to health that are, for the most part, under the control of the individual. The use and abuse of drugs and alcohol, smoking, and even eating are generally related to an individual's outlook and ability to cope constructively with daily frustration. The better a person learns to cope with the inevitable frustrations of life, the less likely he is to abuse his body while seeking escape from his problems.

Most people learn to accept those things that they cannot change, to confide in a sympathetic friend, or to reorder their lives to constructively cope with the difficulties and challenges of life. Frustration is a normal response to a difficult situation, and each person's ability to cope with such frustration will depend on his health and his personality. Healthy forms of coping with frustration include—

- Reevaluating life activities and allowing more time for rest and relaxation
- Devoting more time to quiet meditation and spiritual growth
- Communicating openly with others
- Improving the living environment
- Planning for change in activity

The person who lives in harmony with himself and his environment is said to have an ordered life. Many factors in today's living tend to work against such harmony, including the growth of technology, the "work ethic," and changes in family structure. Circumstances of daily living often lead people to feel that they just cannot cope with changes, tension, and the pace of living. The person who has exceeded his frustration tolerance may not be able to find constructive solutions to his problems or to find release for his tensions. He may become overly anxious, emotionally upset, or depressed. He may seek to protect himself against conflict, anxiety, failure, and loss of self-esteem by various methods that may endanger his health. He may turn to drug abuse, excessive drinking of alcohol, or smoking—or perhaps overeating—or he may even entertain thoughts of suicide. It is very easy for these threats to health to become habit-forming. A person who experiences continuing stress and finds himself caught up in practices and habits that are injurious to his health faces the special challenge of reordering his life in a positive manner. He will then, in turn, find it easier to bring the harmful habits under control. The person who learns to cope constructively with the tensions and frustrations of living not only avoids harm to his body but substantially enhances his own happiness as well.

DRUGS

A drug is any chemical that affects the functions of the body or the mind when taken into the body or applied to its surface. Drugs are an important part of the treatment and cure of many illnesses and are prescribed by the health professional with a specific action in mind. Each drug acts in its own way to bring about changes in specific organs or tissues of the body, to control the secretions of glands, or to stimulate or depress the nervous system. Further, each drug is reacted to differently by different people. Drugs such as antibiotics have saved millions of lives. Drugs such as insulin for the diabetic have increased the life expectancy of thousands of people. Drugs such as tranquilizers have made it possible for people suffering from temporary or long-term emotional distress, and people who have psychiatric disorders, to continue to lead full, productive lives without treatment in mental hospitals.

Each type of drug acts in a specific way, and some drugs may cause harmful side effects. A given drug does not affect every person who uses it in the same way. The effects of drugs are influenced by the age, sex, weight, and physical condition of the user and by food or other substances taken at about the same time. It is very important that medicines be used only under the direction of a health professional and according to instructions. Some drugs can be dangerous when used in combination with alcohol or other drugs, and before giving a prescription, the health professional should always be informed of any other medications that a person uses.

Some of the side effects of drugs are predictable, and the user should carefully follow any instructions in regard to the medicine he is taking. Some drugs cause drowsiness and should not be used by people who will be driving cars, operating complex machinery, or acting in any situation that demands speedy reactions and good body coordination. Drugs can also affect personality and ability to perform. Some produce feelings of extra energy, self-confidence, or relaxation, but other side effects of drugs may include nervousness, restlessness, confusion, forgetfulness, apathy, depression, and feelings of persecution. Since drugs do not affect every person in the same way, some persons may experience rash, hives, nausea and vomiting, blurred vision, headaches, or other disturbing side effects. Any unusual physical or emotional changes that occur while taking drugs should be reported promptly to the health professional, who will advise you what should be done.

Although some persons (such as diabetics) are legitimately dependent upon drugs to maintain their physical health, others may find themselves becoming psychologically dependent upon drugs that ease emotional stress as well as physical problems. They may fall into a pattern of using drugs routinely to help them get through the day. There are very real dangers from such misuse of drugs, and the more a person relies on drugs to solve his daily problems, the greater risk he takes. It is important that young people and adults understand how drugs affect the body, know how to use drugs safely, and, whenever possible, seek less artificial, more emotionally sound methods of dealing with the discomforts and stresses of life.

Prescription Drugs

The safe way to take a drug is to make sure that it is prescribed for you. The health professional prescribes drugs for a specific purpose. Each prescription is written according to a person's age, sex, weight, and physical condition. When a drug is prescribed for you, be sure that the health professional is aware of any other drugs you might be using, since some drugs react with other drugs and may cause harm rather than relieve the health problem. Follow all instructions carefully. Call the health professional for instructions if you have any unusual physical or emotional changes such as rash, hives, digestive upset, or any other unexpected sign.

Over-the-Counter Drugs

Drugs that can be bought at a drugstore or pharmacy without a doctor's prescription are called over-the-counter (OTC) drugs. They may or may not be helpful in a particular health situation. *Never take over-the-counter drugs without checking first with the health professional,* especially if you are taking other drugs that have been prescribed for you. Follow instructions carefully and pay special attention to any precautions such as avoiding driving because of drowsiness. If rash, nausea, vomiting, blurred vision, or other unexpected effects occur, stop using the drug immediately and notify the health professional.

The Proper Use of Drugs

When a health condition arises that seems to call for the use of some kind of drug, always consult the health professional. When the health professional prescribes drugs you can be relatively sure that you are using the drug or drugs best suited to your existing health condition. You will be given instructions for the proper dosage and use and will be advised of any specific precautions to be observed. Always observe the following precautions concerning drug use:

- When you are under medical care, tell the health professional about all drugs that you are currently taking. Doing so will help prevent undesirable or dangerous effects from any medication that the health professional may prescribe or from others you are taking.
- Read the label on any drug carefully, and follow any precautions such as avoiding driving if the medicine is expected to cause drowsiness. Some medicines may require storage in a refrigerator. If instructions are unclear or hard to understand, check with the health professional.
- Take the medicine in the prescribed dosage and as often as the health professional prescribes. For example, the effectiveness of a drug that is to be taken three times a day for 10 days is reduced if the medicine is not taken exactly as prescribed. The medicine should not be stopped before the day ordered by the health professional.
- Some medicines do not work properly except on an empty stomach. Some must be taken with a great deal of water. If no instructions are given, check with the health professional.
- Report any unexpected side effects promptly to the health professional.
- Never take medicines prescribed for another person, even if your symptoms are similar to his. Never share your medicine with someone else.
- Never remove medicines from their original container until you take them, unless they are put in a container already correctly labeled. Do not mix medicines in an unmarked container.
- Discard any drugs that are no longer used, especially any prescription drugs. If you have any doubt about what medicine is in a particular container (for example, if the label is unclear, dirty, or missing), don't take a chance—discard the contents by flushing them down the toilet.
- Never leave medicines where young children can reach them. Many drugs are poisonous when taken in large quantities, especially by small children.

Drug Abuse

The misuse of drugs can occur either unintentionally or deliberately. Use of some kinds of drugs over a period of time—or even just occasionally—can lead to either physical or psychological dependence, or both. Psychological dependence exists when a person feels that he cannot do without the effects produced by the drug. The person who has become physically addicted to a drug emotionally resists doing without the effects produced by the drug, and his body resists as well.

Why People Take Drugs

Persons may become dependent on tranquilizers, alcohol, diet pills, sleeping pills, and various other drugs that stimulate or depress the nervous system, dull pain, or ease emotional stress. Some people get into the habit of using one drug to increase their energy in the morning, another to calm their nerves during the day, and yet another to help them get to sleep at night. The wisdom of this procedure is often not even questioned, since our increasingly drug-oriented society seems to believe that there is a pill to solve every problem. Drug abusers include all persons who use drugs in an improper manner, whether they are housewives dependent on diet pills or tranquilizers, business and professional persons who cannot get through the day without a martini or two, or persons who are addicted to any drug, whether obtained legally by prescription, over the counter, or illegally.

Many people deliberately take drugs to change the mental atmosphere in which they exist. They may be trying to escape from some form of pain—unhappiness, feelings of alienation or depression, or the inability to resolve personal or interpersonal conflicts—or they may be trying to be like their friends or to defy authority. Marihuana, which produces feelings of contentment and well-being, is often smoked as an antidote to emotional pain. Drugs that help people to forget their troubles by depressing the central nervous system include barbiturates and alcohol, as well as morphine, codeine, demerol, and other narcotics. Stimulants (such as coffee and amphetamine) may give a person a surge of energy and a feeling of being able to respond to his problems with self-confidence and without worry about consequences. They may also cause nervousness and feelings of persecution.

How Drug Users Begin

There are several ways in which persons may obtain drugs: (1) through the prescription of a physician, (2) over the counter of any drugstore or pharmacy, and (3) illegally through a "drug pusher." At this writing, marihuana is still illegal in most of the states. Sometimes a person will experiment with the smoking of marihuana or the inhaling of fumes of glue, paint thinners, gasoline, and other solvents, or he may experiment with other people's medicines. The effects of most drugs last only a short time, and the person may soon be using drugs more frequently as an escape from his problems, perhaps spending a lot of money or even resorting to crime to obtain money for more.

How To Prevent and Treat Drug Abuse

Education and a rewarding pattern of life are the most effective methods of preventing drug abuse. A child—in addition to being taught the danger of taking any drug not prescribed for him by a health professional and the danger of inhaling fumes from solvents, glues, etc.—needs to grow up in an atmosphere of love and understanding, with plenty of encouragement toward physical activity and other forms of recreation, creative endeavors, reading, and discussions and meditation on the meaning of life.

Praise and reward are better than punishment for encouraging desirable behavior, and they help to provide positive experiences and to minimize frustration in daily life. Emphasis on the value of maintaining good human relationships and on constructive activities and volunteer service in the community will lead the child to a pleasant, rewarding outlook on life. Because the adolescent's friends will also influence him, they should be chosen carefully. Since drug abuse is becoming more common, it is good for everyone, especially parents and adolescents, to be well informed about the use and abuse of drugs. Drug education materials are available from local health departments and libraries and can be used as a basis for discussion by parents and children.

Behavior changes are associated with many kinds of problems: the problems of growing up for a young person, the problems of increasing age for the older person, or the problems that result at any age from unusual changes in the environment. It is often difficult to determine the cause of such behavior changes, and the possibility should not be ruled out that the following behavior changes may be related to drug abuse:

- Change from being an expressive, talkative, clear-headed individual to being one who is withdrawn, silent, and confused

- Change from being a vital, healthy, energetic person to being one who is nervous, tense, and restless
- Change from being a confident, self-assured person to being one who feels oppressed, tormented, and persecuted
- Change from being a helpful, attentive, and dependable individual to being one who is vague, forgetful, and disinterested
- Change from being an eager, active, enthusiastic individual to being one who is passive, apathetic, and hopeless
- Change from being an open, friendly, trusting individual to being one who is suspicious, antagonistic, and alienated

The following suggestions are for people who suspect that a family member or a friend is taking drugs:

- Avoid panic. Seek professional help such as that from your physician, who may refer you to a mental health center, a public health department, or a local hospital or clinic that has a drug treatment program.
- Keep the lines of communication open. Encourage the person to feel free to talk with you and discuss his problems.
- Maintain an atmosphere of trust. If your child is using marihuana, remember that the majority of youngsters who experiment with marihuana do not continue to use it.
- Avoid stereotyping. Do not assume that departure from normal styles and standards of behavior indicates that a person is using drugs. Such suspicion may encourage the very action you are trying to get the person to avoid.
- Avoid scare or threat tactics. Help the person to become aware of the possible long-term effects of drug abuse. Give honest and accurate answers to his questions.

Alcohol

Alcohol is actually a depressant, although its use in moderation often has a stimulating effect because the individual is less aware of fatigue and discomfort. One effect of alcohol is the reduction of the individual's ability to control his behavior, with a greater tendency to act on impulse. The more alcohol that he consumes, the greater will be the decrease in his judgment and in the control of his emotions and behavior. The individual who drinks moderately often seems more lively than before he had a drink. Excessive use, however, can cause slowing of the body functions to the point of stupor and even death.

When alcohol is consumed often, in large quantities and over long periods of time, there is often both physical and psychological damage to the user. The person may also become addicted. Nerve and brain damage, stomach irritation and ulcers, painful inflammation of the pancreas, and damage to the liver can result from excessive alcohol intake. Prolonged overuse may disrupt social relationships and will often interfere with job performance. Problems with alcohol are found throughout our society—among men and women, the rich and the poor, the young and the old. Of an estimated 9 million alcoholics in this country, only five percent are the "skid row" characters commonly thought of when we think of alcoholics. The majority of alcoholics cannot be distinguished from our neighbors or members of our own families. Even teenagers and younger children can have problems with drinking.

Alcohol should be suspected as the problem when a person—

- Drinks alone
- Drinks in the morning before going to school or work, or just to start the day
- Goes to work intoxicated
- Needs a drink in order to get through the day
- Often drinks to a state of intoxication (loss of control)
- Drinks to the point of "passing out"
- Has blackouts, or periods when he cannot remember events that occurred while he was drinking
- Causes or experiences family arguments because of drinking

Resources are available to help persons with alcohol problems. Some resources are the same as those mentioned for people with drug problems: mental health centers, local hospitals, and clinics. In addition, there are groups run by alcoholics, the most widely known and available of which is Alcoholics Anonymous. Teenagers and families of alcoholics also benefit from the Al-Anon and Alateen groups. Check the local telephone directory in order to contact these organizations.

People who use alcoholic beverages should be careful about setting a good example for children and should never pressure guests or family members to drink. Drinking should never be the purpose of a party or gathering but rather a casual accompaniment at social activities. Soft drinks or coffee should be available for those who prefer not to drink alcoholic beverages, and food should be provided with the alcohol at all times. In addition, the hosts at a party have a responsibility to prevent driving by persons who have had too much alcohol to drink.

SMOKING

Tobacco

The most common form of smoking in the United States is the smoking of cigarettes containing tobacco. Some people smoke for relaxation, for a feeling of well-being, or for stimulation; others continue to smoke simply because smoking is a habit. Many persons develop a psychological dependence on tobacco, and it is thought that there is physical dependence as well. Recent discoveries about the dangers of tobacco use are motivating many older persons to try to break the habit, but teenagers are starting to use tobacco at an alarming rate.

Research has linked cigarette smoking to lung cancer and heart disease. All forms of tobacco—cigarettes, cigars, pipes, and chewing tobacco—are associated with higher rates of various types of cancer. The tar in the smoke is the greatest factor in causing cancer. Because the nicotine in tobacco is a stimulant, smoking causes faster heartbeat and higher blood pressure. Shortness of breath, nagging cough, and other respiratory difficulties are common even among younger smokers. The hazards of smoking can be reduced by choosing a cigarette with low tar and nicotine (a label on the package tells how much is in each cigarette), by smoking fewer cigarettes each day, by taking fewer puffs from each cigarette, and by smoking only half of each cigarette.

If you want to cut down on smoking but do not want to stop abruptly ("cold turkey"), try the following approaches:

- Think about the situations in which you are most likely to smoke, then try to reduce the number of such occasions during the day.
- Carry out a regular schedule of physical activity to help cut down on smoking by reducing tension.
- Have handy some substitute for smoking, such as candy, gum, tea, and raw vegetables.
- Since many people gain weight as they give up smoking, plan your diet carefully to avoid weight gain and the accompanying temptation to revert to smoking.

Marihuana

Some persons smoke marihuana, a drug about which there is much debate. Marihuana is illegal in most states. Research has not proved the degree of physical dependence produced by smoking it, but psychological need for the drug does develop, although it is more moderate with marihuana than with other drugs such as LSD.

Marihuana causes–

- Rapid heartbeat
- Lowering of the body temperature
- Reddening of the eyes
- Changes in the blood sugar level and increased appetite
- Loss of body fluids
- Drowsiness, lack of coordination
- Inflammation of the mucous membranes and bronchial tubes

Also, a state of intoxication, feelings of well-being, hilarity, and confusion, distortion of time and space, and a loss of judgment and memory may result. Other effects may be fatigue, depression, moodiness, fear of death, and panic. Sometimes no mood change is seen.

Driving while under the influence of any mood-altering drug is dangerous. Rapid decisions are more difficult to make while under the influence. A test for marihuana intoxication is available, and drivers can be arrested for driving while intoxicated on marihuana.

OBESITY AND WEIGHT-GAINING

Obesity is a major health problem in the United States. People who are from 10 to 20 percent above their ideal weight for their height and age are considered to be *overweight;* people who are more than 20 percent over their ideal weight are considered to be *obese.* Approximately one fifth of all adults in the United States are overweight to a degree, and this condition may interfere with their optimal health and life expectancy. As people grow older, they find it easier to put on weight and harder to take it off. About a third of the people in the United States over the age of 40 are overweight. Studies show that overweight people die younger than people of normal weight. Overweight people are also more susceptible to high blood pressure, heart ailments, stroke, diabetes, cancer, and diseases of the digestive system.

Causes of Obesity

Overeating, excessive calorie intake, and lack of exercise are the most common factors in weight gaining, since the principle involved is the storing of unused calories as fatty tissue. A very small number of people are obese because of endocrine gland disturbance. There are also people who may have an inherited tendency toward being overweight. People who consistently eat poorly planned meals, often with an excess of starchy foods, fats, and meats and relatively little in the way of fruits and vegetables, tend to have problems with their weight.

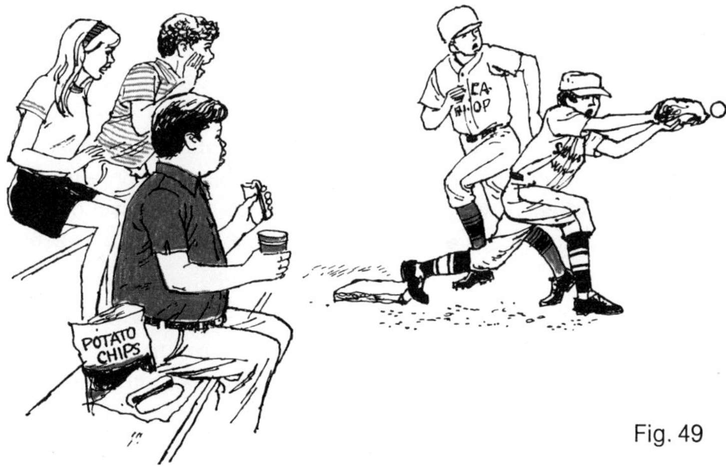

Fig. 49

The obese person has from three to five times as many fat cells in his body as does the person of normal weight. In addition, the fat cells of the obese person are larger. The *number* of fat cells in the body is fixed by late adolescence and does not change with age or even with dieting, although dieting may cause a reduction in the *size* of the fat cells. The fact that extremely obese individuals have many more fat cells makes it especially difficult for them to lose weight.

Overfeeding during infancy and early adolescence promotes an increase in the number of fat cells developed. That is why obese children tend to become obese adults. The most effective method of preventing overweight problems in later years is, therefore, careful attention to diet and weight gain in infants and children. Rapid weight gain in infants should be avoided, and physical activity should be an important part of the child's daily life. Obesity in adolescence may be caused more by lack of exercise than by overeating. Psychological factors are more likely to influence the weight of children than of adults.

Exercise is a very important factor in weight control. Lack of physical exercise encourages obesity, and obesity discourages exercise. In addition, studies show that normal body mechanisms that regulate appetite and the feeling of fullness do not function properly in the person who does not exercise. The individual's eating habits are affected by both "internal" and "external" signals. Persons of normal weight who have adequate exercise are inclined to judge their state of hunger by *internal* signs, such as hunger pangs, loss of ability to concentrate, weakness, lowered body temperature, dryness of the mouth, and irritability, and they will stop eating when they feel full. In contrast, the obese person is relatively insensitive to the internal signals and overly responsive to *external* signs, such as appearance, smell, taste, and nearness of food, time of day, and the environment or surroundings. The obese person who does not exercise often tends to overeat because of these psychological factors and because of a lack of awareness that his stomach is already full.

Advertising of food on television and radio and in newspapers and magazines often tempts people to overeat. We are surrounded with attractive pictures of food. Another encouragement to overeat is provided by the snacks available on most social occasions; these and alcohol add extra calories to the regular daily diet. People also overeat for emotional reasons, and the fatter they become, the more distressed, and perhaps lonely, they become. It becomes a vicious circle as they seek to relieve their stress, anxiety, or depression by eating even more. The young girl or woman who has to wear clothing designed for older adults in order to get the size she needs has even further cause for depression. Fashionable clothing to fit the obese person generally is difficult to find and is more costly than clothes designed for people of normal weight.

Losing Weight

Since obesity is a major health problem, it is the focus of numerous books, fad reducing plans and diets, and often dangerous reducing gimmicks aimed at obese people who have "tried everything" without success. The person who is really determined to lose weight must be ready to change his attitudes and habits; he must establish a specific weight loss goal and stick to it. Any major weight loss program should be supervised by a health professional, who will usually provide a diet plan appropriate to the specific person. It will probably be necessary to count calories as part of the program.

Recommendations for weight reduction dieting usually include eating at regular times and in the same places and following the basic four daily food guide (see page 35). It is not wise to try to lose more than 1½–2 pounds (680.4–907.2 grams) a week, unless otherwise directed and supervised by a health professional. To lose a pound a week, a person needs to reduce his ideal calorie intake by 500 calories a day (3,500 calories a week). Remember that a pound of body fat equals 3,500 calories. Information regarding the calorie value of foods is available from many sources, for example, from health professionals and the local American Red Cross chapter nursing office.

Knowledge of the following characteristics of low- and high-calorie foods may be helpful in dieting:

- Low-calorie foods tend to be—

  Thin, watery, or watery-crisp, such as apples, carrots, citrus fruits, and other fruits and vegetables

  Coarse, with a lot of fiber, such as celery, other greens, and whole-grain breads and cereals

  Puffed or airy, such as enriched cereals

  Bulky but not fat, such as fish, lean meat, and poultry

- High-calorie foods tend to be—

  Thick, oily, or greasy-crisp, such as fried chicken, french fries, and potato chips

  Smooth, thick, and slick, such as milkshakes, sauces, and gravies

  Compact or concentrated, such as jam or stuffings for poultry

  Sweet or sticky, such as candy, cakes, pies, cookies, syrups, and carbonated beverages

Some people do well at sticking to a diet plan by themselves; others do much better if there is a sense of companionship or competition with others. In most communities, there are usually several groups of persons devoted to helping people lose weight. They can be located by asking the health professional or health department or by checking with friends or neighbors.

SUICIDE

Suicide ranks as the second most common cause of death among teenagers, and the rate is increasing. Many more persons, at one time or another, contemplate suicide as a way of coping with frustration and personal problems than actually attempt it. Suicide is more common in males than in females, although the proportion of female suicides has increased. People who have had suicide in their families are more likely to commit suicide than those in whose families no suicides have occurred. Suicide is an increasing threat in the community.

To meet the threat of suicide, individuals and families must know what sort of events may trigger a suicide attempt, what signs of psychological disturbance may lead to suicide, and what guidelines are suggested by health professionals on how to communicate and act with someone who seems suicidal.

Before a suicide attempt, there is usually (but not always) a triggering event, such as a serious crisis involving discipline, punishment that the person considers unfair, jealousy in love, loss of a parent, spouse, or lover by divorce or death, or pregnancy out of wedlock. Suicidal attempts almost always occur when the person feels extremely lonely—isolated by emotional, or even physical, pain.

Signs of severe psychological disturbance leading to suicide are often difficult to separate from typical adolescent expressions of rebellion or from other less severe forms of emotional distress that may occur during a lifetime. Some obvious signs of serious suicidal thoughts are the purchase and hiding of a rope or a gun or other weapon, the giving away of prized possessions, and the disappearance of poisonous drugs. Often the clues are much more subtle, generally involving the three H's: haplessness, helplessness, and hopelessness. People with suicidal tendencies may have a hapless quality: one thing after another seems to go wrong. The person overreacts in a negative and helpless way, failing to see how to get up energy and initiative to get back on track: ("There's nothing that I can do—I'm depressed."). When the feeling of helplessness turns into the last stage of hopelessness ("No one understands me or can help me."), the risk of suicide becomes very high.

The following suggested guidelines for an approach to someone who seems suicidal are adapted, with permission, from *Family Health/Today's Health* magazine, April 1977, ©, all rights reserved:

- Take any threat of suicide seriously, especially if the person has made a previous attempt. It is far better to take a threat seriously and be wrong than to ignore it. Dismissing the threat, or responding with a flip remark such as "Go ahead and try it," may be regarded as a challenge–one that the suicidal person is apt to accept.

- Broach the subject of suicide yourself, at an appropriate time if necessary. Such interest is not harmful. It will be welcomed by a person who is seriously contemplating suicide. He will be grateful for your insight and concern.
- Encourage the person to talk openly and at length. Once he begins, listen and try to fully understand the feelings that underlie the words. Let the person know that you care by asking probing questions. A mere show of sympathy, no matter how well meant, is never enough for someone sorely in need of comfort and attention.
- Don't get involved in life-versus-death arguments. Since your goal is to restore the person's feelings of personal worth and dignity, you should insist that the person concentrate on living. Discuss the effect that the person's suicide would have on surviving family members and friends and stress that everything possible should be done to save the suicidal person's life.
- Act. You must give the impression that you know what you are doing and are taking charge. Make plans for future outings and engagements, for instance, or simply schedule regular telephone calls and visits.
- Seek professional help for the person as soon as possible. Keep in mind that the more definite the plans for suicide, the more acute the problem. Never assume that the crisis is over simply because the person says it is. In a matter of moments, a person on the verge of taking his own life can decide to go through with it. Therefore, arrange for a trusted friend or close relative to stay with the person until you are reassured by a professional that the crucial period has, indeed, passed.

Check the local telephone directory for "hot line" or suicide prevention centers. There are over 2,000 hot lines for suicide prevention in the United States.

Chapter 10

Death and Dying

Willingness to talk about death and dying has grown in the last several years. People have often been uncomfortable with this subject and have considered any talk of death and dying as morbid or abnormal. Several new trends, including caring for the dying at home rather than in an institution and deciding to forego heroic measures to sustain life when there is no hope of recovery, have made people more willing to think about and talk about death. It is now felt that death, which is an inevitable fact of life, should be discussed openly and honestly, that children should not be overprotected from the reality of death, and that persons who may be grieving or who may be thinking ahead to their own deaths should be able to share their feelings with others.

Open and honest discussion about death and grief is important to a person's healthy development from childhood on. Cultural factors, religious belief, and personal life-style will influence each person's attitude toward death; death means something different to each person. Since people tend to live longer now, it can happen that a person can lose a child, spouse, or close friend without ever having faced death earlier through the loss of a parent or older person. If death is accepted as one aspect of living and can be talked about freely, it is easier both to accept one's own death and to care for others who may be dying or grieving.

Few, if any, books in the health field have treated the subject of death in the past. Even the 1963 edition of the American Red Cross *Home Nursing Textbook,* which was a comprehensive home care guide, carried no information about death or the emotional and other factors involved in facing death. Changes in society, however, have led to a need to talk about death and dying and their effect on human behavior.

The purpose of this chapter is to give increased awareness and understanding of death and dying, especially for those who live with or are caring for persons who are facing their own or another's death. The stage-by-stage development of the individual's knowledge and acceptance of death as a fact of life is treated, as well as common reactions to death. Information is also given on hospices, which provide care for the dying patient, and on procedures and options for family and friends after a death has occurred.

THE INDIVIDUAL'S GROWING UNDERSTANDING OF DEATH

The ability to understand death and to finally accept its reality varies with the individual's level of maturity, basic personality, life experiences, and patterns of communication and support. A person who is slow in learning will usually also be slow in grasping the reality of death. Death is not an easily understood concept. The intense grief that usually follows the loss of a person whom one loves and needs often lasts a year or more. A period of grief is necessary while one makes the adjustment to a changed way of life. Experts in thanatology (the study of death and dying) feel that grief is not a sign of weakness but a normal human reaction to separation from a loved person. A person who understands his own responses and his own right to grieve is better able to understand what others are going through.

The Child

Many life experiences provide opportunities to talk with children about death. Death forces its way into a child's world in many ways. The death of a pet, or even of a flower, can be used to help the child develop his thoughts and attitudes on death before he experiences the death of a person.

In general, children go through three stages of development in their thoughts about death. A child under the age of 5 can understand that death means separation but may think of it as being like sleep; he is curious about what happens to the body. Between the ages of 5 and 9, the child begins to understand that death is final, but he does not yet understand that all persons will die sometime—he may think that only unlucky people die. The final stage of the child's understanding of death comes when he realizes that death is final and that everyone will die eventually.

In talking with a child about death, it is wise to limit oneself to answering the child's specific questions in terms that he is able to understand and ready to hear. He should not be told anything untrue—for example, that a dead person is asleep or gone on a trip—because the child may develop a fear of these normal life activities. (One's religious belief will also help determine the approach to explanations of death.)

The death of a pet is often a good opportunity for helping a child understand death and the emotions that people feel on the occasion of death. The child's thoughts may run from denial ("The pet will wake up again.") to guilt ("I should have taken better care of him.") to sadness ("I miss him.") to anger ("Why did he leave me?") and perhaps to asking for a replacement ("Can I get a new one?"). The child will be interested, too, in the disposal of the body; parents can explain burial to him.

Sometimes a child will act out a death in play, perhaps by covering a doll and laying it aside or by trying to bury it. These experiences will give parents an idea of how the child is thinking and some clue as to how he might react to the death of a loved human being. However, in many cases, the child's understanding of death will not be known by his parents, and his thinking may change continuously as he grows.

When a loved person dies, a child may feel angry, hurt, deserted, fearful of being left alone, or even guilty. The child may believe that something he did caused the death. Careful, honest explanations will do much to help the child who may not be able to express this sense of guilt. Like an adult, the child may not show his real thoughts and feelings. He may express joy or relief when he actually feels anger, hurt, or guilt. At such a time the child needs extra cuddling and touching and demonstrations of calm and sincere affection.

When a loved person dies, a child may feel angry, hurt, deserted, fearful of being left alone, or even guilty. The child may believe that something he did caused the death. Careful, honest explanations will do much to help the child who may not be able to express this sense of guilt. Like an adult, the child may not show his real thoughts and feelings. He may express joy or relief when he actually feels anger, hurt, or guilt. At such a time, the child needs extra cuddling and touching and demonstrations of calm and sincere affection.

Adolescents and Young Adults

As a person grows into adolescence and has more ability for abstract thinking, he is more able to understand death. Personal values and social conditions affect his thoughts about death. When a youth has known only discrimination, economic insecurity, inner-city violence, and unemployment, he might think an early and violent death is natural. Where violence is prevalent in a society or where a war exists, an adolescent might think life is of little value. In wartime, deaths of young men are a common occurrence. Some young men disregard the danger, while others may feel very strongly that they do not want to chance being killed.

Middle-Aged Persons

The person of middle age will be influenced in his thinking about death by the experiences he has had with death. If it should happen that he has not already lost a parent or a relative through death, he is apt to be especially stunned by the death of his spouse or child. In the middle-age range, death becomes more common; a person in his forties is twice as likely to die as one in his thirties, and the risk will double again in the fifties. The person in middle age finds himself forced to think about his own readiness and preparations for death, and he will want to be sure that his will is current and that his children will be provided for.

The loss of a parent is a time of special stress for the middle-aged person. Society seems to dictate that the middle-aged person who loses a parent should not display much grief, since the parent was getting older and his or her "time had come." The person who loses a parent with whom he has had a special relationship for many years may be facing the biggest loss he has ever experienced. The parent's age does not necessarily make the grief less painful.

The Older Adult

An older person has many practical reasons for thinking about death. Not only is he feeling the effects of aging on his body but he is also beginning to realize that old age is a time when his chances of dying have greatly increased. When a spouse dies, a major change is brought about in the surviving spouse's life; suddenly the person is facing life alone. About half of the women over age 65 are widows; by age 75, two thirds will be widowed. One man in six over the age of 65 is widowed. The longer a person lives, the more of his friends and relatives will have died. With each death, there is more sense of loss and being alone. Sometimes this grief is more than the person can tolerate, and loss of appetite, difficulty in sleeping, and other physical problems may be a direct result.

The older person is often discouraged from talking about death, since younger persons may have little patience with him and may feel that he is being morbid. Older persons may have a justifiable fear of dying among strangers, since members of their families often live far away. Although most older persons do not want to be a burden on others, neither do they want to be alone, and nowadays, even though the trend is changing, most people still die in a hospital or other institution.

If the older person is able to talk more freely about his fears, his mind is eased, and he is more free to think of living rather than dying; also, those with whom he talks are made more aware of their own attitudes toward death and dying.

WHEN SOMEONE IS DYING

Death is a parting; although it is a physical process, it has very important emotional and social aspects. When possible, there should be a "leave-taking," in which the dying person and those whom he is leaving recognize what is happening and try to be open about its meaning for each of them.

The course of dying is a very individual process. Death may be rapid or it may be slow. The individual and those near to him may be ready to accept death, or they may fight hard against the realization that it is coming. When a person is dying from an illness (such as cancer) that causes gradually increasing weakness and pain, the experience is often traumatic, both for the dying person and for the family. The dying person may feel hopelessness and despair, along with a great fear of the unknown. Normal family routines will be disrupted while the family cares for the dying person and tries to cope with feelings of helplessness and impending loss. It may be even more traumatic if the dying person is the family breadwinner.

Common Responses

There are several common emotional responses that dying persons and their families often experience. Although not everyone may experience them, awareness of these responses will help persons to cope with them when they do exist.

- *Denial*—The dying person or those around him may refuse to think about or discuss the possibility of death, acting as if death does not exist.
- *Anger*—The dying person may be angry that he is dying while those around him will go on living; he wants to know, "Why me?" Or those close to the dying person may be angry at him for leaving them.

- *Bargaining*—The "bargaining" reaction is a very private and personal one in which the dying person or those around him make promises to God or "fate" to do something special or to change their lives if only the dying person can be allowed to live longer.
- *Depression*—The dying person or those around him may be unable to perform even the simplest tasks because of being weighed down with sadness.
- *Acceptance*—The dying person, as well as those around him, begins to accept the fact that death will occur. He begins to take care of any unfinished business and to feel more ready for death. However, this acceptance does not mean resignation, which is a passive and unexamined response to death.

Death of a Child

The death of a child is a tragic reversal of the expected life pattern. The child is often not told of the possibility that he may die, but he may sense it anyway and may want to talk about how he feels. He may even feel that he has somehow caused his own illness. The seriously ill child of 5 or 6 may ask, "Am I dying?" more as an expression of his feeling of sickness than an active realization. Answers to such a question should be honest but might be limited to a discussion of the sickness itself. The hospitalized child tends to be aware of his parents' discomfort and feels their absence keenly; he needs to be reassured that people care and that he will not be left alone.

The slow dying of a child places great demands on the parents and others who care for the child. They must deal not only with their own feelings and needs but also those of the child. If there are other children in the family, the parents will be torn between giving support to the dying child and caring for the other children. Deciding how totally they can dedicate themselves to the dying child is a difficult decision.

Death of a Teenager

The teenager whose dying is a slow, lingering process should be helped to live as fully as possible until actual death. He often has talents and abilities that he can direct toward helping others and would receive great satisfaction from doing so. To the extent possible, he should have the chance to participate in his usual activities, in decisions about his own care and about his final days of life. His reactions to the approaching death will be greatly influenced by the attitudes toward death that he has been forming since childhood. The dying teenager, who has still not fully found his own identity, is often frustrated and ashamed that his body will no longer perform. Death at this age is not expected or easily accepted, and adults will feel the loss acutely, since the young person was just coming into one of the most rewarding phases of life.

Death of a Middle-Aged Person

The middle-aged person often has great responsibilities within his family, his profession, and perhaps his church and community. He has many close relationships, with spouse, children, parents, friends, and coworkers. His children may be in college. His death brings many and varied responses. A very common first response to the death of a middle-aged person is concern for the welfare of the surviving spouse—husband or wife—and dependent children.

Death of an Older Adult

Most people view the death of an older adult as less traumatic than the death of persons in any other age group. This opinion is held partially because death is expected with advanced age and partially because older persons who have already lost spouses and friends through death, and who may be ill or less able to function or to care for themselves, often seem more ready to die. The older adult usually has fewer people depending upon him and has less family and social responsibility. Sometimes continuing to live would be more difficult than dying. Regardless of the realities, the living must be helped to live as long as there is life, and the older person must receive all consideration and must be treated with dignity.

CARING FOR THE DYING PATIENT

Caring for the dying person requires skill and sensitivity. As in caring for any patient, both physical and psychological needs must be met. Whether the person is cared for at home, in a hospital or other institution, or in a special center (hospice) that provides care for the dying, the patient will need a comfortable environment, medication to alleviate pain, some physical exercise, and nutritious food to sustain his energy. Just as important, he needs understanding, concern, support, and reassurance that he is loved. He wants his family to share his burden, and both the dying person and his family may profit greatly from the counsel of either a clergyman or specially trained health professionals, or both.

The challenge of those who care for the dying person is to increase his sense of security through the presence of his family, continuous care, spirtual help if desired, and other signs of sympathy and understanding, and to decrease his fear of being abandoned as death approaches. Many articles and books have been written in the last few years whose overall purpose is to help the dying person cope with his feelings during his remaining days. Also, courses and seminars on dying are becoming more widely available. Family members who are well informed and who can meet the needs of the dying person with compassion will experience less guilt and have a feeling of satisfaction that they have done their best for their loved one.

When there is no reasonable expectation of recovery, the dying person may choose to die in dignity without heroic measures such as continuous administration of oxygen and intravenous feeding. Such a person may prefer to die without special life-saving devices or machines, at home, in the hospital, or in a hospice.

HOSPICES

The term "hospice" once referred to a house or shelter, usually kept by a religious order, that provided rest for pilgrims and strangers. Today, however, it refers to a special kind of care for the dying or the terminally ill. The hospice concept of care is to make the patient physically and mentally as comfortable as possible, with dignity and as much joy as possible. Hospice care may be given in a regular hospital, in a special hospice care facility, or in the patient's home. The hospice care setting is a homelike setting, with care being given by specially trained professionals who know how to control pain without using special lifesaving measures.

The hospice's professional team includes doctors, nurses, sociologists, psychologists, and clergymen, whose goals are to make the dying patient's life more comfortable and to counsel the patient's family on the acceptance of death. The family and friends of the patient are encouraged to be with him as he approaches death. Everyone around him is committed to his care; people listen to him, try to meet his spiritual needs, and help to allay his fear of dying.

For further information on hospices, see the Appendix for the address of the National Hospice Organization.

OTHER MATTERS RELATED TO DEATH

There are several matters a person may wish to consider long before death is expected to occur, such as whether he wishes to have special efforts made to prolong life when death is certain, whether he would like to donate organs such as the eyes or kidneys to those who have need of them, and whether he would prefer that his body be buried, cremated, or perhaps even donated to a medical school for use in research and teaching. A burial plot, if desired, can be purchased years before the need is expected to arise. A funeral home, a specific casket type, and the type of memorial services preferred can also be planned in advance. The person who plans these things in advance of his death can be sure to have his wishes followed, can save money through careful planning, can spare his family the burden of making such decisions during a time of grief, and can ease his own and his family's minds by insuring that everything is taken care of. All concerned are freer to think about the dying person's personal and emotional needs without excessive worry about details to be taken care of once the person has died.

In some states it is now legal to sign a "living will," wherein an individual requests that he be allowed to die without such special life-preserving measures as intravenous feeding and continuous oxygen when it is obvious that there is no reasonable expectation of recovery. Models of such a will and further information are available from the Euthanasia Education Council (see Appendix for address).

A person who wishes to donate his organs and tissues for transplantation can contact the National Kidney Foundation, the American Kidney Fund, or the Living Bank (see Appendix for addresses) or regional Eye Banks. Many hospitals supply "uniform donor cards," which make matters even simpler; if organs are to be removed in usable form, it is essential that they be removed very soon after death. Some states will now put a statement on drivers' licenses to the effect that the person's organs are available for transplant.

A body usually cannot be bequeathed to a medical school without the consent of the family. Donating the body may not be feasible if the medical school is far away or if the school does not have a need for such donations.

If cremation (a process that transforms the remains, by a process of heat and evaporation, into ashes that can be placed in a small container) is desired, be sure to select a funeral director who has the proper facilities.

Information on simple and dignified funeral arrangements is available from memorial societies; reputable ones are members of the Continental Association of Funeral and Memorial Societies (see Appendix for address).

If death occurs at home, the physician who has been caring for the patient should be notified. Regardless of where death occurs, the law requires that a physician sign a death certificate before the body can be prepared for disposition. If the cause of death is not certain, the family may request an autopsy (a nondisfiguring examination of the body to determine the cause of death). Knowing the cause of death brings some comfort to the family and also increases the knowledge of the medical profession and contributes to medical science. The community ambulance service or police should be notified so that arrangements can be made to transport the body.

Families and friends need a time in which to gather to express support for each other in their grief. If an actual funeral service is not held, a memorial gathering would be a good substitute.

Chapter 11

Illness: What It Means and How To Recognize It

An understanding of illness and its impact on both the patient and the family will make those who care for the patient more confident and will improve the quality of their care. Knowing common signs of illness will help them—particularly in knowing what, when, and how to report to the health professional.

Throughout this text, emphasis is placed on the fact that every person is an individual, unique in physical growth and development and having special needs and abilities. A person's response to his illness is also unique. It is usually similar to his response to other kinds of stress that affect his level of wellness (a person's ability to function at his fullest capacity in a given environment).

Since the entire person functions together, physical illness can also affect a person's emotional and psychological health. The home nurse should be aware of the patient's emotional state as well as his physical state.

THE MEANING OF ILLNESS

Illness is often described as the opposite of health. It is even more useful to think of illness in terms of levels of wellness: illness is the degree to which a person is unable to function at his usual level or at his fullest capacity within a certain environment. For example, a person with a broken arm might be able to perform in a singing group as well as usual, but his inability to use a typewriter could be a major handicap in his environment.

Illness may be either general or specific in nature. It may be evident only to the ill person or it may be recognized by others. The ill person may experience loss of energy, pain, blurred vision, and other similar feelings, but until these symptoms cause a change in his behavior or appearance, they cannot be observed by others. Even then, only the changes can be observed, not the actual symptoms.

An individual responds to signs of illness within himself in many ways. He may either pretend that the signs are not present, exaggerate the symptoms, or take reasonable steps to evaluate the situation and to restore health. His perception of his responsibility to himself and to others is a very important factor in his response. The responses of those around him also influence what he does about the signs of illness.

Illness rarely occurs at a time considered convenient in terms of family life, work, or money. (Nonemergency or, "elective," surgery such as the cosmetic kind is one of the few aspects of health care that can be scheduled to cause the least disruption in a person's life.) The ill person tends to have guilt feelings about causing extra demands on his family or others or about not being able to fulfill his work responsibilities. He is also concerned about the cost—both the financial cost of health care and the possible loss of income and the energy cost of catching up in class or at work. All of these factors may make the ill person less likely to admit to being ill or more likely to start back to usual activities before he is actually ready. The impact of this kind of worry may be decreased by an understanding attitude on the part of others, along with efforts to make the adjustments as easy as possible for the recovering person.

HOW TO OBSERVE SIGNS AND SYMPTOMS OF ILLNESS

Signs or symptoms of illness are deviations from what is considered normal for the person. In observing such deviations, obviously it is important to know what is considered usual appearance and behavior for most persons of a given age and similar characteristics. An infant, for example, might usually have three or four soft bowel movements a day. It is equally important to know the usual appearance and behavior of an individual. Some people might have a flushed appearance all the time, while others might usually be pale; a usually pale person who has a bright red face or cheeks might have a fever, might have overexerted himself, or might simply have been out in the fresh air for a change.

The terms "signs" and "symptoms" are often used as if they mean the same thing. However, signs are changes from the usual way that a person looks or acts or a change in vital signs (blood pressure, temperature, or respiration). Symptoms are changes from the usual way that a person feels. The skilled observer will notice such signs of illness as drooping or puffiness of eyelids, a change in the sound of a cough, or uncommon irritability, restlessness, or depression. A sudden change in personality may also be a sign of a serious health problem. Identifying the symptoms of illness requires knowledge and practice.

Since babies and small children are not able to describe their feelings, those responsible for their well-being must learn to recognize the location of pain in children by their behavior. A baby or small child may keep putting his hand on the part of his body that hurts.

Or if there is pain in his abdomen, he may pull his knees up to his chest. A mother learns to suspect illness when her baby cries too much or when her toddler whines and loses interest in his toys.

The observer must be cautious in the process of observation. A child or adult who knows that his condition is being carefully watched might exaggerate every little ache or pain, or he might try to hide it. Usually the sick person does not intend to mislead. He may be unconsciously seeking special attention, trying to deny the presence of a problem, or trying to save others trouble. If possible, signs of illness should be observed without the person's knowledge and without too much obvious concern, to avoid arousing the person's interest or anxiety.

Observation alone may not be sufficient to diagnose illness. Many symptoms of illness can be detected only by scientific laboratory procedures. Even laboratory tests do not always provide enough facts for the health professional to make a definite diagnosis; therefore, the results of such tests must be studied along with the sick person's description of his pain or discomfort, the observations and judgments of those who know him, and a history of past illnesses. In making a diagnosis, the health professional may depend as much on

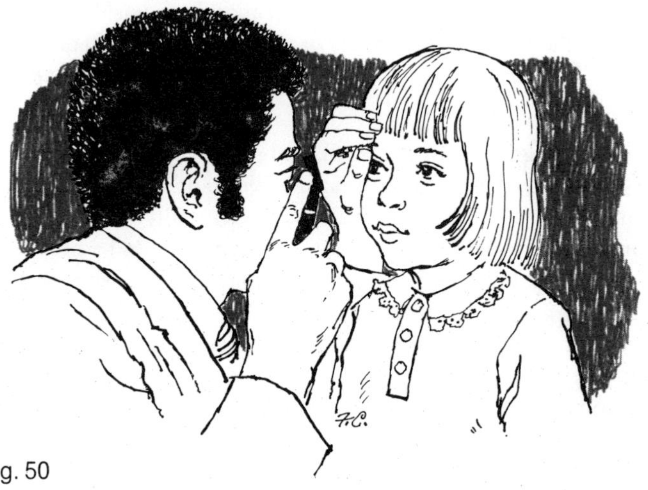

Fig. 50

the absence of certain signs as on the presence of others. For all of these reasons, careful observation and recording of symptoms by the parent or home nurse are important responsibilities.

Early detection of disease is important. Frequently, the earlier the symptoms are noticed and the sooner the person receives good medical care, the more rapid will be the patient's recovery. In the case of communicable disease, prompt treatment reduces the chance of complications such as pneumonia, inner-ear infections, and heart damage; it may also decrease the likelihood of the disease's being spread from one person to another. In the case of chronic (long-lasting) diseases and degenerative diseases (those that reduce the body's functions), it is important to begin treatment before there is severe damage to any body organ and before the person's general health is badly impaired. Most forms of cancer begin in just one part of the body and can be treated successfully if detected and treated *early,* before cancer cells spread to other parts of the body.

HOW TO EVALUATE SIGNS AND SYMPTOMS OF ILLNESS

Once a sign of illness has been observed, it must be evaluated. The experienced home nurse who knows what to observe and what questions to ask to pinpoint the nature of the illness must decide what steps need to be taken and how quickly. First aid or home care procedures such as bed rest, increased fluid intake, or cold or hot compresses may be adequate, or immediate advice from a health professional may be needed. Sometimes it may be advisable to wait and observe the symptoms for a day or two before deciding on a course of action. Whenever there is great doubt, the advice of a health professional should be obtained.

Having a regular source of health care assures the availability of professional advice regarding treatment for colds and other minor ailments, as well as for major illnesses. Generally, the health professional gives guidelines as to what symptoms should be present and as to how long before he should be notified. The health professional may also give suggestions as to the kind of treatment that may be given for common ailments. Such guidelines and suggestions prevent overuse of the health professional's time and allow the parent or the home nurse to be more independent and self-reliant.

Evaluation of symptoms and decisions about actions to be taken are influenced by knowledge of an individual's personality and the manner in which the person reacts to stress. Different persons can tolerate different amounts of pain. A person's mood, his desire to avoid responsibility, or his need for companionship may cause him to complain or to exaggerate symptoms. An adult who is bored or lonely may complain of something a busy person would never notice. A child who wants attention may exaggerate or even imagine symptoms. On the other hand, persons who want badly to engage in previously planned or regular activities may deny their symptoms or say the symptoms are insignificant or not worthy of attention. In addition, some persons may be fearful of a particular diagnosis because their knowledge of the kinds and effectiveness of modern treatments is inadequate; thus they avoid the truth.

In an emergency, there is need for immediate assistance. Emergencies include–

Acute chest pain

New and acute abdominal pain

Broken bones

Profusely bleeding wounds

Extensive burns

Swallowing of poisonous substances

Loss of consciousness that is not relieved within 3 minutes after the individual has been placed flat on his back

First aid for these problems is discussed in chapter 14. The fire department, the police, the volunteer ambulance service, and the local poison control center are all sources of assistance in these kinds of emergencies. Every household should have a list of emergency telephone numbers in a handy place.

WHAT SIGNS TO REPORT TO THE HEALTH PROFESSIONAL

In most cases, the decision to call for medical advice is brought about by a combination of symptoms. In reporting symptoms to the health professional, you should describe the character of the illness, the complaints of the sick person, any first aid or treatment given, and the observations made by the home nurse, the parents, or others with regard to the following signs and symptoms:

- The degree of severity, the duration, and the location of any pain and how the pain is affected by eating or by a change in body position. The pain may be a dull ache or it may be acute, shooting, or stabbing. It may be constant or intermittent.
- The temperature, the pulse, and the respiration rate (see chapter 18).

- The location, color, and amount of any bleeding.
- The character and color of the bowel movement, the material vomited, and sputum, urine, or other body discharges. If a discharge is unusual in appearance, a sample should be saved in a covered container for the health professional to examine. (The container can be a small jar or plastic box with a lid. Any container used will be thrown away.)
- The patient's behavior, his mood (for example, irritability, listlessness), how he says he feels, and the length of time during which any unusual condition has been noticed.
- Any other unusual condition noted, such as a rash, discoloration of the skin, or swelling of any part of the body.

SIGNS AND SYMPTOMS OF ILLNESS

Parents and home nurses should be alert for signs of illness and should record their observations. Important signs of illness are described below, *not* in order of their frequency or importance. The severity of a symptom is not a true guide to its importance, because a mild symptom may precede a serious illness. Parents and home nurses should remember that they observe only the outward change. This change may not tell the whole story or take into account the individual's unique response to his symptoms.

A change that may indicate illness can be a change in appearance or in activity. Changes in general appearance may be observed in the face, eyes, hair, nails, skin, posture, or weight. If the person has a runny nose or a hoarse voice or is sneezing or coughing, the home nurse should ask questions about other possible symptoms such as a sore throat. Complaints of sore throat, difficulty in seeing, headache, dizziness, pain, fatigue, or other unusual sensations in any part of the body could be symptoms of illness.

General Appearance

The appearance of the patient's *face* often gives a clue to the nature of his illness and to how much he is actually suffering. In illness, the facial expression may be drawn and haggard, alert and anxious, or dull and listless. The face may appear swollen or puffy about the eyes, or it may be flushed or pale.

The *eyes* may be watery, glassy in appearance, dull and listless or unusually bright, or unusually sensitive to light. The white part of the eye may be bloodshot, yellow, or have a yellowish tinge. The eyelids may seem heavy, or the area around the eye may appear puffy or inflamed. Because disturbance of vision characterizes some diseases, the home nurse should be alert to complaints of spots before the eyes, halos around lights, seeing double, or not being able to see clearly. All of these signs should be brought to the health professional's attention.

Dull, limp *hair* with broken ends may indicate poor health or poor health practices. Extreme brittleness or discoloration of the nails can also be a sign of a low level of wellness.

Other Conditions

Running nose, sneezing, coughing, hoarseness, difficulty in breathing, and sore throat are all symptoms of the common cold. They could also mean the onset of more serious illness. When these symptoms persist and are accompanied by fever, it is a matter of concern.

Sore throat is one sign of many disease conditions, including the common cold and many communicable diseases. Throat conditions that should be reported to the health professional immediately include severe sore throat, painful throat conditions that persist and are accompanied by fever, a throat that shows yellow or grayish patches on the inside or is red and spotted, and a throat that is raw and bleeding inside. The most common type of sore throat is caused by an infection and is characterized by an inflamed, raw throat with or without whitish patches. Abscessed or infected tonsils usually cause pain and difficulty in swallowing.

It is wise to know how to inspect the throat quickly and skillfully. A good practice for parents is to accustom their children to throat inspection when the children are well so that they will accept the throat inspection when they are ill. This practice also allows the parent to know what the child's throat normally looks like. (See "Throat Inspection," chapter 18.)

Any person with a sore throat should keep away from others, go to bed if he has a fever or any patches in the throat, drink plenty of fluids, eat a light or soft diet, and get plenty of rest. His toilet articles and dishes should be kept separate from those of others until the possibility of communicable disease has been ruled out.

Voice

The voice is often changed in sickness; it may be hoarse, weak, or reduced to a whisper. In extreme weakness, speech may be difficult.

Take note of any unusual moaning, groaning, or crying. Persistent huskiness or a change in the tone of the voice may be a symptom of serious illness.

Skin

The skin acts as a protective covering for the body and a barrier against disease. Breaks in the skin may allow the entrance of bacteria and therefore should receive first aid and care to insure cleanliness of the area. Rashes and other eruptions may be signs of allergic response or of disease. Eruptions that persist should be brought to the attention of the health professional. Coloring of the skin (pale, red, yellowish, bluish), its oiliness, dryness, or moistness (clamminess) are also clues to the person's level of wellness.

Swellings

Swellings of fingers, wrists, or ankles may indicate a serious condition and should be reported to a health professional.

Posture

Posture, the way in which an individual carries his body, often reflects such emotions as anxiety, anger, or dejection. Changes in posture—droopiness or increased tension in the legs, arms, or body—may be symptoms of serious illness.

Weight Gain or Loss

Unusual gain or loss of weight in a short period of time that is not the result of a weight control program may indicate serious illness. Such a change may be caused by disease, improper functioning of the internal organs, emotional tension, or the wrong kind or insufficient amounts of food. (See chapter 2 for discussion of good diet.) Because most people lose weight in a severe illness, it is especially important that nourishing foods be provided for the ill person. Such foods protect the body from too great a weight loss, help maintain normal functions, and promote healing. (See chapter 2 for more information.)

Sensations

Sensations of the skin and body can indicate illness. Persons with fever often notice a feeling of chilliness or a special sensitivity or a tingling of the skin. Strange sensations in any part of the body, or loss of feeling, should be reported *at once* to a health professional. Difficulty in controlling the movements of any part of the body is also significant and may be a symptom of stroke or other serious illness.

Headaches

Recurrent headaches may be signs of emotional tension, high blood pressure, response to poisonous substances in the air, or other significant conditions. Self-medication for headaches is often dangerous because it may cause the person to postpone seeking professional help needed to discover the cause. Also, the medicine itself (for example, common aspirin) can cause serious problems for some persons.

Dizziness

Dizziness is often related to blood pressure. It may occur when the blood pressure is elevated or when there is an abrupt change in posture such as standing up after lying down, or it may occur as a side effect of medication. Dizziness should always be reported to the health professional. If dizziness or fainting is the result of low blood pressure or abrupt posture change (causing a lack of oxygen supply to the brain), have a sitting person place his head between his knees, or have the person lie down and raise his legs on pillows or some other support.

Pain

Pain is always a sign that something is wrong, but it is not always a sign of a serious problem. Pain in the arms, legs, or back muscles may be due to unusual exercise. Different persons have different "pain thresholds." The person with a high pain threshold can tolerate more pain than a person with a lower threshold. Older persons are usually much less sensitive to pain than are younger people; therefore, when an elderly person complains of pain, the complaint has greater significance. A sudden, acute pain in the chest should be reported to the health professional at once. When any pain is being reported, the health professional will want to know the location and intensity of the pain, whether the pain is sharp, dull, or throbbing, when it began and whether it hurts some of the time or all of the time, whether a change of position helps, and whether it is worse or better after eating or when sleeping.

General Malaise

General malaise is a feeling of general body discomfort, weakness, fatigue, and listlessness. Malaise at the start of an infectious illness may be accompanied by headache, fever, or loss of appetite. The patient who has been in bed for some time experiences weakness, physical fatigue, and loss of muscle tone and strength caused by lack of exercise. It may take several days of gradually increased activity before the feeling of weakness and fatigue disappears. (See chapter 22 for more discussion.)

Menstruation

Women should be alert during menstruation for change in frequency of periods or in amount of flow and for the occurrence of unusual discomfort. Such symptoms should be reported to the health professional. Itching, pain, and discharges in the genital area are often signs of vaginal infections. Women who are being treated for these infections should ask the health professional if it is necessary for their sexual partners to receive treatment, since a symptomless infection may also be present in the male.

Temperature, Pulse, and Respiration

The individual's temperature, pulse rate, and rate of breathing are important indicators of illness. Every family should own a fever thermometer and know how to use it and care for it. Further information is in chapter 18.

American Red Cross chapters teach people how to take temperature, pulse rate, and respiration rate with a self-instruction workbook, *Vital Signs: Module I.*

The healthy human body maintains an internal temperature that varies only slightly with the time of day or the amount of physical exercise. The normal temperature is most likely to be lowest in the early morning hours (3:00 to 5:00 a.m.) and reaches its maximum in the late afternoon (4:00 to 7:00 p.m.). The low and high readings are generally within 1 degree Fahrenheit (.50 centigrade) of each other.

Age can influence the normal temperature. The normal temperature of infants and young children tends to be slightly higher than that of an adult. The normal temperature of older people is often slightly lower than that of younger adults. It may be helpful to keep a record of each individual's normal temperature so that deviations from the normal can be recognized when they occur.

Fever

Fever, a temperature higher than normal for a person, is a sign that something is out of order in the body, although a person may be ill without a rise in temperature. For many years, a change from the normal body temperature has been used by health professionals as a basis for judging whether a person is sick, for diagnosing and treating illness, and for noting the progress of the patient's recovery from illness. One of the first questions the health professional asks when consulted about someone's illness is, "What is his temperature?"

Temperature should be taken under the following circumstances:

- Whenever a person complains of feeling ill or shows signs of illness.
- Whenever there is headache, pain in the chest or abdomen, sore throat, chills, vomiting, diarrhea, or skin rash.
- During illness, once or twice a day, at the same time each day (usually in the morning and the evening). Temperature may be taken as often as every 4 hours or only once a week, depending on the condition and age of the patient.

Whenever there is a fever, check for other symptoms. If the temperature is over 99.6°F (37.6°C) orally, or over 100.6°F (38.1°C) rectally, and there are chills, stiff neck, marked pain (especially abdominal pain), or vomiting, seek medical advice. If the accompanying symptoms are more vague than those just mentioned, the patient requires extra fluids and rest and continued observation. Children often run higher fevers than adults, even though the cause may be minor and their temperature rises more rapidly. If the fever of a child reaches 101°F (38.3°C), or higher rectally, a health professional should be consulted even if the child does not seem very ill. If sponge baths are recommended to bring down the temperature, follow the procedures and cautions outlined in chapter 23.

Pulse

The pulse rate is the number of times the heart beats in a single minute. All persons have different pulse rates. Age and sex account for some of the wide variation. A child's pulse rate, for example, is faster than that of an adult. The pulse rate may also increase for such reasons as fever, exercise, eating, fright, emotional tension, dehydration, and extreme heat or cold. The pulse rate decreases when a person is resting or is asleep. The beat should always be regular, unless a health professional has said that an irregular beat is normal for a particular individual.

Respiration

The act of breathing may be affected by illness. The parent or home nurse should observe the *rate of respiration* (the act of moving air in and out of the lungs) and the degree of *difficulty in breathing* experienced by the individual. Breathing is more rapid with a fever or after exercise and is slower, deeper, and often irregular during sleep. Continual difficulty in breathing accompanied by a cough may be associated with chronic irritation due to smoking or air pollution or may indicate more serious conditions. Noisy, labored breathing, often accompanied by coughing, may occur during acute infection, may be an allergic response, or may be due to chronic lung disease. Shortness of breath when lying flat in bed, upon climbing stairs, or after other normal activity may be a sign of heart disease or other illness.

Patterns of Food Intake and Elimination of Wastes

Patterns of food and fluid intake influence health. Persons who are experiencing stress may occasionally develop enormous appetites or strong cravings for certain foods. Illness is often accompanied by loss of appetite or prolonged thirst. If a problem is suspected, keep a record of what the person is eating and how much. Since the amount and kind of fluid in the body influences fever and recovery, keep a record of water and other liquids taken by the ill person.

Pica (A Craving for Unnatural Food)

Pica, the desire to eat unusual things such as dirt, plaster, starch, paint chips, hair, or grass, is experienced by some children and, more rarely, by adults. The cause might be an emotional reaction, a social custom, or a special need of the body for something missing from the diet. In any event, pica is a fairly serious matter and should always be called to the attention of a health professional.

Abdominal Distress

Abdominal distress includes nausea and vomiting, heartburn, pain, and other problems or discomforts due to change in frequency or consistency of bowel movements. In some individuals, the cause of such discomforts could be certain foods. Milk is an example of a food that is soothing to many but may cause distress and discomfort to others. Nausea is a feeling of distaste at the thought of food, or an actual sensation that precedes vomiting. If nausea and vomiting are accompanied by severe cramps or abdominal pain, notify the health professional, because the patient may have appendicitis, bowel obstruction, or some other serious illness.

Pain in the stomach or abdomen may result from food poisoning, improper eating, appendicitis, or some other serious condition. Abdominal pain resulting from food poisoning is commonly accompanied by nausea, vomiting, and diarrhea. If abdominal pain is not relieved promptly by rest and withholding food, the patient should be seen by a health professional. Abdominal pain accompanies so many serious conditions that it should always be reported, and the patient should be carefully observed. *Do not give a laxative or an enema. Do not apply heat.*

Vomiting

If vomiting is caused by indigestion, tension, or mild food poisoning, the patient will often feel much better after vomiting has occurred. Support the patient's head during vomiting to prevent his falling or choking. Cool cloths on the forehead and the use of mouthwash may provide comfort after vomiting. Fluids may be taken if the person wants them and can retain them. Begin with water, tea, or carbonated beverages.

The amount, color, and general appearance of the vomitus (material vomited) should be observed. If vomiting is continuous, is severe, or is accompanied by blood, or if the material has a very offensive odor, report the condition at once to the health professional and save the vomitus for him to see. Blood in the vomitus may be either dark or bright red. In some cases, blood that looks like coffee grounds may appear in the vomitus and indicates bleeding in the stomach.

Diarrhea

Diarrhea is characterized by frequent bowel movements that are watery or slimy. Infection, poisonous or undigested food, and emotional strain are the most common causes. In babies and small children, diarrhea is often the result of improper feeding or of consuming contaminated water, milk, or other food. Sometimes it is caused by a disease process such as colitis or cancer, in which there is irritation of the mucous membranes. Careful attention to hygiene measures such as hand-washing help prevent the spread of infection. Widespread epidemics of diarrhea can be prevented by using good hygiene.

Diarrhea may have serious results because it exhausts the patient and dehydrates his body tissues. Severe or persistent diarrhea should be reported to the health professional. For children, particularly, even one day of diarrhea is serious and must be reported immediately. The individual experiencing diarrhea should be encouraged to increase his fluid intake.

Bowel Movement Changes

Changes in color, shape, or consistency of feces (stools, products of bowel movement) and changes in patterns of elimination should be noted. If stools are black-colored, tarry, or clay-colored, samples should be saved for possible testing in cases of abdominal distress or diarrhea. Measures to prevent constipation are discussed in chapter 2.

Urinary Disturbances

The following urinary disturbances are all critical danger signals:

Inability to urinate
Incontinency (inability to delay urination)
Urinating too frequently
Pain or burning sensation when urinating
The presence of blood in the urine

Note any change from the usual amber color of the urine (such as rust color or cloudy coloring with particles of sediment that settle to the bottom of a container after a period of time) and whether there is more or less urine than usual. Symptoms should be reported to the health professional.

MENTAL FUNCTIONING

The person who is mentally healthy is one who is awake and alert at appropriate times, who engages in conversation that makes sense in terms of the situation at hand, and who is capable of activity directed toward some constructive purpose. Generally, the person whose mental health is not disrupted can answer the following questions correctly:

What is your name? Where are you (we)?
What year, date, day of the week, and time of day is it now?

Undesirable Behavior

Undesirable behavior or mixed-up thinking may be a warning that something is wrong. Frequently occurring symptoms are anxiety, depression, brooding, inability to concentrate, sleeplessness, restlessness, and lack of interest in friends, family, job, or accustomed recreation. Other observable symptoms are obsessions or fixed ideas, physical complaints of an imaginary nature, undue sensitivity, reluctance to mingle with others or to go to new places, confusion as to one's identity or that of others in the family or as to one's surroundings, recurrent daydreams or hallucinations of an impossible nature, and resentment toward a person without apparent cause.

Side Effects of Illness or Medication, or Both

Some mental symptoms are temporary—they may accompany physical illness or may result from the use of certain medications. The mental condition of the patient who has a high fever or a severe infection of any kind should be carefully watched, because the very ill patient may become delirious (in a temporary state of mental excitement) or disoriented (not know who or where he is) and may try to get out of bed. The very ill patient who has become delirious or disoriented is not responsible for what he may do and should never be left alone. Elderly patients, especially, may become confused or disoriented because of medications (particularly sedative drugs) that they have been given. Any talk of suicide should be taken seriously, and the help of persons trained to handle such problems should be sought (see chapter 9).

Sleep

Sleep is nature's way of resting the body and mind and is essential both in sickness and in health. Some of the body changes that occur during sleep are not entirely understood, but sleep comes primarily as a result of lessened activity of the nervous system. Breathing slows down and may be irregular, heart action is slower and is accompanied by a lowering of the blood pressure, muscles relax, and the energy requirements of the body are lessened. The amount of sleep needed varies with age and the individual. An infant may sleep from 18 to 20 hours a day, children from 12 to 14 hours, adults from 7 to 9 hours, and old people perhaps no more than 5 hours at night because they take short naps during the day.

Pain or fever may disturb sleep. Emotional tension may make falling asleep difficult or may cause early awakening. A person who is in bed all the time may not need as much sleep as he does when he is up and about. Regular, light physical activity may help a person to sleep better by promoting fatigue or contributing to relaxation. The establishment of a nightly routine of pleasure-giving activities just before sleep may also be beneficial.

SYMPTOMS OF CANCER

The "Seven Warning Signs of Cancer" listed below are publicized by the American Cancer Society. Since the presence of any *one* of these symptoms could indicate the possible presence of cancer, the person who has such a symptom should seek the advice of a health professional.

1. *Change in bowel or bladder habits.* Many things cause changes in elimination habits—what the person eats or drinks, for example—but take action if the changes seem too extreme or last for any length of time.
2. *A sore that does not heal.* Although it may not be painful, the sore may signal an early, curable mouth or skin cancer, particularly if it lasts a long time.
3. *Unusual bleeding or discharge.* Never ignore this serious sign. See the health professional immediately.
4. *Thickening or lump in the breast or elsewhere.* Eight out of ten breast lumps are not cancer. If it is cancer and is found before it spreads, chances of cure are excellent.
5. *Persistent indigestion or loss of appetite.* Indigestion is a common complaint, but persistent indigestion, heartburn, nausea, or loss of appetite demands medical advice.
6. *Obvious change in a wart or mole.* Take action if a wart or mole gets bigger, blacker, or scaly.
7. *Nagging cough or hoarseness.* If such a symptom persists—especially if you smoke any form of tobacco—don't wait, make an appointment with a health professional.

Chapter 12

Common Illnesses

Most illnesses can be prevented—or at least the effect on the victim can be made much less severe—by the effort a person puts into promoting his own high level of physical well-being. Personal hygiene, rest, exercise, good nutrition, and keeping immunizations current do much to help the body fight off communicable and even some chronic diseases. Research and experimentation have resulted in new ways to prevent and cure many diseases and have caused changes in the treatment of persons with illness or infection.

Deaths due to communicable diseases have decreased markedly in the United States in the last 25 years. There is great concern, however, that because of the low incidence of childhood communicable diseases, families and most public and private agencies have neglected to take the critical step of keeping immunizations current for all persons, especially children. Serious outbreaks (epidemics) of such diseases can occur when large portions of the population are not properly protected by immunization.

This chapter gives information on the ways in which infections spread and on how to prevent spreading. Information is also given about the more common communicable and chronic diseases.

COMMUNICABLE DISEASES

Illnesses that spread from one person to another are called communicable (infectious) diseases. Germs (micro-organisms) that cause disease are spread from the body of one person (or animal) to another by a variety of methods. Infection begins when the germs enter the body and begin to reproduce. Usually it takes a large number of germs to produce the symptoms of a disease.

Germs that cause disease may enter the body directly, through contaminated water or foods, or by being breathed in with air containing germ-laden dust, or indirectly, through contact with material contaminated by body discharges. There may be disease germs in infected wounds and in the discharges of the nose, mouth, bowels, and sometimes the bladder. Milk that has not been pasteurized or boiled may transfer diseases like undulant fever or tuberculosis. In some diseases, the infection is carried in the bloodstream and may be transmitted by unsterilized needles or blood transfusions from an infected person. The bite of an infected insect such as a wood tick or dog tick may cause Rocky Mountain spotted fever. The bite of an infected animal may cause rabies.

Infection can also be transferred by a well person who, although he does not have symptoms of the disease himself, carries the disease-causing germ in his body. Such a human carrier may have had the disease at some time and recovered, or he may be suffering from such a mild case of the disease that the characteristic symptoms are not noticeable. The human carrier serves as a breeding place for the disease-causing germs, which take up temporary or permanent residence in his body but are harmless to him because his body defenses are able to keep them under control. The carrier poses a threat to the health of other persons who have no immunity and whose body defenses may be less able to ward off illness. Diseases most often carried in this way are diphtheria, scarlet fever, and typhoid fever.

The organisms thrive in a specific part of the body of the carrier or the ill person. The part of the body in which they thrive determines the symptoms of the disease and the way in which the disease is spread from one person to another. Examples are given below.

The germs of colds, influenza (flu), tuberculosis, and the so-called children's diseases (measles, whooping cough, chickenpox) live in the soft mucous membranes that line the nose, throat, and lungs. They leave the infected person's body and enter another person's body through the mouth and nose. Germs are in the droplets of moisture that spray out when a person talks, laughs, coughs, or sneezes. They are in the handkerchiefs or tissues the person uses to blow his nose; they may be on his hands, on things he has touched, or on things that have been in his mouth.

The germs of hepatitis A, typhoid fever, dysentery, and salmonellosis are found in the intestinal tract. They leave the body in the stool (bowel movement). These diseases spread when an infected person is careless about washing his hands after going to the toilet and then handles food that will be eaten by others. Water contaminated with stool may cause disease when it is used to wash food that is to be eaten raw. Flies may carry germs to food from uncovered sewage or unclean toilet areas.

The organisms causing venereal diseases such as syphilis and gonorrhea live in the mucous membranes of the genitals, anus, and mouth. These diseases are spread by sexual intercourse or other very close body contact.

Germs of hepatitis B live in the bloodstream. Sources of infection include transfusions of blood taken from infected persons and inadequately sterilized syringes and needles such as those used for ear piercing, injections, and tattooing.

Germs are present in infected wounds and in the skin eruptions or open sores that appear with some diseases such as impetigo, scabies, chicken pox, and one stage of syphilis. The infection can spread if any material from the rash or sore enters another person's body through a break in the skin.

Preventing the Spreading of Disease

Preventing the spreading of disease is an important contribution to public health. There are two major ways of carrying out such prevention: by protecting oneself and by isolating or destroying the germs. The first method, personal care aimed at protection, includes having a well-balanced diet, maintaining good personal hygiene, getting adequate rest and exercise, and not taking unnecessary risks (such as drinking unpasteurized dairy products or water that may be contaminated, or going unnecessarily to crowded places when many cases of flu or colds are known to exist). The second major way to prevent the spread of disease involves isolating carriers and germs, sanitizing objects exposed to germs, carefully disposing of contaminated items, and destroying germs.

The methods of preventing the spread of communicable diseases depend on how the disease leaves the body of the infected person and how it enters the body of another person. The following measures to prevent spreading of communicable disease are listed according to how the germs leave the body of the infected person.

When germs are in the nose and mouth—

- Keep the patient away from people who are likely to become ill from his disease.
- Encourage the patient to cover his mouth and nose with a tissue when he coughs or sneezes. Soiled tissues should be placed in a waste container lined with a plastic or paper bag.
- Dispose of soiled tissues by removing the plastic or paper bag lining the waste container, close the bag tightly, and discard it according to the advice of a health professional. Depending on the circumstances, the preferred method may be burning or burying, flushing down the toilet, or simply placing the tightly closed bag in the trashcan. Careful hand-washing should follow.

- Keep the towels, washcloths, toothbrushes, and soap of the patient in his room, away from those of other family members.
- Wash your hands before and after caring for the patient or handling soiled clothing or linen.
- Have the patient wash his hands often.
- Do not allow the sick person to prepare food for others.
- Immediately after removing dishes from the patient's room, wash them with soap, rinse them with hot water (boiling, if possible), and place them in a rack to dry. (Disposable dishes may be useful if they are available and can be afforded.)
- Air the room daily. Keep it as dust-free as possible.
- Occasionally, a health professional will advise you to use a mask to cover your nose and mouth. In that case, wear a fresh mask each time you enter the patient's room. Masks can be made or can be purchased from the drugstore. Check with a health professional.

When germs are in the stool (bowel movement)—

- Encourage the patient to wash his hands well, with warm water and soap, after he uses the toilet.
- Keep the patient's towels and washcloths in his room, away from those of others.
- Wash your hands before and after caring for the patient or handling soiled clothing or linen.
- Follow specific instructions of a health professional concerning the care of soiled linens and clothing, as well as the use of a protective gown or apron.
- If the water is not from a certified safe source (or when the water supply is disrupted in a disaster), boil water 20 minutes before using it for drinking, for ice, or for brushing teeth. Do not eat raw fruits and vegetables that have been watered or washed with contaminated water.

When germs are on the skin—

- Wash your hands thoroughly before and after caring for the patient or handling his soiled linen or clothing.
- If the infected area is covered with a dressing and the secretions soak through the dressing, add an additional layer to the dressing and allow a health professional to change the dressing. If instructions on how to change the dressing have been given, careful hand washing before and after the procedure is extremely important (see "Changing Dressings," chapter 23).

- Follow specific instructions of the health professional concerning the care of the infected area and the disposal of soiled dressings, linen, and clothing.
- If you have an infected hand, do not prepare food.
- If you have a break in your skin, such as a cut on the hand, avoid any contact with the patient's infected area, since your own cut could become infected.

Local news media usually serve the public by giving information about communicable diseases that are affecting people in a community. The public health department tries to control the spread of such diseases by warning people through the news media of precautions that should be taken. Persons needing more information can usually get it from their regular health professional, the health department, or sometimes from the health professionals in the schools.

A chart with detailed information about the communicable diseases most prevalent in the United States is in the Appendix. Some communicable diseases, such as colds, influenza, venereal disease, and food poisoning, occur frequently enough, particularly in childhood, to deserve the additional information presented below.

The Common Cold

The common cold is not a disease in the regular sense of the word "disease." It is, rather, a set of signs and symptoms affecting the respiratory system and may include such symptoms as runny nose, swelling of nose and throat passages, watery eyes, sore throat, general discomfort, and, sometimes, low fever. Infants may run high fevers, from 102° to 104°F (38.9°–40°C). Symptoms of a cold may be caused by a wide variety of microorganisms from virus to fungi. Even though the symptoms may be mild, as they often are, they sometimes lead to more serious diseases.

Because the common cold is not a specific disease and at the same time its symptoms are common to diseases, some of which can be serious, caution should be observed for both the patient and the home nurse. This is particularly true in the case of infants, young children, older adults, and persons with generally low levels of health. The most common and universally accepted treatment includes extra rest, increased fluid intake, and moderate eating. These steps help the body fight off the disease by improving circulation and by building up the body generally. Although aspirin and other pain relievers reduce fever when fever exists, it is not wise to use them unless advised to do so by the health professional, especially for the higher-risk groups mentioned. Antibiotics are considered to be of little value in relation to the cold symptoms but they are sometimes used to prevent or destroy organisms that may cause other infections, such as pneumonia.

Recent research on the use of large doses of vitamin C has received public attention, both as a preventive measure and as a treatment for common colds. There is not yet enough conclusive research to determine the possible negative effects of very large amounts of vitamin C (such as the possibility of causing stones in the bladder or the urinary tract). As with any new scientific theory, caution should be exercised.

Prevention of the common cold, and all other common illnesses, is the keystone to a high level of physical well-being.

Influenza

Influenza (flu), another illness caused by viruses, is an acute infection of the upper respiratory tract bringing on a sudden set of symptoms that may include fever, chills, muscle and joint pains, headaches, and weakness. Often there may be a severe cough, which continues long after the other symptoms disappear. There is even danger of such complications as pneumonia.

Influenza can be a very serious disease for some people, particularly for the elderly or those who are generally not in good health. Great care should be taken to prevent influenza, including the following of general good health practices and the avoiding of crowds to the extent possible when influenza is common in the area. Vaccines are available that *may* confer protection (immunity) against specific types or strains of influenza. The type of influenza that develops in a person's community, however, may not be the same type against which he has been vaccinated.

There is no specific treatment for influenza. Treatment is focused primarily on easing the discomfort of the symptoms. Most viral infections are self-limiting: they clear up of their own accord when the body's defense mechanisms bring about the isolation and destruction of infected cells.

Pneumonia

Pneumonia is an inflammation involving one or both lungs. When both lungs are infected, the condition is called bilateral pneumonia. The onset of pneumonia is often sudden, with shaking chills, sharp pains in the chest, cough, expectoration of a rusty-colored sputum, fever, and headache. The person may also have shortness of breath, with rapid and often painful breathing. There may be profuse sweating or bluish coloring. A person with these symptoms is acutely ill and needs immediate medical attention.

Pneumonia is usually caused by bacteria, but it may be caused by a virus or by inhaling either solid or liquid materials into the lungs. Inhaling irritating or poisonous fumes such as chlorine or ammonia can cause *chemical* pneumonia, and may be severe enough to cause death.

Pneumonia is more likely when a person's body has low resistance to infection, particularly in elderly or terminally ill persons. Influenza, measles, and whooping cough weaken the respiratory passages so that pneumonia may develop. In children with measles, pneumonia may be suspected when fever and difficulty in breathing continue after the acute phase of the disease. Chronic conditions such as heart ailments, anemia, and hardening of the arteries may make a person more susceptible to pneumonia.

The home nurse can do much to help the patient with pneumonia. The patient needs—

- Physical and mental rest, with as little exertion as possible
- Extra fluids, to aid circulation and elimination
- A diet that is light and easily digested, and foods that are high in proteins
- Frequent changing of his position in bed
- Protection from other diseases

Other persons around the patient should be protected from the possibility of pneumonia by use of the very best hygienic measures: encouraging the patient to cover his mouth when coughing, carefully disposing of dirty tissues, and taking extreme care to insure the cleanliness of eating utensils.

Venereal Diseases

Diseases classified as venereal diseases are those that are transmitted from one person to another by sexual contact. Most infections occur from germs transmitted in the pus from a sore and from body fluids and secretions in the infected areas—sex organs, anus, mouth, and throat—to similar areas of the noninfected individual. Transmission of infection to a developing baby may occur during pregnancy (in syphilis) or during delivery (in gonorrhea). *Very rarely* is there transmission from contaminated articles, such as toilet seats. Venereal diseases are highly communicable: easily spread from one person to another during sexual contact. The effects of these diseases can be harmful and irreversible if the diseases are not treated adequately.

Treatment for syphilis and gonorrhea is available through health department clinics and private sources of health care. One dose of medicine may be all that is needed. If repeated doses are advised, it is to make certain that all of the germs are killed. Public clinics, where treatment is generally free, are very good sources of treatment because of their experience and readily available laboratory facilities. They also maintain careful procedures to insure confidentiality, as do all health professionals. Laws in most states permit treatment of teen-agers *without* parents' consent *or* knowledge. All persons with whom the infected individual has had sexual or close body contact should be examined so that the disease is not transmitted to others.

The best protection against venereal disease is to be sure that both partners are free from the disease. A health professional can provide that information after performing a physical examination and certain blood tests or cultures. Because there are no home remedies for venereal diseases, and because the symptoms may be confused with those of other diseases, it is necessary to seek health care whenever there is an unusual discharge, itching, or burning sensation in the genital area.

For answers to questions about venereal disease, including consultation about treatment, call the local health department or call the United States Center for Disease Control at this toll-free number: 800-523-1885.

Poisoning and Infection Caused by Contaminated Food

Contaminated food can cause many illnesses in the digestive system, including food poisoning, infection, and the growth of parasites in the body. The common symptoms of food poisoning are nausea, cramps, vomiting, and diarrhea—all of which start suddenly and often occur in all members of a household or all persons sharing a common source of food.

Improperly processed or cooked foods, poorly stored foods, foods exposed to rodents and flies, or foods served on unclean plates or handled by persons with infections are all possible sources of infection. Foods that commonly cause food poisoning if not properly refrigerated include custards, salads and salad dressing, and sandwiches. Meats and meat products, if handled by persons with infected wounds on the hands, infected eyes, abscesses, etc., may also cause illness.

CHRONIC DISEASES

The term "chronic disease" is used to describe illnesses that are not communicable and that last or persist over long periods of time. This section gives brief descriptions of the chronic illnesses that occur most frequently in the United States and that often respond to good health practices and nursing care. Three points about chronic illness are particularly important:

- Early detection promotes either cure or control, or both, with fewer disabilities.
- Each person with the disease has his own individual symptoms and treatment regimen. Symptoms and good treatment for one person may not be the same for another.
- Education regarding the disease should be part of the treatment.

It is possible for the person with the chronic illness, and his family, to learn to modify activities so that a full and meaningful life can be achieved. Patients and their families should demand, from the health professionals caring for them, explanations about the disease process, the alternative treatments, and the benefits and possible side effects of the proposed treatment. This information will allow informed consent to and participation in treatment. When persons have questions about any particular disease, the health professional or the specific organization interested in the disease should be consulted. (See Appendix for list of organizations.)

Diseases of the Heart and Blood Vessels

(Cardiovascular Diseases)

Diseases of the heart and arteries are so interrelated that they should be considered together. It is common for conditions of the blood vessels or the circulatory system to be referred to as "heart disease" or "a bad heart." A more accurate medical term is "cardiovascular disease."

The heart is the body organ that by action of its muscles pumps blood through the arteries and veins to all parts of the body. One side of the heart pumps blood to the lungs, where oxygen is added to the blood and carbon dioxide is removed from it. The other side of the heart pumps blood through the arteries to the whole body. When the heart beats, it forces blood through the arteries and against their walls. This pressure of the blood within the arteries is commonly called *blood pressure.* The pumping action of the heart is known as the heartbeat, or *pulse.* The pulse can be counted at places where an artery is near the surface of the body, such as at the wrist. (See page 393 for information on counting the pulse.)

Blood pressure and pulse are important clues to the functioning of the heart and the health of the whole body. Blood pressure increases when a person is excited, afraid, or exercising. It goes down when the person is relaxed or sleeping. Any factor that makes the heart work harder, such as obesity, causes an increase in blood pressure.

Any illness that causes impairment of the heart's action as a pump can result in congestive heart failure. That is not a specific disease but rather a set of symptoms of various types of heart disease.

Arteriosclerosis is a condition of hardening of the arteries that increases with the age of the person and results from a deposit of salts on the artery walls.

Atherosclerosis is a condition occurring when fats are deposited on the artery walls, making them rough, thick, and hard. It is this condition that is usually the cause of a "heart attack." Sometimes the blobs of fatty material can close off an artery. If the closed artery is in the heart, a *heart attack* occurs. If the artery is one that takes blood to the brain, a *stroke* occurs.

Stroke

A stroke (cardiovascular accident, or CVA) is a condition occurring when the blood supply to the brain is cut off. This lack of oxygen in the brain may cause brain tissue to die. A stroke may be the result of a blood clot, the closing of an artery because of fat deposits, or the rupture of a blood vessel. The bleeding that occurs when a blood vessel in the brain ruptures is referred to as *cerebral hemorrhage.* Because the brain controls body functions, any part of the body may be affected, depending on where in the brain the damage is done. The extent of the damage in the brain influences the kind of problem the person will have and the severity of it. Sometimes speech is affected, sometimes leg and arm muscles, and sometimes memory. Often, only one side of the body is affected.

The person may or may not have warnings, or "little strokes." He should seek the advice of a health professional at once if the following signs of these little strokes occur:

- Sudden, temporary weakness or numbness of the face, arm, or leg
- Temporary difficulty with speech or loss of speech, or trouble in understanding someone else's speech
- Brief dimness or loss of vision, particularly in one eye
- Double vision
- Unexplained headaches or a change in the kind of headaches the person formerly had
- Temporary dizziness or unsteadiness
- A change in mood, personality, or mental ability

These signs may also be signs of other illnesses. The health professional will try to determine the specific illness. Early treatment of little strokes can often prevent more serious strokes later on.

Treatment for a person who has had a stroke is primarily rehabilitation in the form of exercise of the affected parts. The extent of recovery of motion is influenced by the extent of damage in the brain and the quality of rehabilitation. Health professionals, usually physical therapists, recommend specific exercises to be done by a person with assistance from others. The home nurse or other person caring for the patient who has had a stroke must realize that the future independence of the patient may be a direct result of how well the exercises are carried out. Since the patient may give up easily, the home nurse must have patience and perseverance to help him reach his greatest possible recovery of motion.

Hypertension (High Blood Pressure)

Hypertension is known as the greatest silent killer, because many people who have high blood pressure do not know it. If a person's blood pressure consistently stays at a level of 149/90 or above, he should be checked by a physician. Some common signs of high blood pressure are headaches, dizziness or tiredness, flushed face, or a ringing in the ears. Because these are also signs of other illnesses, the person may not know he has high blood pressure unless he is checked with a sphygmomanometer and stethoscope. Usually a health professional takes blood pressure, but the American Red Cross has a self-instruction workbook *(Vital Signs: Module II—Blood Pressure)* to teach other persons to take and monitor blood pressure also.

Hypertension can usually be controlled with the use of medication. It may be necessary for certain persons to continue taking such medication throughout their life. A major problem in the control of hypertension is that persons who take medication for hypertension do not feel symptoms and may therefore stop taking their medication because they feel well. Their blood pressure may then rise once more to unsafe limits without their realizing it, *unless* they have been monitoring it regularly. (See page 397 for instructions on taking blood pressure.)

Cardiovascular diseases are a major threat to life and happiness. All persons need to take special precautions against them—especially persons who have a family history of such diseases.

The good health habits given in chapter 2 give a general picture of good health maintenance. The following specific practices can reduce the risk of heart diseases:

- Do not smoke.
- Avoid becoming overweight.
- If you are overweight, consult a health professional regarding sensible weight reduction. *Avoid fad diets.*
- Avoid eating large amounts of fats—especially animal fats, whole milk, butter, and eggs.
- Exercise regularly. Walk, jog, or run if advised to do so by a health professional.
- Avoid stressful situations when possible. If involved in a stressful occupation, take shorter and more frequent vacations.

The American Heart Association (see Appendix for address) provides free pamphlets that give information about heart disease and that assist individuals in making alterations to their usual patterns of life in order to lessen the risk of such disease.

Cancer

Cancer is the name given to diseases in which there is uncontrolled and disordered growth of cells. The cause of cancer is unknown at this writing, but it is known that the cancer cells invade the tissue that surrounds them, causing pain and disruption of normal function. Cancer may spread in the body by way of the lymph channels and blood vessels—a process called metastasis.

Treatments for cancer include surgery to remove the cancerous tissue, medications to kill the cancerous cells or prevent their spread, and radiation to kill cancerous cells. Because some kinds of cancer can be cured if detected early, it is important that treatment be sought promptly.

The American Cancer Society (see Appendix for address) provides information about cancer, and many of its local chapters sponsor detection clinics, distribute supplies, and provide services such as transportation for patients with cancer. The local chapter may help a patient or family get in contact with persons who have had cancer and who know about rehabilitation techniques and equipment to assist patients following surgery on the breast, larynx, or intestine.

Mental Illness

The term "mental illness" generally refers to patterns of behavior that prevent a person from functioning at his level of capacity or at commonly expected levels consistent with his age, sex, and other personal characteristics. In general, mental health and mental illness may be identifiable by a very small degree of difference in behavior.

Emotional health involves a kind of self-confidence, freedom from guilt, and a solid, positive relationship with family, friends, co-workers, and others. The ability to get along with oneself and with others and the ability to adjust to changing situations without undue physical stress are important signs of mental health. A person who is considered to be mentally healthy also—

- Has a fairly good understanding of himself and his personality
- Can relate to other people and has the ability to love and to accept love
- Feels and expresses positive emotions more frequently than negative emotions such as hate
- Adopts a code of behavior that has positive effects on himself and on others
- Strives for new experiences from which he obtains satisfaction and gains new skills—experiences that enable him to give satisfaction and pleasure to others

- Has a life goal and works toward it
- Is able to cope with stresses of life without damage to his body or his mental functioning

Some undesirable symptoms in behavior that should be a warning, especially if they continue over long periods of time, are—

- Anxiety, depression, brooding
- Lack of interest in friends, family, job, or regular recreation and reluctance to mingle with others or to go to new places
- Sleeplessness
- Inability to concentrate
- Oversensitivity or resentment toward a person without apparent cause or with fears that are baseless
- Obsessions or fixed ideas
- Confusion as to one's identity or that of others in the family or confusion as to one's surroundings
- Headaches not attributable to usual causes
- Physical complaints of an imaginary nature
- Recurrent daydreams or hallucinations of an impossible nature
- Suicidal threats. (*Any* suicidal threat is an undesirable symptom that should *never* be disregarded.)

Symptoms of mental ill health may be evident to both the sufferer and the observer, but neither may recognize the signs as anything serious. Because the symptoms may develop slowly and the changes may occur gradually, a problem can be quite severe before it is detected. Assistance should therefore be sought as soon as any concern is felt about the behavior of an individual. A health professional should be contacted, who can help define the problem and start treatment.

Mental problems can be difficult to diagnose and to treat. Sensitive listening and careful observation of physical, emotional, and social factors are therefore required before a diagnosis can be made. Treatments include medication, individual counseling, and, sometimes, family counseling.

Information regarding sources of help in the community can be obtained from the Mental Health Association, a voluntary organization with local chapters throughout the country. There are mental health clinics in many communities, some of which may be sponsored by the public health department. There are also "hot lines" or crises centers, which may be advertised in the local news media, telephone books, or hospitals. When a person poses a danger to himself or others, the police can often be very helpful.

Diabetes

Diabetes (more properly known as diabetes mellitus) is a disorder in the body's metabolism: the body cannot handle sugar and starches normally, and high glucose levels occur in the blood and urine. This condition results from insufficient insulin in the body. Special diets, oral medication, or injections of insulin usually can keep diabetes under control. Persons who have had the disease for a long time may develop complications involving blood vessels, kidneys, heart, eyes, and nerves.

There is a hereditary tendency to diabetes. Persons with a history of diabetes in their family should have regular checkups with their health professional. Obesity creates a higher risk of developing diabetes.

Persons with diabetes need to have complete information about the disease and about their own condition, since a person's daily pattern of living, including food intake, exercise, and stress, has a great effect on the functioning of the body and the progress of the disease. Regular and continued supervision by a competent health professional is essential to help the person maintain his highest possible level of physical well-being.

The American Diabetes Association (see Appendix for address) provides literature and educational programs for diabetics and their families. Additional services such as counseling, detection programs, and special camps for children may be available in some communities.

Persons with diabetes (or other similar diseases) are advised to wear or carry a bracelet (Fig. 51) or card indicating that they have the disease. In emergencies, such information could save their life.

Arthritis and Rheumatism

Arthritis and rheumatism are terms that refer to a variety of disorders. There are about 50 rheumatic diseases. They all have in common pain and stiffness that is attributable to the muscles, bones, and

Fig. 51

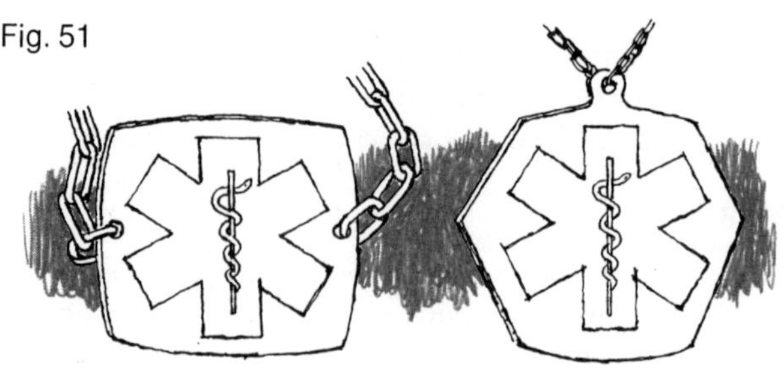

associated connective tissues. More specifically, the term "arthritis" is used to describe diseases in which there is abnormality within the joint itself. The pain and stiffness associated with osteo-arthritis (the arthritis that affects most persons as they grow older) results from changes in the joints that bear weight—often the spine and hips. Inflammation causes the pain and limitation of movement associated with rheumatoid arthritis, which is a more difficult disease to control. Gout is a special form of arthritis. The term "rheumatism" refers to a more severe pain with difficulty in movement.

Proper use of medication and heat, and appropriate balance between rest and exercise, good posture, and weight control can greatly relieve the pain and discomfort of arthritis and rheumatism. Since medical treatments can also be effective, individuals with symptoms in their joints should seek health care. Arthritis often "goes into remission," which means that there are periods of spontaneous improvement (lessening or disappearance of symptoms). Such remissions make it easier for quacks to claim cures from their expensive and useless treatments.

The Arthritis Foundation (see Appendix for address) provides free literature and recommends readings for those who want further information.

Chapter 13

Alternatives and Supplements to Home Care

Maintenance of the highest possible level of wellness of family members often requires the services of health care institutions, agencies, and organizations in the community. Some of the needs that must be provided for by community health resources include surgery and testing with highly technical equipment to diagnose and treat illness, close professional supervision to regulate medication as in the case of diabetes, and care that cannot be given in the home or by family members. Knowledge about how persons can prepare themselves and family members to obtain the best possible care is essential. The financial and human resources of the individual, the family, and the community need to be used to the greatest advantage.

In many cases, special responsibilities fall to the home nurse or responsible family member in preparing the person for care outside the home, and again for care upon return to the home. To help the person responsible, information is presented in this chapter regarding hospitalization and the selection of nursing homes and care in such homes. In addition, information is given about other community resources that provide important types of assistance for home care that cannot otherwise be provided.

HOSPITALIZATION

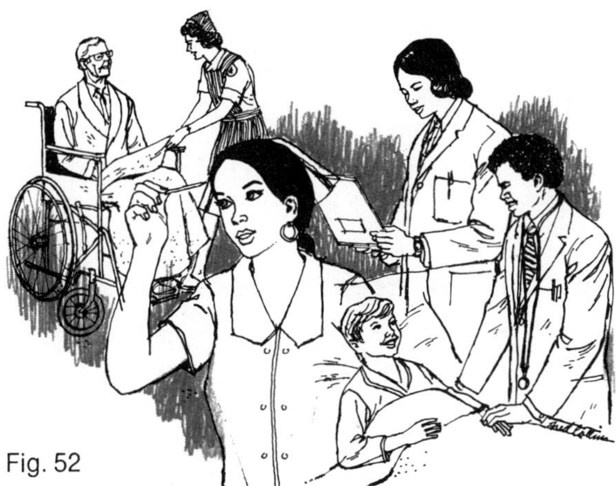

Fig. 52

Hospitals provide the kind of care that usually cannot be provided in the home, in the health professional's office, or in a nusing home. Hospitals are centers for the delivery of a wide variety of types of care for the sick and injured, including surgery and intensive care for the seriously ill. Although they vary greatly in the kinds of care provided, they have the highly technical equipment, staff, and expert health professionals needed for the most complex emergencies and illnesses.

Many hospitals have emergency rooms staffed by skilled health professionals, outpatient departments where persons can be tested and treated without admission to a patient care room, and special educational programs such as preparing for childbirth or managing the care of diabetics.

Hospitals are licensed by the states and must meet basic minimum standards. In addition, they may be accredited by a national commission representing selected health care professionals. Such accreditation means that the hospital meets national standards with respect to education of its staff, management, and other aspects of quality health care.

Preparation for Hospitalization

Many hospital admissions are planned, or at least allow enough time for some action to be taken that will reduce stress for those involved. A general understanding of the information in this section will be helpful to all concerned in the event of an emergency admission for which there can be no advance preparation.

Preparation for hospitalization should be a joint effort of the individual, his family, the primary health professional, and the hospital. Such preparation should include discussion of financial arrangements, admission procedures, and discharge plans. Plans may need to be made in regard to carrying out the patient's responsibilities during his absence from home, particularly in the case of a mother with young children.

Preparing a Child for Hospitalization

Many adults have had some firsthand experience with hospitals or they may have visited hospitalized friends and relatives and therefore may have some idea of what a hospital is like. A child who has not been prepared may have no idea of what to expect. Hospital surroundings will be new and strange, and the child may be left in the hospital without a family member close by. Hospitalization can be especially frightening for a child. To reduce fear, it is important that the parents tell the child as much as possible about what to expect.

Parents should discuss the coming hospitalization with the child shortly before the event so that the child does not have too long to worry, but enough in advance to allow him to prepare for it as much as possible. The parents should explain to the child what to expect and what will be done to help him, in an honest, straightforward manner. The child needs help in trying to understand why hospitalization is necessary.

It may be possible to "rehearse" some of the expected activities. Some hospitals have special programs whereby children who are scheduled for admission can visit the pediatric (children's) section of the hospital before the actual admission. Books or pamphlets that prepare the child for his hospital adventure may be available from the hospital or from the local library. The U.S. Department of Health, Education, and Welfare has a booklet that lists and describes some books that might be helpful. This booklet, *Books That Help Children Deal With a Hospital Experience,* can be ordered from the Superintendent of Documents, U.S. Government Printing Office, Washington, D C 20402.

The child may feel more secure if he is allowed to take one or two special toys or books to the hospital. His mother may be able to sleep on a cot or in a chair in his room.

Advance Arrangements

When hospitalization is planned in advance, some of the admission routine may be completed before the day of entry into the hospital. Information that will be needed by the hospital can be gathered, and perhaps a preadmission form can be filled out. Financial arrangements can be discussed. The admission procedure is usually completed more quickly and easily if the needed information is handy, and the hospital can function more efficiently when it has time to get records and charts labeled before they are needed by medical and nursing staff.

Hospitals' policies vary in regard to payment plans. At the time the patient is admitted, the hospital will request information about the hospitalization insurance available: the name of the company, the type of policy, and the policy number. If the patient is eligible for Medicare or Medicaid, the claim or identification number will be requested. Insurance claim forms will have to be filled out. If there is no hospitalization insurance or other medical coverage, the hospital should be informed before admission. Some hospitals will require a deposit on or before the admission date; some require proof of ability to pay; and some set up a schedule for later payments. Because hospitals are concerned about the patient and his financial problems, many have social workers or other persons who can suggest ways of organizing payment or outside sources of financial help for those who qualify. In cases of emergency, hospitals usually provide the necessary care as needed and work with the family regarding payment.

Sometimes laboratory tests will be performed during the week preceding admission to the hospital.

What To Take to the Hospital

Hospital policies vary as to what patients should bring with them for an overnight stay or a longer period of hospitalization. The degree of illness of the patient also makes a difference. Most people like to have their own sleepwear and toilet articles. A basic list of useful items includes—

Pajamas, nightgowns, or bed jackets (ones that are easily laundered and that fasten down the front, since they are easier to put on and take off in bed).

Slippers and bathrobe.

Toothbrush, toothpaste, and dental floss.

Hairbrush and comb and any necessary hair equipment such as hair clips and curlers.

Toilet articles, shampoo, lotion, shaving equipment, etc.

Coins for purchasing newspapers, to use in a pay telephone, etc.

An inexpensive watch or clock. (Most patients' rooms do not have clocks.)

Books and handiwork in small quantities. (Light reading materials or easy crafts are most appropriate. The patient should not expect to get caught up on correspondence and all the latest books and magazines.)

Take as few things as possible, since most rooms are small and have little storage space and no security. *Do not bring valuables* of any kind, especially money and jewelry. Most hospitals will insist that valuable jewelry and large amounts of cash be kept in an envelope in the hospital safe. Two or three dollars is usually enough to keep in the room. If a patient changes rooms during his stay, extra articles to move become a problem. The street clothes worn to the hospital may be put in a closet or may be taken home by a relative or friend and brought back when the time of discharge is near.

Persons should check with their physician about bringing their medicines to the hospital. Any medicines brought (such as those for heart disease, hypertension, diabetes, or birth control, or any steroids or hormones) should be stored in their original containers so that the health professionals will be certain what medicine a person is taking. *Do not use medicines brought from home* while in the hospital unless advised to do so by the health professionals. If the physician has not been informed of these drugs, there is danger of overdosage or of a dangerous reaction with other drugs that may be ordered for the patient.

Admission Routine

The hospital needs several kinds of information in order to serve the patient well. It will usually request the following information during admission procedures:

The patient's full name, address, and telephone number.

The patient's age, date of birth, and birthplace.

The parents' names and places of birth (or death). (This information is useful for the numbering system used by hospitals, as well as for identifying children.)

The name and address of the patient's employer.

The closest relative or other person to be called in case of emergency.

Insurance information. (Most hospitalization plans have a wallet-sized card that has all the necessary information, including type of policy and policy number.)

Religious preference.

Whether the patient has been treated at the hospital before (with date, if possible).

After the admitting office procedures are completed, the following steps are common:

1. An identification bracelet with name, etc., is usually attached to the patient's wrist (Fig. 53).
2. The patient is taken to his patient care room and is assigned a bed.
3. Room equipment, especially the call button, is explained.

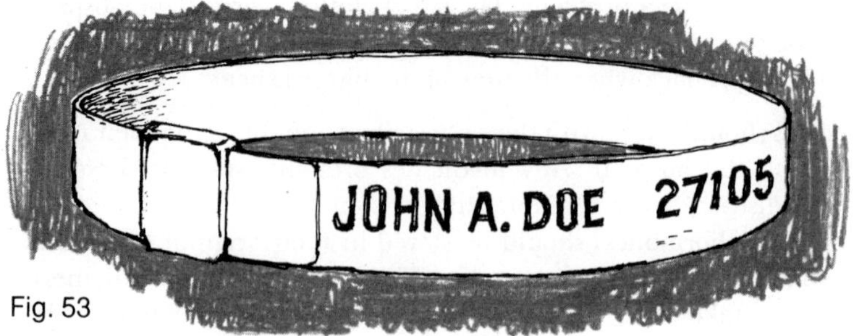

Fig. 53

4. Policies and schedules (mealtimes, visiting hours, etc.) are explained.
5. Vital signs (blood pressure, pulse, respiration, temperature) are taken, and a sample of urine may be requested.
6. The patient is asked (or helped) to undress and get into bed.

A complete physical examination will be given, and a medical history may be taken at this time. Laboratory tests, including X-rays and blood tests, may be done.

Learning To Identify Hospital Workers

There are many different kinds of hospital workers. Since most wear the traditional white uniform, or colored uniforms or smocks, it is often difficult to distinguish which persons are physicians, nurses, dieticians, technicians, or volunteers. Registered or practical/vocational nurses wear caps in some hospitals but not in others. Many hospitals now require all personnel to wear name pins. Such pins usually state the name and function of each person, such as: Nancy B. White, R.N., Head Nurse.

Consent for Procedures

Discussion of procedures to be performed and their consequences should ideally precede hospitalization, although this discussion is not always possible in cases of emergency or diagnosis of disease during hospitalization. Such discussion gives patients and their families an opportunity to "digest" the information and to think about the consequences. The patient has a legal right to information about procedures and consequences, and this information must be presented in a way that he can understand and that will allow him to ask questions and to give *informed* consent.

In order to fulfill legal requirements, the patient must consent in writing before certain diagnostic tests and most surgical procedures are done. Parents may sign for minors, except in cases where adolescents must have certain kinds of treatment. Signing of the consent form often occurs immediately before the performance of the procedure.

The Patient's Rights

The American Hospital Association has adopted a "Patient's Bill of Rights" to guide patients, hospitals, and health care professionals in effective patient care, with the greatest possible satisfaction of all concerned. These rights are presented here with permission of the American Hospital Association:

- The patient has the right to considerate and respectful care.
- The patient has the right to obtain from his physician complete current information concerning his diagnosis, treatment, and prognosis in terms the patient can be reasonably expected to understand. When it is not medically advisable to give such information to the patient, the information should be made available to an appropriate person in his behalf. He has the right to know, by name, the physician responsible for coordinating his care.
- The patient has the right to receive from his physician information necessary to give informed consent prior to the start of any procedure and/or treatment. Except in emergencies, such information for informed consent should include but not necessarily be limited to the specific procedure and/or treatment, the medically significant risks involved, and the probable duration of incapacitation. Where medically significant alternatives for care or treatment exist, or when the patient requests information concerning medical alternatives, the patient has the right to such information. The patient also has the right to know the name of the persons responsible for the procedures and/or treatment.
- The patient has the right to refuse treatment to the extent permitted by law and to be informed of the medical consequences of his action.
- The patient has the right to every consideration of his privacy concerning his own medical care program. Case discussion, consultation, examination, and treatment are confidential and should be conducted discreetly. Those not directly involved in his care must have the permission of the patient to be present.

- The patient has the right to expect that all communications and records pertaining to his care should be treated as confidential.

- The patient has the right to expect that within its capacity a hospital must make reasonable response to the request of a patient for services. The hospital must provide evaluation, service, and/or referral as indicated by the urgency of the case. When medically permissible, a patient may be transferred to another facility only after he has received complete information and explanation concerning the needs for and alternatives to such a transfer.

- The patient has the right to obtain information as to any relationship of his hospital to other health care and educational institutions insofar as his care is concerned. The patient has the right to obtain information as to the existence of any professional relationships among individuals, by name, who are treating him.

- The patient has the right to be advised if the hospital proposes to engage in or perform human experimentation affecting his care or treatment. The patient has the right to refuse to participate in such research projects.

- The patient has the right to expect reasonable continuity of care. He has the right to know in advance what appointment times and physicians are available and where. The patient has the right to expect that the hospital will provide a mechanism whereby he is informed by his physician or a delegate of the physician of the patient's continuing health care requirements following discharge.

- The patient has the right to examine and receive an explanation of his bill, regardless of the source of payment.

- The patient has the right to know what hospital rules and regulations apply to his conduct as a patient.

- No catalog of rights can guarantee for the patient the kind of treatment he has a right to expect. A hospital has many functions to perform, including the prevention and treatment of disease, the education of both health professionals and patients, and the conduct of clinical research. All these activities must be conducted with an overriding concern for the patient, and, above all, the recognition of his dignity as a human being. Success in achieving this recognition assures success in the defense of the rights of the patient.

The Patient's Responsibilities

A patient is responsible for being considerate of other patients and hospital personnel by—

- Assuring his roommate's privacy
- Limiting visitors to the number allowed during the hours allowed
- Reminding visitors to maintain a quiet atmosphere and to observe smoking regulations
- Using television, telephone, radio, and lights in a manner that does not disturb others

The patient's additional responsibilities include—

- Supplying accurate and complete information about medications, past illnesses and hospitalizations, and other matters relating to his health.
- Notifying the doctor or the nurse of any unexpected change in his health.
- Advising the doctor or the nurse immediately if he does not understand instructions or if he feels that instructions are such that they cannot be followed.
- Keeping appointments. If an appointment cannot be kept, the health professional concerned should be notified.
- Using hospital equipment appropriately, thereby assuring its availability to future patients. (The patient is responsible for loss or damage of equipment.)
- Fulfilling the financial obligations for health care as promptly as possible.

Intensive Care

When a patient is acutely ill and needs constant, specialized care, he may be placed in an intensive-care unit, or special section of the hospital. Expert personnel and special equipment for monitoring his vital signs are easily available. The unit is arranged in such a way that all patients are close to immediate help. Smaller hospitals that may not have a special care section may keep patients needing constant care in rooms close to the nurses' station. As recovery occurs, the patient will usually be returned to a regular patient care room.

Visitors are usually allowed for limited periods in intensive-care units, several times a day.

Surgery

Preparation for surgery should include an explanation to the patient and his family of what should be expected before surgery, in the recovery room, and after the patient returns to his room. It should include a discussion of anesthesia, how the recovery room functions, what (if any) tubings, attachments, and dressings to expect, and their purposes. If there is to be general anesthesia, the patient should have the opportunity to practice the deep breathing and coughing exercises that will help keep his lungs clear following surgery. Patients should feel free to ask questions and should expect answers.

The patient scheduled for major surgery usually arrives at the hospital a day or two before surgery. For minor surgery, the patient may arrive as late as the morning of the surgery. For any surgery, there are certain procedures to be followed beforehand, some of which may begin at home or in the doctor's office:

- Blood testing (a complete blood count, determination of blood type, and cross matching of blood in case a blood transfusion is needed).
- Urinalysis (examination of a sample of urine, when the patient is admitted to the hospital).
- Fasting from food and water for 6 to 12 hours before surgery.
- Shaving of the area for surgery (to keep the area as clean as possible, since hairs can carry germs).
- Special cleansing procedures. (Special washing, douches, or enemas may be required.)
- Preoperative medications.

A sleeping pill is often given the night before surgery and may also be given the morning of surgery. About an hour before the actual operation, an injection (shot) is given to relax the patient and to make it easier for anesthesia to take effect.

Planning for Discharge

Planning for discharge can begin before the patient enters the hospital and certainly should occur during the last part of a patient's stay. Considerations in planning for discharge include—

- The patient's safety and continued progress in recovery.
- What kinds of treatment, if any, will need to be continued at home. (These may include medications, exercise programs, physi-

cal therapy, changing of dressings, injections, special provisions for elimination, and respiratory treatments.)

- The patient's ability to manage his own hygiene and personal care.
- Whether help will be required for meal preparation, laundry, shopping, and housecleaning, and if so, for how long.

The patient, the family, the medical and nursing staff, and other hospital personnel (such as social worker and dietitian) should work together in planning for the patient's discharge. The plans should be acceptable to both the patient and the family and wherever possible should make use of existing community resources so that the patient and the family need not bear the whole burden of care.

At the time of discharge, the patient should be given information regarding particular treatments, diet, follow-up visits, etc. The instructions should be clear, should be given in writing, and should be checked by the health professional before the patient leaves. There should also be instructions about what to do and whom or where to call in case an emergency arises.

NURSING HOMES

A nursing home may be needed when a patient requires medical, nursing, or other professional attention that the family cannot provide at home. Such occasions may arise following hospitalization for a major illness, when special rehabilitation is required, or when recovery will be slow. A nursing home can provide the needed care for a patient who might otherwise have been cared for at home but who cannot be because—

- There are no community resources to help the family provide care
- The patient needs skilled services on a 24-hour basis but does not need hospital care
- The necessary services either are not available or are too costly to provide at home
- Caring for the patient at home would be too disrupting to family life or because the patient has no one at home to care for him

Some nursing homes specialize in medical and nursing services, others in personal care service. Not all nursing homes are able to provide skilled nursing care after hospitalization. The kind of facility needed must be determined by the patient, the family, and the health professional. Health professionals will often know which nursing home in the community provides the type of service required. Other sources of information include the local health department, welfare or family assistance offices, senior citizens or social work groups, clergymen, relatives, and friends.

Not all nursing homes qualify for payment under whatever insurance coverage the patient carries. Medicare, for example, will pay for care only in a skilled nursing care facility. Both Medicare and Medicaid programs encourage home care whenever possible. However, because government and other programs are constantly changing, be sure to obtain up-to-date information.

It is a good idea to find out as much as possible about nursing homes before the need is expected to arise. The U.S. Department of Health, Education, and Welfare publishes a booklet, *Nursing Home Care,* that explains the various kinds of nursing homes, describes what to look for and how to do it, and gives information on how they operate. The booklet is available free from the U.S. Government Printing Office, Washington, D C 20201. (Ask for SRS 76-24902.)

What To Look For in a Nursing Home

A nursing home should fit the patient's needs and preferences. A specific diet or type of therapy may be required. Convenient location is also important—within a reasonable distance not only of family, friends, and other potential visitors but also of an accredited hospital with which there is a transfer agreement in case of patient need. After making a list of possibilities, telephone the nursing homes to ask if they provide the necessary services and whether they qualify for payment under the system that will be used.

The next step is to visit the nursing homes that appear to meet the patient's needs. At the time of the visit, look for documents indicating that the facilities meet the following minimum standards:

- Having a current license issued from the state to the home *and* to the administrator
- Having received a certificate of compliance with federal or state fire codes, or both, within the past year
- Having a certificate of participation in government or other financial programs for which the patient is eligible

For nursing homes participating in Medicare and Medicaid, inspection ratings can be seen at the local social security district office. The local health department, the hospital social worker, or senior citizen groups may be sources of further information.

During the visit to the nursing home, you should look for the following desirable characteristics:

- A cheerful atmosphere, where each staff member, from administrator to janitor, is pleasant and shows genuine, personal interest in each of the persons living in the home. (Staff should address residents by their names, calls for assistance should be answered promptly, and courtesy, respect, and affection should be demonstrated at all times.)
- A good appearance and adequate living arrangements. (Beds should be well spaced and no more than four to a room. Curtains should draw around each bed. Toilet facilities should be convenient and in sufficient number. Bathrooms should have bars to help the patient sit on the toilet or use the tub or shower. Rooms and hallways should be well lighted. Hallways should have handrails. Furniture should be appropriate for the residents, sturdy and arranged for easy use.)
- A clean environment, free of unpleasant odors. (A slight smell of urine may be acceptable, but the heavy scent of deodorizing sprays should arouse suspicions of uncleanliness.)
- Alert and active residents who wear their own clothing, which is neat, clean, and in good repair. (Residents should be allowed to bring in their personal belongings: photographs, pillows, a favorite chair, etc.)
- Attractively served meals that are appealing to look at, tasty, and as stated on the menu. (Snacks should be available to those who are allowed to have them.)

Be sure to talk with the residents, staff, visitors, and volunteers and ask their opinions of the nursing home. There should be no reports of interference with mail, and there should be good access to communication outside the nursing home, such as by telephone. If there are no visitors or volunteers around, ask why not. Ask to write to family members of residents to hear what they think of the home, or call the health department. The "Patient's Bill of Rights" statement should be posted in clear view in the lobby, along with the certificate of Medicare participation.

Be sure that financial charges are clearly specified. Determine what the basic rates include. Add extra charges, such as those for laundry and disposable supplies, to figure the total charges. Residents should not be required to have their prescriptions filled in the nursing home's pharmacy. Compare nursing homes on the basis of the total cost.

In selecting a nursing home from those that meet the minimum criteria and are suitable to one's financial situation, it may be necessary to make the final decision on the basis of which qualities are most important to the prospective resident.

OTHER RESOURCES TO SUPPLEMENT HOME CARE

For many years, nursing homes were looked to as the best and almost the only alternative to hospital care for persons with chronic diseases and elderly persons who could not be cared for in their own homes without outside assistance. More recently, it has been realized that for many persons, nursing home care is not necessary. Various community agencies exist that can often supplement home care with full- or part-time health-care assistance.

Before deciding that nursing-home care is the best approach to caring for an individual, think carefully about whether nursing-home care is being considered mainly because—

The person needs help in personal hygiene (toileting, bathing, dressing, hair combing, etc.) or habits of daily living (preparing meals, doing household chores such as laundry and cleaning).

Special therapy or treatments are needed that might not be obtainable from community resources or in the home.

Family or friends can give necessary help or care only during the evening and night.

If these or similar problems exist, people should check their community resources carefully. Many communities have developed a variety of services to assist the ill and the elderly so that they will be able to manage in their own homes. The person with special care needs should be involved to the fullest extent possible in any discussions and decisions about his care. He may prefer to continue living in his own home or his family's home rather than going to a nursing home. With the variety of forms of assistance now available, this is often a workable decision.

Visiting Nurse Associations

The services of a professional nurse in the home can often be obtained either through a visiting nurse association (a voluntary, nonprofit agency) or through a public health department. Such service might include personal care, special treatments, health-care advice, and supervision that cannot be provided by the family. The nurse's services may be supplemented with care by practical/vocational nurses, physical therapists, social workers, home health aides, homemakers, and others. The services available may vary greatly in different communities. Further information is presented in chapter 11.

Other Home Care Agencies

The types of services commonly provided by proprietary (for profit) home care agencies vary greatly from one agency to another and from one community to another. Services most commonly provided include home health aide or homemaking services, or both. Some agencies provide different levels of nursing care, and others also provide a kind of "chore," or handyman, service.

Proprietary agencies are often referred to as profit-making organizations. Some home health-care agencies operate all over the nation and are owned and operated by large business enterprises. As in most "for profit" businesses, the practices of the owners vary greatly; some have very high standards for quality care, while others seem much more interested in making a profit than in providing quality care. The educational preparation of the workers, control of their practices, and their supervision in the home to which they are assigned are matters of critical concern.

Proprietary agencies have been the focus of much debate in the federal government and among others concerned with health care in their efforts to promote home health care, to protect consumers, and to control the quality of services provided by any agency, public or private. State and federal laws have not developed fast enough to control the development and operation of proprietary agencies, which are growing at an alarming rate. Caution in selecting home health-care agencies is therefore very important.

Most communities have one or more types of home health-care programs or services available. They are often listed in the telephone directory yellow pages under "nurses," "nursing services," or "home health services." Good sources of information about the existence and reliability of these agencies are—

The person's regular health professional

The nursing or social service department of the local public health department

The social service department of a hospital

The local medical or nursing organization

The local chamber of commerce or Better Business Bureau

In selecting a home health-care agency, give careful attention to the type of workers in the agency and the financial arrangements for the services to be provided. In particular—

- What are the educational or personal qualifications of persons providing the care? Can the qualifications be checked?
- Are the workers bonded (a protection against theft)?
- Do the workers have malpractice insurance?
- Are the workers supervised, and if so, what are the qualifications of their supervisor?
- What steps can be taken if their services are not satisfactory?
- What does each type of service cost? Is there a minimum number of hours?
- Are charges figured on an hourly, weekly, or monthly basis?
- Are there extra charges for transportation of workers, for overtime, or for any other reasons?
- When and to whom is payment to be made, and in what form (cash, check, credit, insurance)?
- Does the agency explain for what and for how long the Medicare and Medicaid benefits may be used?
- Will the person's health insurance cover home health care of the type needed, and if so, who will be billed, the customer or the insurance company?
- Is the cost of the health-care services tax deductible? (If certified necessary and approved by a physician, most home health care is deductible from federal income taxes.)

Adult Day-Care Programs

Adult day care is a relatively new alternative to hospital or nursing home care in the United States, although it has existed in England since the 1950s. Adult day-care programs may be the ideal solution for a person whose family cannot provide the full range of care that he needs or can care for him only in the evening and at night. Adult day care may also follow hospitalization or nursing home care. Most adult day-care centers provide lunch, general nursing supervision, social work, and help with personal hygiene; some will provide special diets or dietary counseling, or both, to participants and their families; some provide physical, occupational, and speech therapy.

Adult day-care programs vary greatly from one community to another and from one agency to another. Some are able to help with a variety of problems, while others are directed toward helping persons with a specific kind of health problem. The programs might be located in a local health department building or in an unused building. They also vary in the number of persons they can care for each day.

Families having need for day-care services for handicapped, elderly, or otherwise infirm persons might be able to locate such services through their regular health professional, the local health department, the local hospital, social service professionals, or other health-care agencies. Questions regarding cost and type of payment accepted for this kind of care should also be investigated.

Ambulatory Care

There are many health problems that do not require admission to a hospital or a nursing home or confinement to bed. Ambulatory patients (persons who can get to sources of care without special assistance) can now receive care in many types of settings. The health professional's office is the best-known ambulatory care setting, but recently there has been much expansion in the amount and type of care available to ambulatory patients. Ambulatory care is now available also in outpatient departments of hospitals (sometimes through their emergency rooms), in neighborhood health centers and outreach facilities, and in medical buildings. Some hospitals have "satellite" clinics, which are located in places where significant numbers of people have special health-care needs.

Neighborhood health centers may be run by a variety of agencies: hospitals, labor unions, governmental agencies, and consumer groups. They try to provide a broad range of health services. In meeting his own health needs, the individual may also find employment and an opportunity for involvement in the community.

Outreach facilities offer health services in areas of special need, such as housing units for the elderly. The idea is that if people cannot come to a medical center, the medical center should be brought to the people. This type of care may be provided by different kinds of groups—for example, the health department or a voluntary agency such as the American Red Cross—and the extent of their services varies considerably.

Chapter 14

First Aid for Home Emergencies

When someone is suddenly taken ill or is injured, it is important to know what to do as well as what not to do. If there is the slightest doubt about the seriousness of the illness or the accident, call a health professional *immediately.* Tell him what has happened and what first aid, if any, has been given. Or get the patient to a hospital at once. If the emergency is of a serious nature, the patient will require immediate first aid to keep the condition from growing worse, or to keep him alive. Because of this, it is advisable that someone in the home knows how to give first aid.

THE VALUE OF FIRST AID TRAINING

First aid is the immediate and temporary care given to a person who has been injured or has suddenly become ill. It includes self-help and home care if medical assistance is not available or is delayed. It also includes well-selected words of encouragement, evidence of willingness to help, and promotion of confidence by demonstration of competence. The person who has been properly trained to give this care is able to assist people when they need help the most, particularly at the time of disaster.

The purposes of first aid training are to develop safety awareness, to train people to do the right thing at the right time if an accident does occur, to prevent additional injury, and to provide safe and proper transportation for the injured.

The American Red Cross has developed several practical courses in first aid that are offered by its chapters throughout the country. It has also published textbooks that cover the prevention and treatment of common emergencies that are likely to occur in the home. Its first aid training is of value in training individuals to provide care in case of accidental injury, sudden illness, and injuries resulting from natural disasters or other catastrophes, and in handling a variety of emergency situations. In any such situation, it is important to know what to do and what not to do.

The information in this chapter is not intended as a substitute for a first aid course but as a review and an aid to the home nurse in meeting and preventing common home emergencies.

EMERGENCY AND FIRST AID SUPPLIES

Every family should have on hand a small supply of medicines and first aid supplies. A list of preferred drugs and supplies can be obtained from the family health professional. He may suggest specific medicines that might include a pain killer and fever reducer, an antacid for indigestion, an antidiarrhea remedy, a laxative, a decongestant, an antiseptic such as rubbing alcohol, an emetic (to cause vomiting), and a lotion for the treatment of poison ivy or insect bites.

Some drugs deteriorate with age and become either ineffective or unsafe to use. For that reason, attention should be paid to the expiration date stamped on the bottle, if there is one. If no expiration date is indicated, the pharmacist or other health professional can tell you how often certain medicines should be replaced.

There should be a first aid kit in every household. Avoid keeping first aid supplies in a medicine chest in the bathroom, where small children can get to them. It is difficult to keep track of first aid supplies kept at random on medicine chest shelves. Keep them together in a convenient place. A covered box makes a good first aid kit, whether made of plastic, cardboard, or metal, and keeps first aid supplies together and convenient to get at. Such a box makes it possible to see at a glance when a particular item is running low or needs to be replaced. It is a good idea to organize the contents of the first aid kit so that a needed item may be chosen quickly, without unpacking everything in the container. Unused materials should be wrapped carefully so that they remain clean.

A first aid kit should include the following items:

- A variety of dry, sterilized gauze squares in different sizes—2, 3, and 4 inches (5.1, 7.6, and 10.2 centimeters)
- Three gauze roller bandages—one 1 inch (2.5 centimeters), one 2 inches (5.2 centimeters), and one 3 inches (7.6 centimeters)
- Two plain absorbent gauze pads—one 18 x 18 inches (45.7 x 45.7 centimeters) and one 24 x 72 inches (61 x 182.9 centimeters)
- One eye dressing
- Three triangular bandages
- A packet of assorted adhesive dressings
- A small roll of adhesive tape, ½ inch or 1 inch (1.3 or 2.5 centimeters) wide
- A small pair of sharp scissors
- A pair of tweezers
- One tourniquet
- Two clinical thermometers, one oral and one rectal, with cases

- Tongue blades and wooden applicator sticks
- A tube of petroleum jelly or other lubricant
- Safety pins—large and small
- A cleansing agent as recommended by the health professional

The family may need additional equipment such as an ice bag, an electric heating pad, or a hot water bottle. Any electrical device should be inspected to make sure that it is safe and in good condition and it should be stored and used according to the manufacturer's directions.

A copy of the American Red Cross *Standard First Aid and Personal Safety* textbook should be on hand.

A list of emergency telephone numbers should be readily available at all times. It should include the numbers of the rescue squad or emergency ambulance service, your family physician or other source of medical care, the hospital emergency room, your pharmacist, the poison control center serving your area, and the local police and fire departments.

COMMUNITY RESOURCES

In case of sudden illness or injury, it is important to know what facilities for immediate help are in your community.

Ambulance Service

Ambulance service may be provided by the city or county or through a privately owned service.

Rescue Squads

In many communities, police departments or fire departments, or both, have rescue squads. Most of these squads are trained to handle emergencies and carry life support and rescue equipment. Other communities may handle emergencies with the help of privately owned ambulance services. Find out what local rescue services are available in your community, what they are called, and where they are. Note the names and telephone numbers in your list of emergency numbers.

Emergency Rooms and Trauma Centers

The trauma center in a hospital is an emergency treatment room containing highly specialized equipment that meets certain standards set up to give immediate care to the severely injured person.

Some communities have special trauma centers (for example, special burn trauma centers). Everyone in the family should know where the nearest emergency room or trauma center is located. Find out in advance the name, location, and telephone number, and record this information in your list of emergency numbers. When calling, give the following emergency information:

- Describe the problem and indicate what is being done.
- Give your name, the location of the accident, the number of persons involved (their sex and age), and the telephone number where you can be reached.
- If the patient will be transported by you, indicate when you expect to arrive at the emergency room.
- Do not hang up the receiver until after the treatment center hangs up, because the center may wish to have further information.

Poison Control Centers

Poison control centers have trained personnel who will give immediate information on emergency first aid treatment for poison victims. When a poison control center is called, certain information is required. The person calling should, therefore, be prepared to answer the following questions:

- What is the name of or type of poison suspected?
- Who manufactures it?
- If the container is available, what are the listed ingredients?
- When and how much of the poison was taken?
- What symptoms were present when the victim was found?
- What action has been or is being taken?

Once the center has the information it needs, it can advise what antidote to use (if there is an antidote for the specific poison involved) or can suggest other immediate emergency measures to be taken.

There are several hundred poison control centers across the nation. Look in the telephone book to see if you have a center serving your area and include the telephone number in your list of other emergency numbers. The number is often listed with other emergency numbers in the front of the telephone book and can also be found under "Poison Control Center" in the white pages. If there is no listing in your telephone directory, check with your local hospital or health professional for the number of the nearest poison control center. Post telephone numbers at all telephones.

GENERAL PROCEDURES FOR SEVERE INJURIES

When there has been an injury or sudden illness, prompt action may be needed to save a life. At other times, there is no need for haste, and efforts can be directed toward preventing further injury, obtaining help, and reassuring the victim, who may be frightened and worried as well as in pain.

Carefully observe whether or not an emergency exists. In cases of serious injury or sudden illness, arrange for help to be called, and give immediate attention to the following first aid priorities:

1. If necessary, rescue the victim from any dangerous environment.
2. If breathing has stopped, provide the victim with an open airway and give mouth-to-mouth or mouth-to-nose artificial respiration. A person who has been trained will know how to give first aid for an obstructed airway and how to give cardiopulmonary resuscitation (CPR).
3. Control any severe bleeding.
4. If necessary, give first aid for poisoning or for swallowing of harmful chemicals.
5. If the victim is unconscious and there are no indications of a neck or back injury, place him on his side so that fluids can drain from the mouth and the air passages can remain clear.
6. If the person is in shock, be sure to maintain normal body temperature and get medical help immediately.

After these priorities have been carried out, if they were needed, you should consider the following points as you administer first aid:

- **Do not move a victim unless it is necessary** for the safety of the individual (for example, if the room is filled with gas or if there is a fire). Keep the victim in the position best suited to his condition. Do not permit him to get up or walk about. Do not allow the victim to be overhandled or disturbed. Keep him comfortably warm by using blankets or covers as necessary. If the victim is lying on a cold, damp floor, place a blanket or a coat or other clothing under him if possible. Check his pulse at the carotid artery at the side of the throat.

- **Examine the victim carefully for injuries.** If he is unconscious, try to find out what happened from another member of the family, a friend, a neighbor, or any witness who may have been present at the time of the accident or sudden illness. Look for evidence of a head injury. Check for any medical emergency identification. Check all signs that may give a clue to any injury or illness.

If the victim is conscious, find out exactly what happened (including the surrounding circumstances) so that you may report this information to the health professional who has been called to give assistance. Also look for paralysis of one side of the victim's face or body.

Check the victim's general appearance, such as skin discoloration. Skin color changes may be difficult to note in persons with dark skin; it may be necessary to depend upon changes in the color of the mucous membrane on the inner surfaces of the lips, mouth, and eyelids. Check for evidence of a recent convulsion (for example, the victim may have bitten into his tongue). Check the size of the victim's pupils and any other changes in his eyes, such as a dull or glazed expression. Check to see whether a surgical opening has been previously made in the neck for breathing; if it has, make sure it is open and that the patient is breathing. Examine his body and arms and legs for open wounds and bruising and for signs of fractures.

If poisoning is suspected, check for odors and for stains or burns about the patient's mouth and for a source of poisoning nearby, such as pills, medicine bottles, household chemicals, or pesticides. Look for *all* injuries and treat minor as well as major illnesses in the following order of lifesaving priority: (1) stopped breathing, (2) bleeding, (3) poisoning, and (4) shock.

- **Carry out the necessary first aid.** Act according to the nature of the injury or sudden illness. Apply emergency dressings, bandages, and splints, or give other first aid as indicated. Remain with the victim and provide comfort until he can be turned over to some qualified person or persons (for example, a doctor, an ambulance crew, a rescue squad) or until he can care for himself. If a victim is revived by cardiopulmonary resuscitation (CPR), obstructed airway care, or other artificial means, he must be examined by a physician.

- **Know the limit of your capabilities.** Provide the patient with whatever appropriate first aid care you can give him. Using your best judgment based on first aid or emergency care knowledge, do what you think is necessary to cope with the particular emergency. Never, however, try to do more than you know you can do safely. It is as important to know *what not to do* as well as what to do.

FIRST AID FOR SPECIFIC PROBLEMS

If Breathing Stops

When breathing stops for any reason, begin mouth-to-mouth respiration immediately and continue until the person begins breathing for himself or until medical help arrives. Have someone else send for help as soon as possible. Follow these steps:

1. Tip the person's head back so that his chin juts up (Fig. 54). In this position, the tongue cannot block the throat so as to shut off

Fig. 54

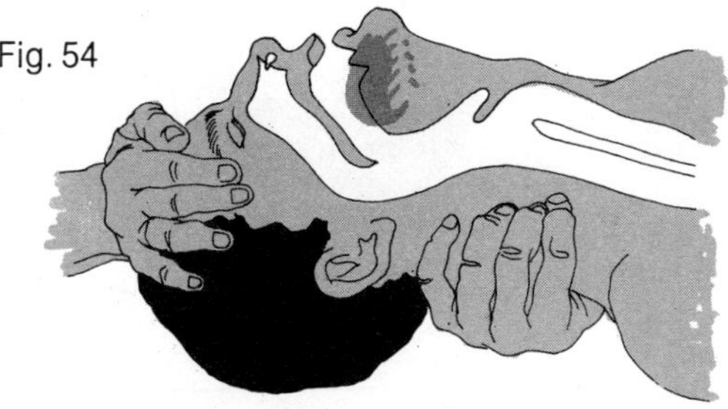

the flow of air. Place your ear close to the victim's mouth, listening and feeling for breathing. At the same time, watch for the rise and fall of the victim's chest for at least 5 seconds.
2. Pinch the victim's nose shut (Fig. 55A).
3. Take a deep breath, seal your mouth around the victim's mouth, and blow air into his lungs (Fig. 55B). You should be able to see or feel his chest rise. Start with four quick, full breaths, one after another, without allowing your lungs to completely empty between breaths.
4. Stop blowing and watch to see if the victim's chest falls as air leaves his lungs (Fig. 56).
5. Take another breath and repeat the cycle. Give at least one breath every 5 seconds (12 breaths per minute) for an adult.

If the victim is an infant or a small child, cover both his nose and mouth with your mouth and blow only small puffs of air (one breath every 3 seconds, or about 20 breaths per minute) as needed to make the chest rise and fall.

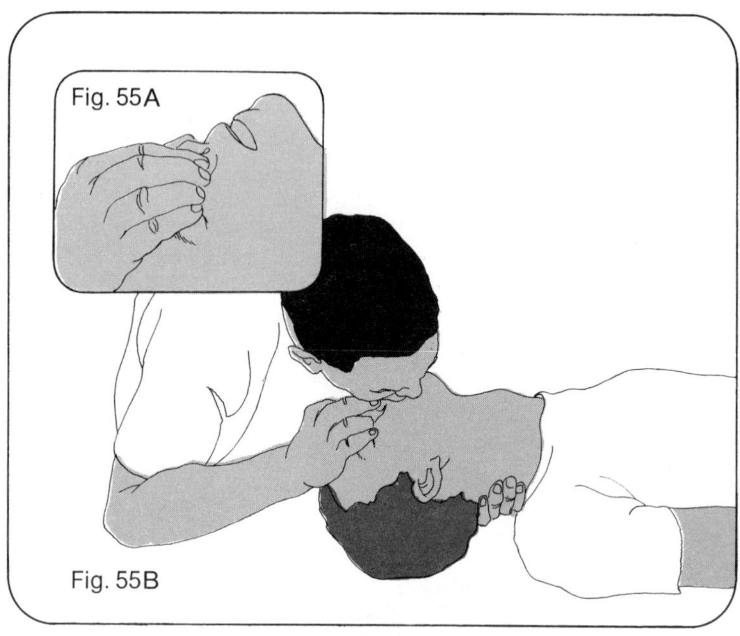

Fig. 55A

Fig. 55B

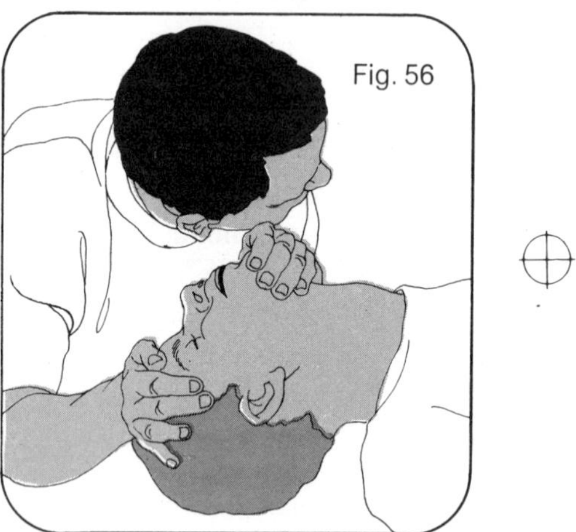

Fig. 56

If you cannot see the chest rise and fall or cannot hear the return rush of air, reposition the victim's head and attempt the breathing process again. Check to make sure that there is no food or other object stuck at the back of the victim's mouth.

If something is blocking the airway, use the procedures described on pages 312–319 to remove the material and restore breathing.

Wounds and Bleeding

Types of Wounds

A wound is an injury that causes either an internal or external break in body tissue. An *open* wound (as in a knife cut) is a break in the skin or the mucous membrane. The most common accidents that result in open wounds are falls, mishandling of sharp objects, accidents with tools and machinery, and car accidents. A *closed* wound (also referred to as a "contusion" or internal bleeding) is a bruise that occurs as a result of an injury that damages the underlying tissues without breaking the skin (as in a black eye).

There are five different types of open wounds:

- *Abrasions.* An abrasion (Fig. 57) is a skin wound caused by rubbing or scraping the skin against a hard, rough surface. Bleeding in this type of wound is usually limited, but it is important that the skin be cleaned in order to guard against infection.

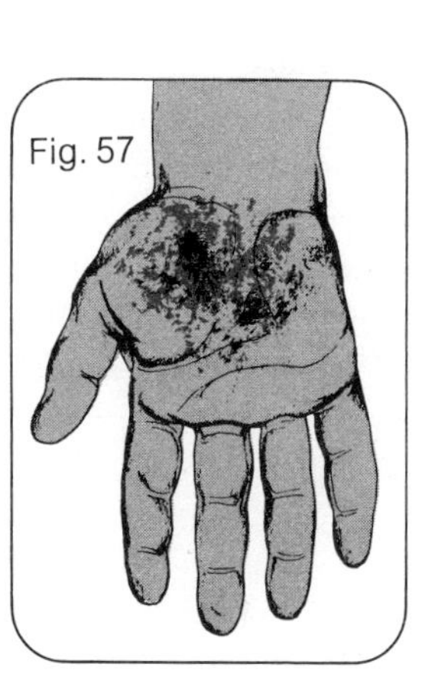
Fig. 57

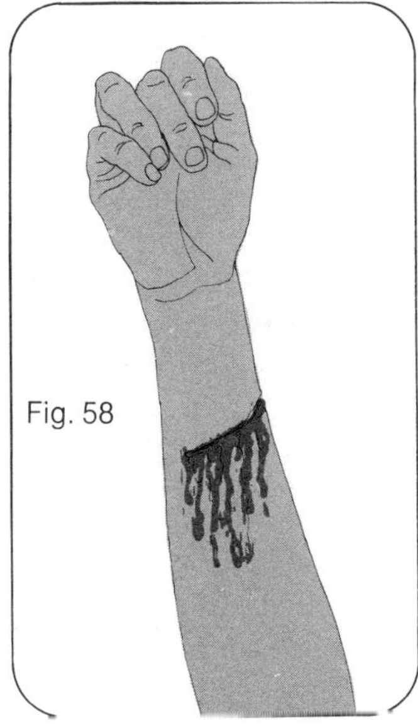
Fig. 58

- *Incisions.* An incision (Fig. 58) is a cut caused by a knife, the rough edge of metal, broken glass, a razor blade, or some other sharp object. This type of wound generally bleeds rapidly and heavily. If the cut is deep, muscles, tendons, and nerves may be damaged.

- *Lacerations.* A laceration (Fig. 59) is a jagged, irregular, or blunt breaking or tearing of soft tissues, often resulting from mishandling tools and machinery or other accidents. Bleeding from a laceration may be rapid and extensive.
- *Punctures.* A puncture (Fig. 60) is a piercing wound that causes a small hole in the tissues. Such objects as nails, needles, ice picks,

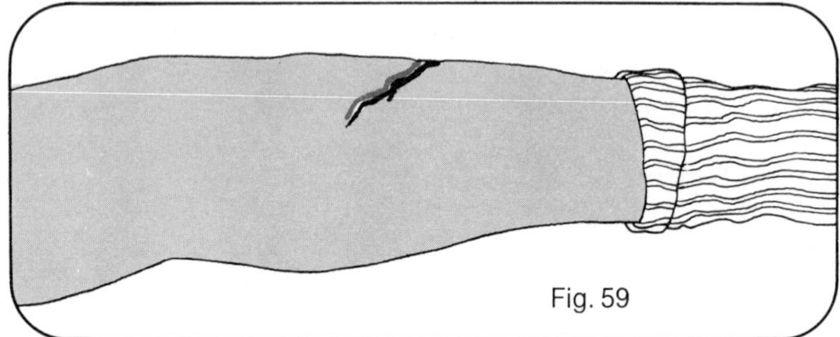
Fig. 59

and other pointed objects can produce puncture wounds. Even if external bleeding is slight, there may be serious internal bleeding resulting from internal damage to an organ (as in a gunshot wound). All puncture wounds require the attention of a health professional because of the danger of tetanus.

- *Avulsions.* An avulsion (Fig. 61) is a forcible tearing or partial tearing away of tissues. It occurs in such accidents as gunshot wounds, explosions, animal bites, or other body-crushing injuries. Bleeding is heavy and rapid. If a body part (a finger, tooth, or toe, for example) has been torn away in an accident, it should always be sent along with the victim to the hospital, since it can sometimes be reattached.

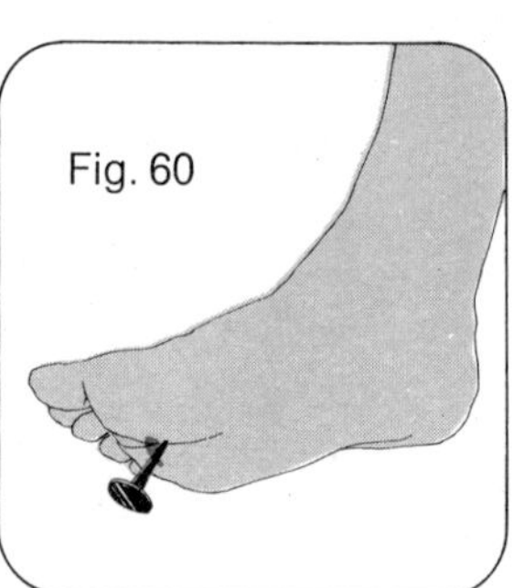
Fig. 60

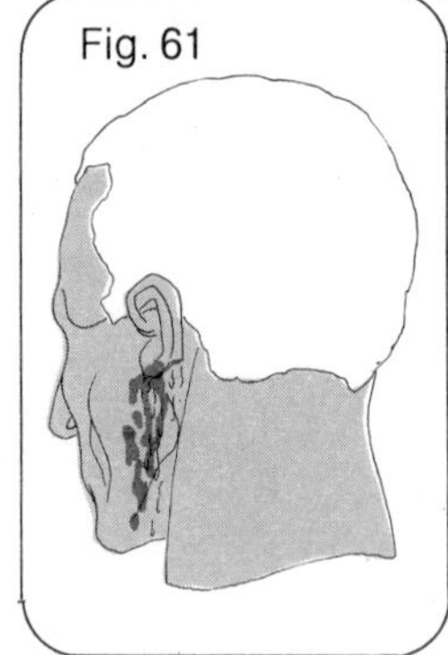
Fig. 61

First Aid for Minor Wounds

Small cuts and bruises generally do not require a great deal of attention. If a dressing (compress) is required to protect the wound and keep out infection, cleanse the wound with water as well as possible before applying a sterile dressing. Minor cuts, however, often heal more quickly if left uncovered. The health professional should advise whether stitches or further treatment will be needed.

Puncture wounds that stop bleeding rapidly present special problems. Such wounds can become infected easily and provide breeding areas for tetanus bacteria (lockjaw). They are difficult to clean because the flushing action of external bleeding is limited. Regardless of the amount of bleeding, a health professional should be consulted to determine whether a tetanus shot is needed.

First Aid for Severe Bleeding

It is urgent to stop any large, rapid loss of blood immediately. Shock and loss of consciousness may occur from the rapid loss of as little as a quart of blood. Direct pressure, by hand, should be applied over the wound with a clean dressing such as a thick pad of gauze, a folded clean cloth, or a sanitary napkin (Fig. 62). This prevents loss

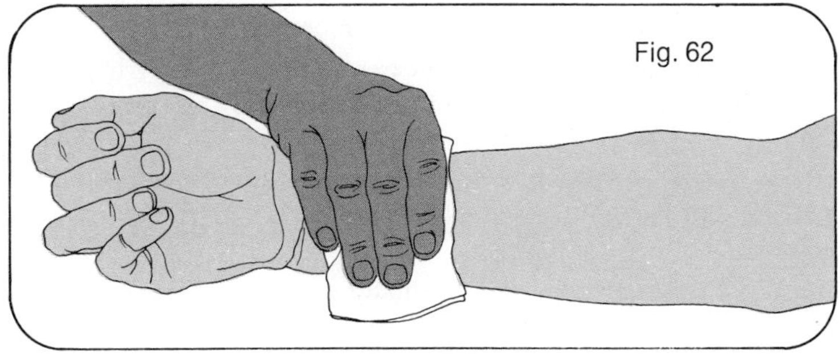
Fig. 62

of blood from the body without interfering with normal blood circulation. If a dressing is not available, pressure may be applied with the palm of the bare hand or the fingers, but only until a dressing can be obtained.

A dressing will help control the bleeding by absorbing the blood and permitting it to clot. If blood soaks through the dressing without clotting, leave the dressing where it is, add additional thick layers of cloth, and continue the hand pressure as firmly as possible. Do not apply absorbent cotton directly to the wound, since cotton fibers would be left in the wound. Do not apply adhesive directly to the wound, since that may cause additional bleeding when the adhesive is removed.

Pressure bandages, nylon hose, or a clean towel can also be used to hold a pad of cloth over a severely bleeding open wound. Place the center of the bandage directly over the pad on the wound and wind both ends of the bandage around the body part and then tie the bandage with the knot directly over the pad. Since pressure bandages and nylon hose restrict circulation, particular care should be used in applying them so that they are not too tight.

If there is no sign of fracture, a severely bleeding open wound of the hand, neck, arm, or leg should be raised above the level of the patient's heart. Apply pressure against the arterial pressure points first. These are located as follows:

For scalp wounds, in front of the ear (temporal artery)

For neck wounds, at the side of the windpipe (carotid artery)

For face wounds, at the jawbone (facial artery)

For shoulder and high arm wounds, at the inner part of the collarbone (subclavian artery)

For arm wounds, at the middle of the upper arm (brachial artery)

For leg wounds, at the mid-groin (femoral artery)

Never use a tourniquet except in cases of massive hemorrhaging (as with a severed limb) that cannot be controlled by any other means. The decision to use a tourniquet is in reality a decision to risk sacrifice of a limb in order to save a life. Once a tourniquet is applied, care by a physician is absolutely necessary. If a tourniquet must be applied, follow these steps:

1. Apply the tourniquet (which should be at least 2 inches, 5.1 centimeters, wide) immediately above the wound, taking care that it does not touch the edges to the wound. If the wound has occurred in a joint area or just below, the tourniquet should go just above the joint.
2. Wrap the tourniquet band tightly around the limb twice and tie a half knot (Fig. 63A).
3. Place a short, thick stick (or some similar object that will not break) on the half knot. Tie two half knots (or one full knot) on top of the stick (Fig. 63B).
4. Tighten the tourniquet by twisting the stick until the bleeding stops (Fig. 63C).

5. Secure the stick in place with the loose ends of the tourniquet (Fig. 63D), a strip of cloth, or other improvised material (Fig. 63E).
6. Attach a note to the victim's clothing giving the location of the tourniquet and the time it was applied. *Loosen the tourniquet only on the advice of a physician.* Never cover a tourniquet.

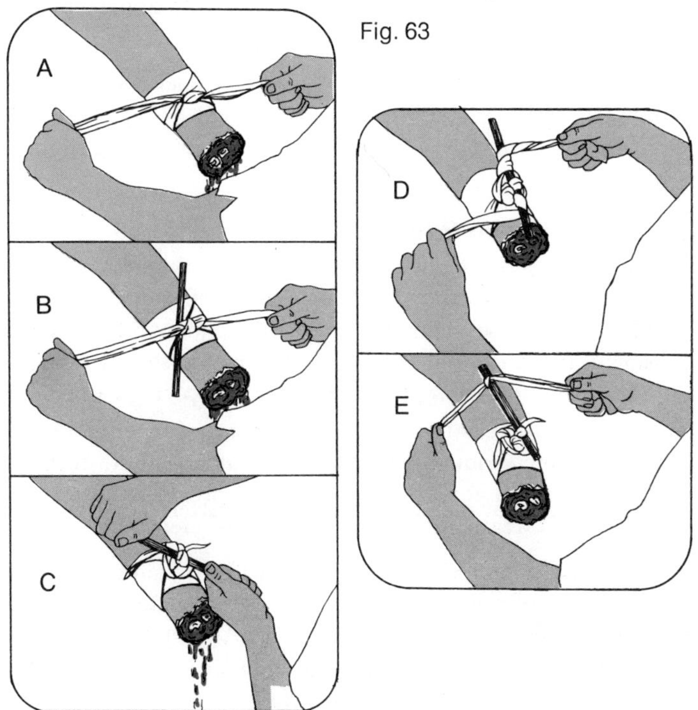

Fig. 63

First Aid for Closed Wounds and Internal Bleeding

Many closed wounds are relatively small injuries involving soft tissues, such as a black eye. Other closed wounds may involve internal bleeding plus severe physical damage to the tissues or organs.

Internal bleeding may occur with a wound or several other problems. Such problems might include a bleeding ulcer, a rupture of the bowel, a miscarriage or other pregnancy-related problem, or a bleeding condition. Some internal bleeding is visible (for instance, blood vomited from the stomach or expelled from the vagina); other internal bleeding signs are more difficult to determine (for example, a ruptured spleen).

When internal bleeding is severe, symptoms of shock (cold, moist skin, restlessness, and severe thirst) will often set in. The patient experiencing severe bleeding should be treated for shock and taken to the nearest emergency center at once. When internal bleeding is less severe, the patient should remain in bed and follow the advice of the health professional. Have a patient who is pregnant and has vaginal bleeding go to bed and call the health professional for advice immediately.

When a relatively small closed wound such as a black eye occurs, put cold applications (wrapped or covered) on the injured area to prevent additional swelling of tissue and to slow down internal bleeding.

Animal and Human Bites

A major danger associated with any bite that breaks the skin is infection. For this reason, the care of a health professional should be sought in all such cases. However, before the patient sees the health professional, first aid should be given, which consists of thoroughly washing the wound with soap and water and applying a dressing.

Human bites that break the skin are particularly dangerous because they may become seriously infected. The human mouth normally has many germs in it at all times. The health professional can order medications and treatments to prevent serious infection.

The bite of any animal, whether it is a pet or a wild animal, carries a great danger of infection. Rabies and tetanus are added dangers in animal bites from warm-blooded animals. Although a dog bite is likely to cause more extensive damage than a cat bite, the cat bite may be more dangerous. A wider variety of bacteria is usually present in the mouth of a cat.

Many wild animals, especially bats, raccoons, and rats, may transmit rabies. Rabies can even be transmitted when a rabid animal licks an open wound on a human or on a nonrabid animal.

Every effort must be made to capture any suspected rabid animal so that it can be determined by health authorities whether or not the animal has rabies. Do *not* kill the animal unless it is absolutely necessary to do so. If killing is necessary, take precautions not to damage the animal's head, because it should be examined by public health authorities.

If the animal proves to be rabid, vaccine therapy must be given to the infected person to build up body immunity in time to prevent the disease. If a suspected rabid animal cannot be caught or found and thus cannot be identified and observed, arrange for immediate medical care for any person it has bitten. Injections are effective in preventing rabies in 95 percent of patients. While waiting for the care of a health professional, administer first aid and advise the patient to avoid moving the affected part.

Nosebleeds

Nosebleeds may be the result of injury or of disease such as high blood pressure, or they may occur without known cause. Nosebleeds sometimes occur at high altitude, following athletic activity, or as the result of a cold or the lack of humidity in the house. Ordinarily, they are not serious. If the bleeding persists or is severe, however, the care of a health professional should be sought. Frequent nosebleeds should be investigated to determine the cause.

A person with a nosebleed should remain quiet, preferably sitting up and leaning forward. If it is necessary for him to lie down, his head and shoulders should be elevated. To stop the bleeding, press the bleeding nostril toward the center. Apply cold dressings to the victim's nose and face.

If bleeding is not controlled by pressure and dressings, a small, clean pad of gauze (not absorbent cotton) should be placed into one or both nostrils, and pressure should be applied on either side of the nostril with the thumb and index finger.

Poisoning

Poisoning by Mouth

Most victims of accidental poisoning are small children who have not been adequately protected from the dangers of the environment. Common household items that should be kept out of the reach of children include bleaches, detergents, soaps, water softeners, waxes, polishes, lighter fluid, cosmetics, kerosene, insecticides, and all types of drugs and medicines. Nearly all cases of accidental poisoning could have been prevented if parents of preschool children kept medicines and all other poisonous substances either locked away or out of climbing reach of children.

First aid for poisoning victims involves diluting or neutralizing the poison as quickly as possible with water or milk. *Do not attempt to induce vomiting* unless specifically advised to do so by the poison control center or physician. While one person administers first aid, another should call the area poison control center, if there is one nearby, or the family physician or an emergency room for further instructions. Treat the victim for shock and maintain an open airway. Note first aid instructions on the label of the container and read them to the poison control center or doctor. Be aware that the information on the label may be incorrect. Take the container to the hospital, because it will be helpful in identifying the poison. Save a sample of any vomitus (vomited material) to take to the hospital for evaluation.

Poisoning by Insect Bites or Stings

Stings from bees, wasps, hornets, and yellow jackets are generally painful and cause some local swelling. In some victims, death can occur because of acute allergic reactions. Bites of certain spiders (the black widow or the brown recluse) and some scorpions can cause severe illness as well. A person who is very allergic to insect bites or stings should carry such information where it can easily be found, such as on a bracelet or in a wallet.

First aid for minor reactions includes removing the stinger with tweezers if it is still in the skin, applying soothing applications such as baking soda or calamine lotion, and applying cold dressings. (See Chapter 23, "Special Nursing Measures.")

If the victim has a history of severe allergic reactions to insect bites, take him immediately to the nearest location where medical treatment is available, such as an emergency room. If he has medicine to combat the effects of the sting, he should take it immediately. Give artificial respiration if the victim is having trouble breathing.

If a severe reaction develops, place a constricting band above a bite (between the bite and the heart) that is on the victim's arm or leg. Keep the affected part below the level of the heart. Apply an ice bag to the area and consult a health professional about further treatment.

Contact Poisons

When the skin comes in contact with certain poisonous plants, a rash, itching, and redness will often appear within a few hours or within 1 to 2 days of exposure.

When exposure to a poisonous plant such as poison ivy is known to have occurred, washing the area with soap and water soon after the exposure can sometimes decrease the severity of the reaction or prevent it.

When a rash occurs, wash all exposed areas with soap and water, then with alcohol. If the rash is mild, apply calamine or other soothing lotion. Avoid scratching. Seek the advice of the health professional for severe reactions.

Shock

Shock is a condition in which many vital body functions are seriously depressed because of injury or illness. In all cases of shock, the normal supply of blood to the vital organs is reduced. Because the patient in shock has very unstable circulation, he should be handled gently and moved no more than absolutely necessary.

Shock may occur after a severe injury, from lack of oxygen, hemorrhage, or loss of body fluids other than blood (as in prolonged vomiting or diarrhea). It may result from food or chemical poisoning, heart attacks, strokes, or severe pain. The severity of shock is increased by abnormal changes in body temperatures and by the patient's exposure to more stress than he can tolerate.

Signs of Shock

When a person is in shock—

- His skin is pale or bluish. If the victim has dark skin, it may be necessary to rely primarily on the color of the mucous membrane on the inside of the mouth or of the eyelids, or the color of the nail beds.
- The skin is cold and may be moist to the touch if perspiration has occurred.
- The pulse is quite rapid and often too weak and faint to be felt at the radial artery at the wrist (Fig. 64) but it can be felt in the carotid artery at the side of the neck (Fig. 65).
- The rate of breathing generally increases and may be irregular.
- Breathing may be shallow or possibly deep. If there has been injury to the chest or abdomen, breathing will almost certainly be shallow because of the pain.
- The victim may be restless, anxious, weak, or dizzy, and he may thrash about.

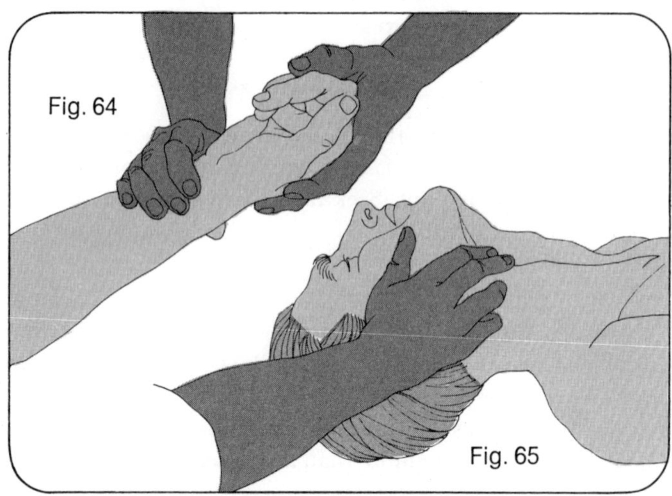

Fig. 64

Fig. 65

- The victim may complain of severe thirst.
- The victim may be nauseated and may vomit.

If the victim's condition worsens, the pupils of the eyes will become widely dilated, and the eyes may have a vacant look (Fig. 66). The

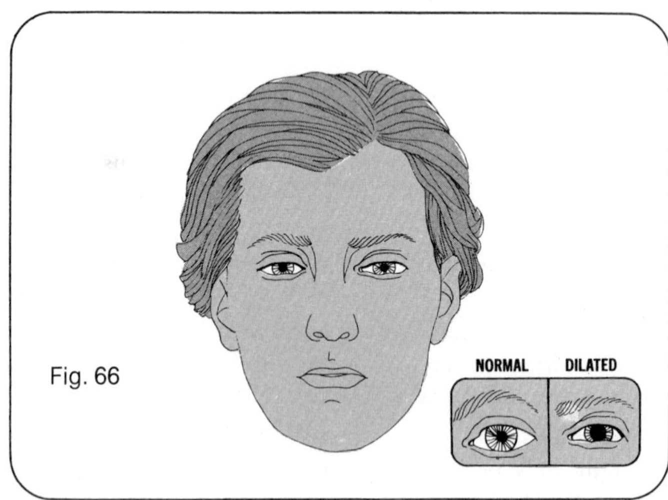

Fig. 66

victim may become unresponsive and uninterested in anything. If his skin develops a mottled appearance, it is an indication that his blood pressure has fallen to a low level. If not treated promptly, the person may become unconscious, his body temperature will drop, and he may die.

First Aid for Shock

1. *Get medical help at once.*
2. While waiting for help, reassure the patient. A calm attitude on the part of those around the patient can often help relieve some of the person's fear.
3. Loosen the victim's clothing gently and cover him *lightly,* depending on the environment. The point is to *retain* body heat but *not to add to it.* Place material such as a blanket or a coat under the victim to prevent chilling. Do *not* apply a heating pad, a hot water bottle, or an electric blanket, since it can make the victim's condition worse.
4. The preferred position for the patient in shock depends on his condition. If in doubt concerning the proper position for the patient, keep him lying flat. The unconscious patient should be placed on his side with his head turned to one side to prevent choking on fluids, vomitus, or blood. If the patient has a head injury or is experiencing trouble in breathing, slightly raise his head and shoulders unless other injuries make doing so unwise. If there is an abdominal injury, leave the patient lying flat. Some patients benefit by having their feet elevated from 8 to 12 inches (20.3–30.5 centimeters) as they lie flat. However, if elevating the feet increases difficulty in breathing or causes pain, the feet should be lowered.

Fluids are valuable in the treatment of shock but *should not be given when medical assistance is available within an hour.* Fluids should *never* be given to the patient who is unconscious, who is vomiting, or who is having convulsions, since choking may occur. Nor should fluids be given to someone who may need surgery or who has brain or abdominal injuries, because doing so could be harmful. *If medical care is delayed for an hour or more, fluids should be given,* except when the patient has any of the conditions mentioned above. A salt-soda solution—1 level teasponful of salt and ½ level teaspoonful of baking soda to each quart (.946 liter) of water or two pinches of salt to one pinch of soda per glass (8–10 ounces), or 226.8–283.5 grams—may be given as follows:

For an adult, about 4 ounces, or 118.3 milliliters (½ glass) every 15 minutes

For a child, 1 to 12 years old, 2 ounces, or 59.2 milliliters (½ glass), every 15 minutes

For infants under 1 year old, 1 ounce (29.6 milliliters) every 15 minutes

Stop giving fluids immediately if the victim becomes nauseated.

Specific Injuries

Head Injuries

Following any head injury, attention should be paid to the mental state of the victim. When changes such as unconsciousness, confusion, or drowsiness occur, medical attention is needed immediately because of the danger of brain damage. If progressive drowsiness and unconsciousness occur, they could indicate swelling of the brain or bleeding inside the skull. The victim should be taken immediately to the nearest emergency clinic or trauma center.

Wounds of the scalp, even if small, tend to bleed profusely. The severity of the wound may be concealed by thick hair. Scalp wounds may be complicated by brain injury, skull fractures, or contamination by foreign materials.

Do not attempt to cleanse scalp wounds, because more serious bleeding may result. Bleeding should be controlled by raising the victim's head and shoulders and applying a snug, sterile dressing to the wound. Excessive pressure should not be used, because there could be a skull fracture. When bleeding is under control, wrap a bandage around the head to hold the dressing in place and to provide continuing pressure.

Broken Bones

A fracture is a break or crack in a bone. It can occur from a fall or an automobile or sports accident. A simple fracture does not involve an open wound on the body surface. A compound fracture does include an open wound. Simple fractures are more common than compound ones and must be diagnosed by the health professional with the help of X-ray examinations. Fractures are generally accompanied by pain and difficulty in moving the injured part. There may be swelling, discoloring, or an obvious deformity.

First aid for fractures depends on which body part is injured. In general, the injured part and the joints next to it should be immobilized.

If it is possible, elevate a broken arm or leg (after it has been splinted) without disturbing the suspected fracture. (When an injury of the neck or the spinal cord is suspected, *never* move the victim without a rigid support for his back, neck, and head.) Do *not* attempt to straighten a limb or push a protruding bone end back in.

In a serious accident, unless the victim is in danger, do not attempt to move him. Let the ambulance or rescue squad personnel move the victim. In situations when there is a delay in transportation, or when ambulance service is not available, splints may be applied according to the directions in the *Standard First Aid and Personal Safety* textbook published by the American Red Cross.

In a compound fracture (with an open wound), control bleeding by applying pressure through a large sterile dressing over the wound. Cover the entire wound with the dressing or with freshly laundered sheets or towels in such a way as to provide mild pressure on the wound.

Injured persons with suspected fractures should be examined by a health professional as soon as possible to prevent possible complications. If a fracture is found to be present, prompt treatment of the injury can prevent permanent deformity of the injured body part.

Burns

Burns, frequently the result of unsafe practices in the home, can be caused by dry heat (such as from electrical equipment), wet heat (scalds from steam or hot liquids), or chemical agents (lye, strong acids, and detergents).

In general, an adult who has suffered burns over 15 percent of his body surface (with a child, 10 percent) requires hospitalization. The area of the burn may be a crucial factor. Burns of the face are often associated with injury to the respiratory tract and may obstruct breathing as swelling increases. Burns on the hands and feet can be very painful and may involve loss of functioning. Prompt medical attention is necessary.

Burns are classified according to depth or degree of skin damage:

- *First degree burns* (Fig. 67) are characterized by redness, mild swelling and pain, and rapid healing. They may be the result of overexposure to the sun, scalding by a hot liquid or steam, or light contact with a hot object.

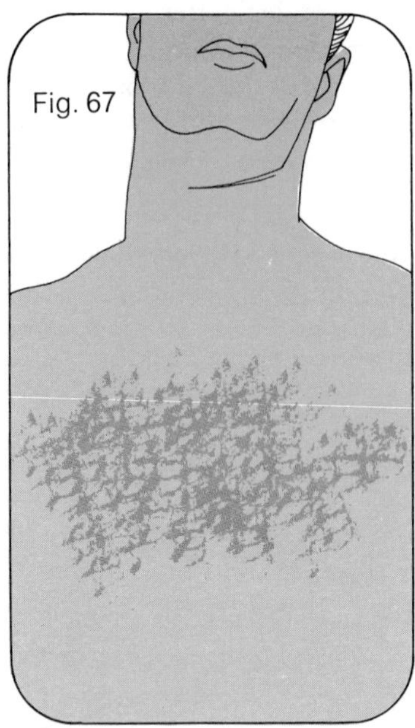

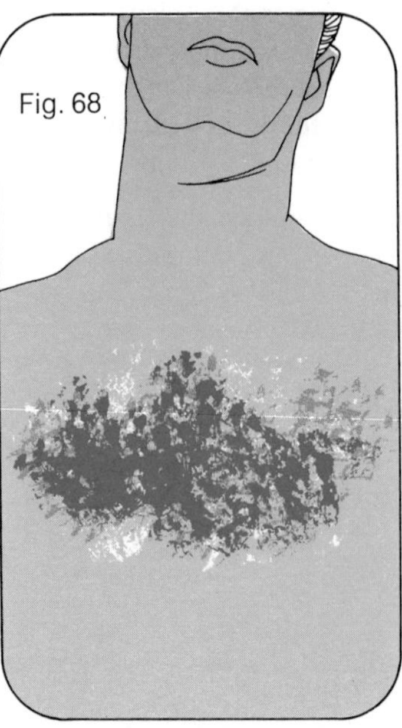

First aid consists of immediately putting the burned area in cold water or applying cold, wet dressings. If it is necessary for protection, apply a dry dressing. Do not apply other preparations unless advised to do so by the health professional.

For sunburn, a cool bath or cold, wet dressings can bring relief from pain. A severe sunburn requires medical treatment.

- *Second degree burns* (Fig. 68) are characterized by a red or mottled appearance, blisters, pain, and either swelling or a wet appearance on the surface of the skin or both. They may be the result of deep sunburn, contact with hot liquid, or flash burns from gasoline or kerosene. First aid is as follows:

  If the skin is not broken, immerse the burned area in cold water for 1–2 hours, or apply clean cloths that have been wrung out in cold water.

  Blot the area dry gently, then cover the area with dry, sterile gauze or a clean cloth for protection.

  Do not apply antiseptic preparations, sprays, ointments, or other home remedies to severe burns.

  Do not open blisters and do not remove burned tissue.

If arms or legs are affected, keep them elevated.

Consult a health professional for advice on further treatment.

- *Third degree burns* (Fig. 69) are characterized by deep tissue destruction, white or charred appearance, and loss of all layers of the skin.

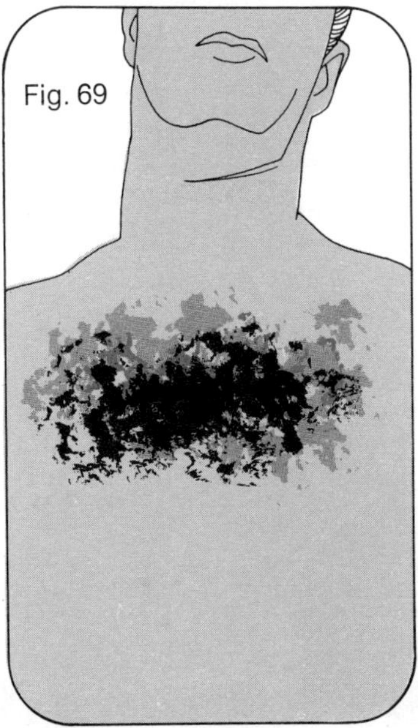

Fig. 69

They can be caused by flame, burning clothing, very hot water, contact with hot objects, or electricity. Skin grafting is usually necessary for healing. First aid is as follows:

Protect the burned area from the air with a thick, sterile, dry dressing or gauze, ironed or laundered sheets, or other household linens.

Immediately arrange for transportation to the hospital.

Make no attempt to strip away clothing from charred areas until help arrives.

Elevate burned feet or legs. Keep burned hands above the level of the victim's heart.

Make sure that persons with face burns either sit up or are propped up and are constantly observed for difficulty in breathing.

Do not immerse large areas of the body in cold water or apply ice water over large areas, because cold may intensify any shock reaction.

Apply a cold pack to the face or to the hands or feet after bandaging.

Do not apply any sprays, ointments, or other remedies.

Have the victim sip fluids slowly if medical help will not be available for an hour or more and if he is conscious and not vomiting. Give him 1 level teaspoonful of salt and ½ level teaspoonful of baking soda to each quart (.946 liter) of lukewarm water, or mix two pinches of salt to one pinch of soda in one glass of water (8–10 ounces, or 236.6–295.7 milliliters).

- *Chemical burns* require special treatment. Wash away the chemical with large amounts of water at once, using the shower or a hose, if either one is available, for at least 5 minutes (Fig. 70). Remove the

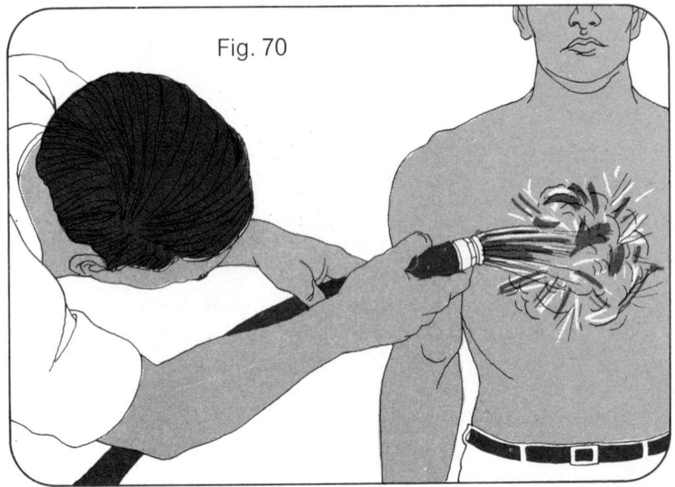
Fig. 70

victim's clothing from the involved area. Cover the burned area with a clean, dry dressing. If the chemical container is available, follow the first aid instructions given on the label. Get medical help at once.

Chemical burns of the eyes should be treated immediately with large amounts of water. The face, eyelid, and eye should be washed for at least 15 minutes. If the victim is lying down, turn his head to the side, hold the eyelid open, and pour water from the inner corner of the eye outward, making sure that the chemical does not wash into the other eye. Cover the affected eye with a dry, sterile dressing and bandage it to hold it in place. Do not permit the patient to rub his eyes. Rush him to the emergency room of the nearest hospital.

Sunburn

The most effective preventive measure against sunburn is to limit the length of time you are exposed to the sun the first time, especially if you are sensitive to the sun. For swimming and sunbathing, the first exposure should not exceed 15 minutes, with gradual increases of from 5 to 10 minutes.

During the summer, especially when participating in water sports, children and adults should avoid long exposure to the sun from mid-morning until midafternoon, when the rays of the sun are most direct. People involved in outdoor work or sports should wear protective clothing during this critical period.

People with light complexions should use sunburn prevention preparations. Commercial preparations are available for sunburn protection; however, all are not equally effective, and some may cause individual allergic reactions. You should test small samples on your skin before applying very much.

Your eyes should be protected from overexposure to the glare of sun, sand, water, ice, and snow. You can achieve protection by using sunglasses and hats or caps with visors.

A cool bath or cold, wet dressings can bring relief from the pain of sunburn. A severe sunburn requires medical treatment.

Foreign Bodies

Foreign Bodies in the Eye

Any object that gets into the eye is potentially harmful because it may become embedded in the eye or may scratch its surface. The eye should not be rubbed. If you think something is embedded in your eye, you should see a physician.

If a foreign body is on the surface of the eyeball or on the inner surface of the eyelid, the following first aid steps should be taken:

1. The lower lid should be pulled down to determine whether the object is on the inner surface. If it is on the inner surface, the object should be lifted off gently with the corner of a clean handkerchief or paper tissue, but never with dry cotton.

2. If the object is not visible on the inner surface of the lower eyelid, grasp the lashes of the upper lid gently (the patient should look down) and pull the upper lid forward and down over the lower lid. Tears may dislodge the object.
3. If the object is still in place, a matchstick may be placed against the outer part of the upper eyelid (Fig. 71A), and the eyelid should be turned up and over the matchstick (Fig. 71B). While

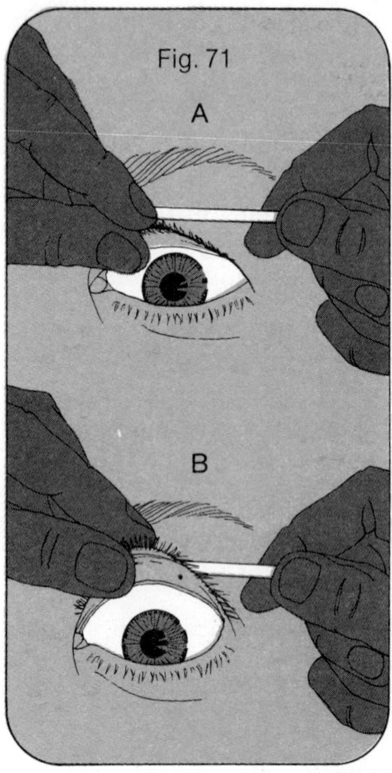

doing this, tell the patient to continue to look down. The foreign body may then be visible and may be removed gently with the corner of a handkerchief. The eyelid will return to normal when the patient looks upward, or it may be returned to place by pulling gently downward on the lashes. The eye should then be flushed with water.

4. If the object still remains in the eye, or if the object has in any way damaged the eye, cover the injured eye, or both eyes if possible, with a dry, protective dressing and take the patient to a doctor immediately.

Foreign Bodies in the Throat or Air Passage

One of the leading causes of death in the home is obstruction of breathing due to foreign objects trapped in the throat or in the air passage. Two thirds of such deaths occur among children under the age of 4, who either place objects in their mouth out of curiosity or are given food (such as nuts, raw fruits, or chunks of meat) before they have enough teeth to chew food well. Airway obstruction in adults may occur when unchewed meat or food is swallowed or when an object is breathed into the air passage.

Foreign bodies that enter the airway are often successfully removed by coughing. Foreign bodies that block the air passages, however, create an extreme emergency. If someone who has been eating is suddenly unable to speak, cough, or breathe, if his face turns blue, or if he uses the "distress signal" (clutching at his throat), he is choking (Fig. 72).

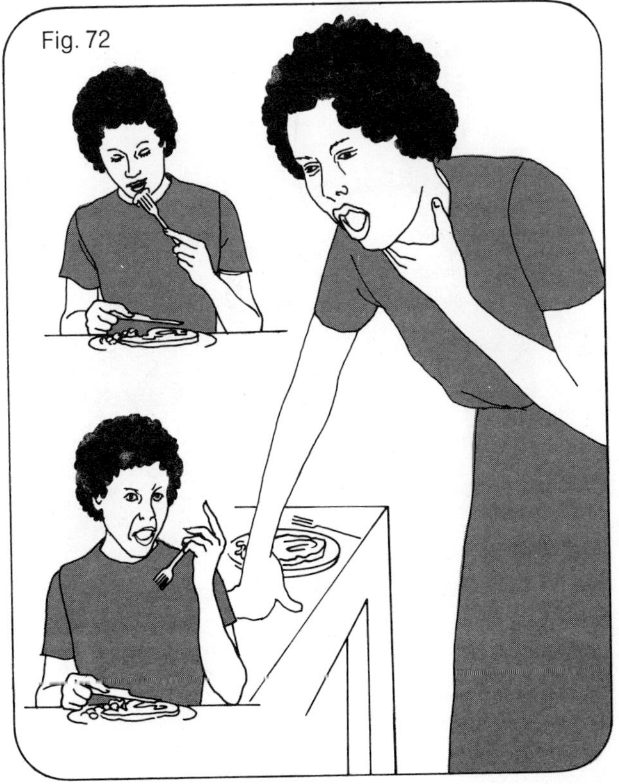
Fig. 72

Removal by Thrusts

For a conscious choking victim, the steps that follow should be performed at once, with no hesitation or interruption, in an attempt to dislodge the foreign body. The procedure may be carried out while the victim is in either a sitting, standing, or lying position. The procedure is as follows:

1. Position yourself slightly behind the victim and at one side. The victim's head should be level with or lower than his chest, if possible.
2. *If the victim is standing or sitting,* deliver four sharp, forceful blows in rapid succession with the heel of your hand between the victim's shoulder blades, over his spine, while placing your other hand on the front of his chest to provide support (Fig. 73).

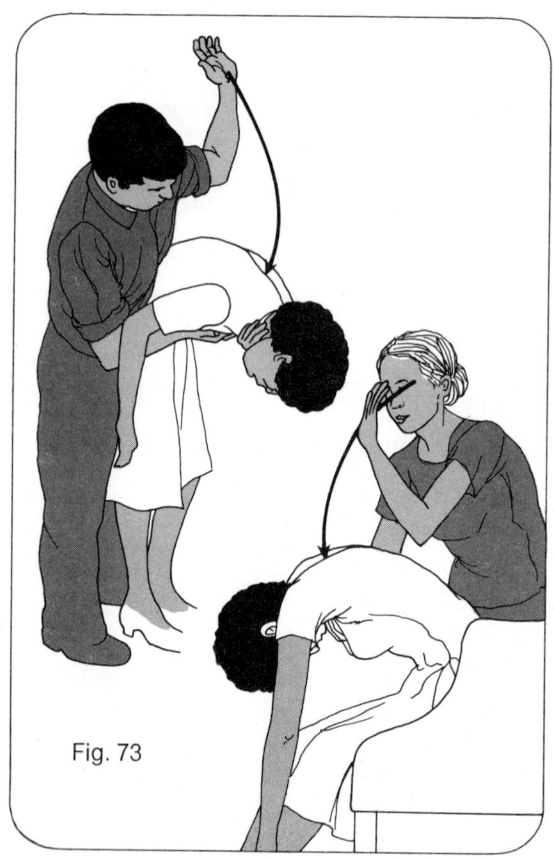

Fig. 73

3. *If the victim is lying down,* kneel and roll him onto his side, facing you with his chest against your knees, and deliver four sharp blows as described above (Fig. 74).

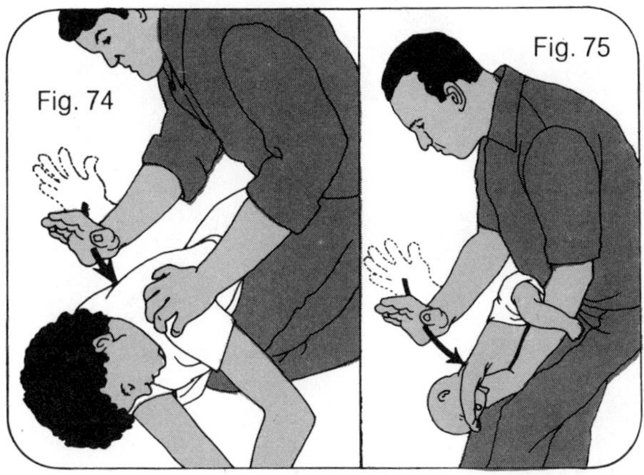
Fig. 74
Fig. 75

4. If the victim is an infant or a child, place him face down on your forearm, with his head down, and deliver four sharp blows (not as hard as for an adult) as described above (Fig. 75). Do not place an infant or a child in a head-down position if his breathing is only partially obstructed and if he is able to breathe adequately in the upright position.
5. Proceed to the use of manual thrusts, as described below, without hesitation.

Manual thrusts are a rapid series of movements, directed to the victim's upper abdomen or chest, that force air from the lungs. Either an abdominal or a chest thrust may be used.

The abdominal thrust procedure varies with the victim's position:

- When the victim is standing or sitting (Fig. 76)–

  Stand behind the victim and wrap your arms around his waist. Place the thumb side of your fist against the victim's abdomen, palm down, and exert a *quick* upward thrust.
- When the victim is lying down (Fig. 77)–

  Place the victim on his back and kneel beside or astride him. Place the heel of one of your hands in the middle of the victim's abdomen, slightly above the navel and below the rib cage, and place your other hand on top of it.

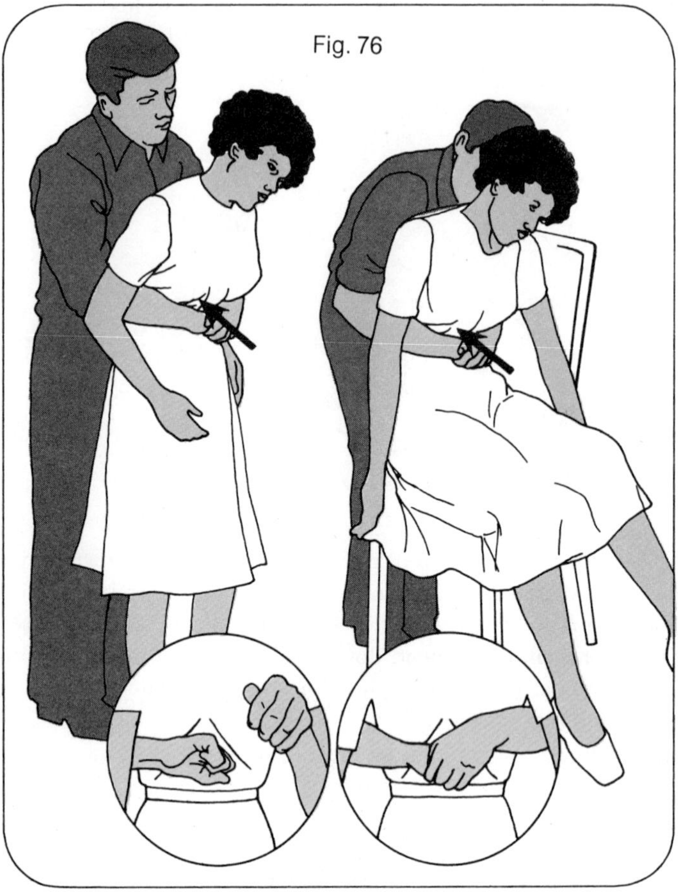

Fig. 76

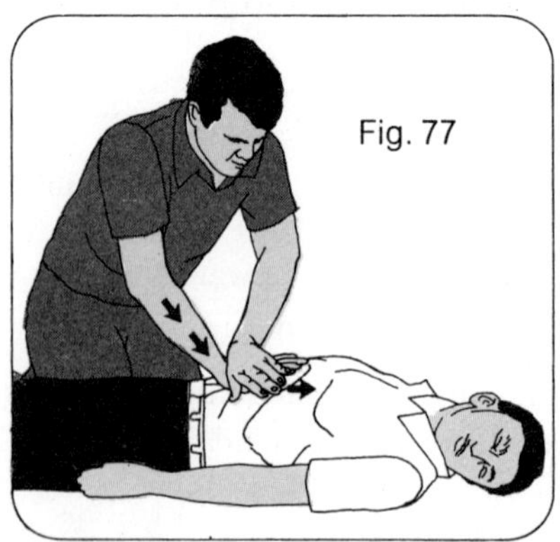

Fig. 77

Rock forward so that your shoulders are directly over the victim's abdomen and press toward the diaphragm (Fig. 78) with a *quick upward thrust.*

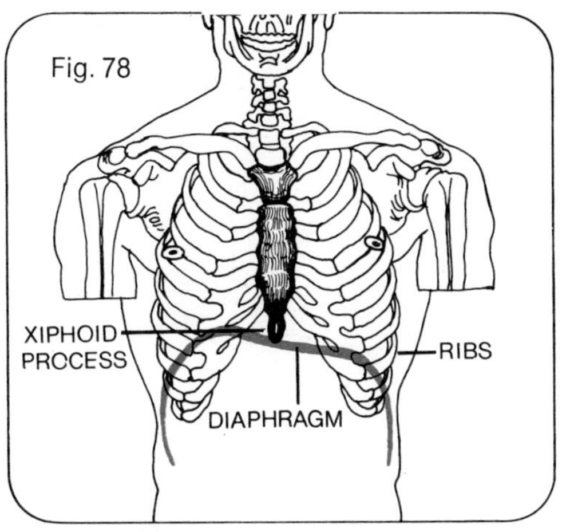

Fig. 78

Do not press to either side.

Repeat the thrust four times, if necessary.

The chest thrust is done as an alternate to the abdominal thrust. It is especially useful if the victim is excessively fat or is in a condition of advanced pregnancy, when the rescuer's arms cannot reach around the victim's abdomen. To give chest compression correctly, great care must be taken to apply pressure on the proper area of the breastbone. *Never push directly on the lower end of the breastbone,* because doing so will injure the victim. The breastbone runs down the front of the chest, and the ribs join it in front. The correct place to apply pressure is from 1 to 1½ inches (2.5–3.8 centimeters) or about the width of three fingers, from the lower tip (also called the ziphoid) of the breastbone.

- When the victim is standing or sitting (Fig. 79)—

  Stand behind the victim, place your arms under his armpits, and reach around his chest.

  Place the thumb side of your fist on the victim's breastbone, but not on the lower tip of it, or place it on the lower edge of the rib cage.

  Grasp your fist with your other hand and exert a quick backward thrust.

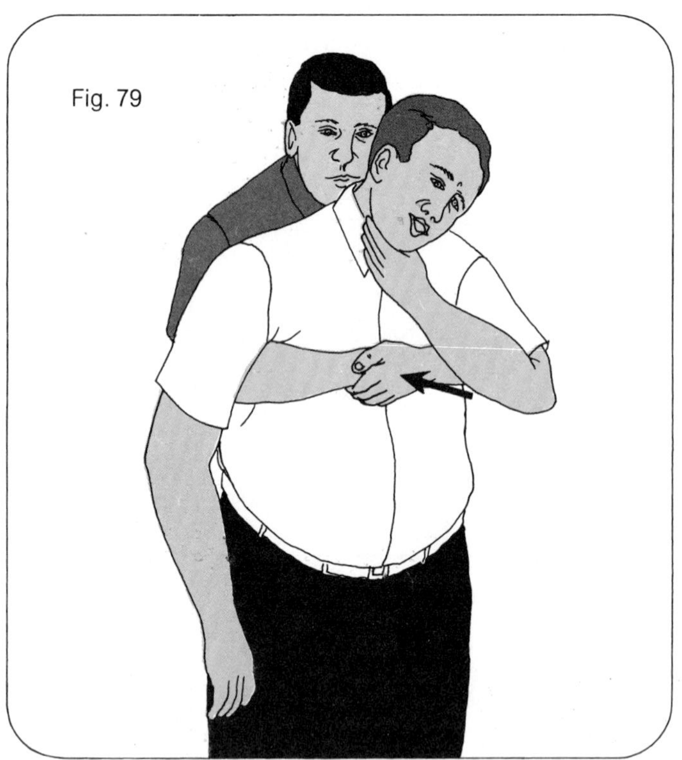
Fig. 79

- When the victim is lying down (Fig. 80)–

  Place the victim on his back and kneel close to his side. Stand on your knees; don't sit on your heels.

  Locate the lower tip of the victim's breastbone, using your hand that is nearer to his feet. Measure up 1 to 1½ inches (2.5–3.8 centimeters) from the lower tip of the breastbone, about the width of three fingers.

  With your shoulders directly over the breastbone, and with your fingers pointing across the victim's chest away from you, push with your arms and shoulders straight down. Do not push when you are moving forward. Do not put your hand at an angle, because you will push too much on the ends of the ribs where they join the breastbone. Doing so can injure the victim.

Manual Removal

If the presence of a foreign body in the mouth is strongly suspected

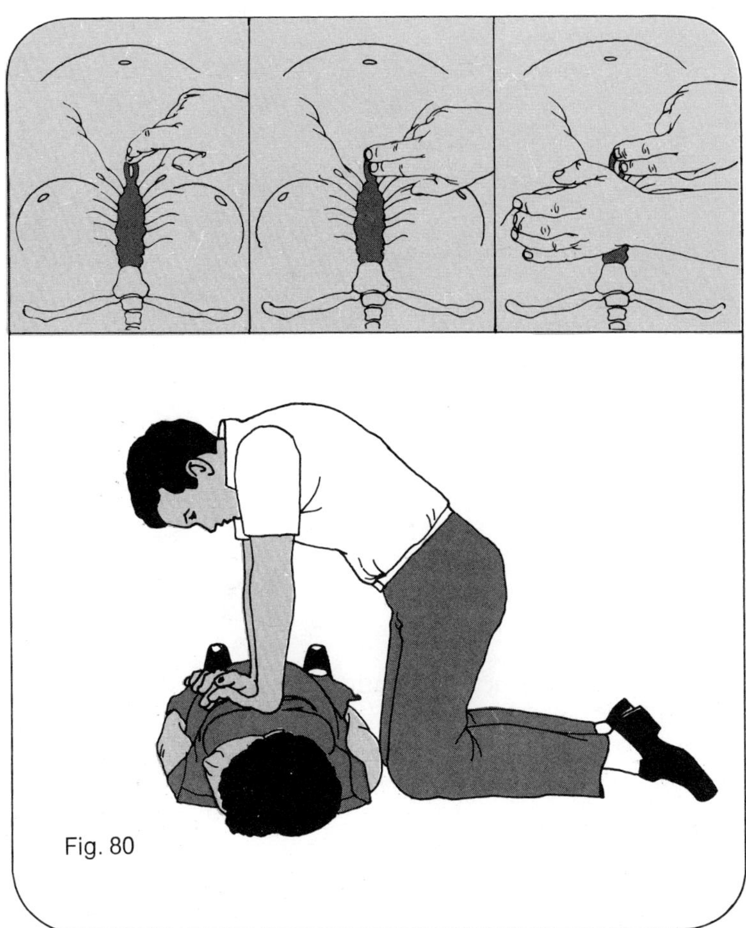
Fig. 80

or can be seen, the object should be removed with the fingers. If it cannot be seen, the combination of back blows and manual thrusts may expel it or dislodge it so that it can be more easily removed by the fingers.

If the patient has good air exchange with only partial obstruction and is still able to speak or cough effectively, do not interfere with his attempts to expel a foreign body.

It is difficult to remove foreign bodies from the airway with your fingers, and in most cases it is impossible to open the mouth of a conscious person.

For the unconscious victim, the following procedures are used after the manual thrusts:

1. Tongue-jaw lift.
   To try to open the victim's airway and sweep with your finger, grasp both the tongue and lower jaw between your thumb and fingers and lift (Fig. 81).

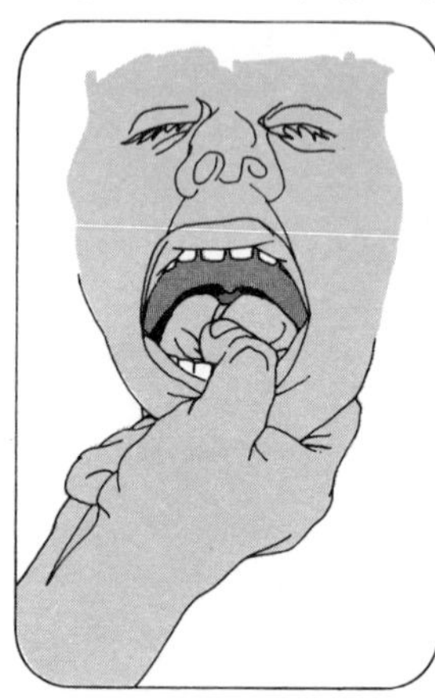

Fig. 81

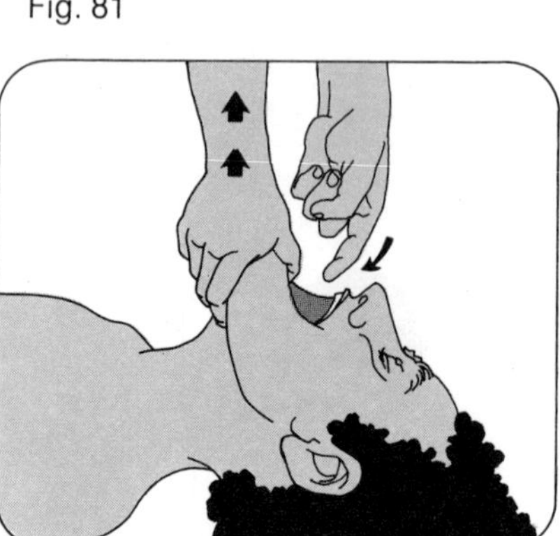

2. Finger sweep.
   After opening the victim's mouth, insert the index finger of your other hand down the inside of the victim's cheek and deeply into the throat to the base of the tongue (Fig. 82). Next, use a hooking action with your finger to dislodge the foreign body and get it into the mouth for removal (Fig. 83). Be careful not to force the object deeper into the airway.

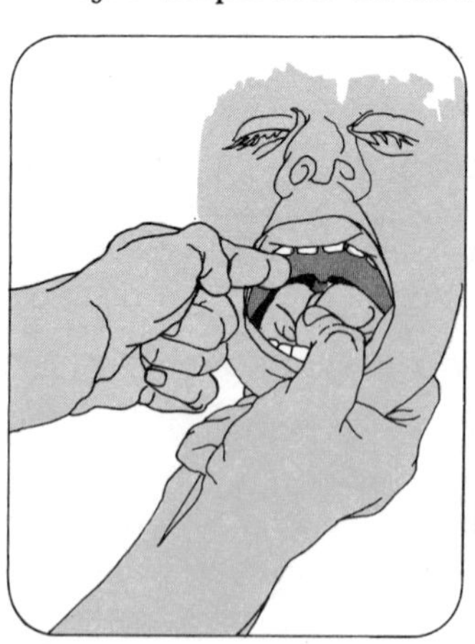

Fig. 82

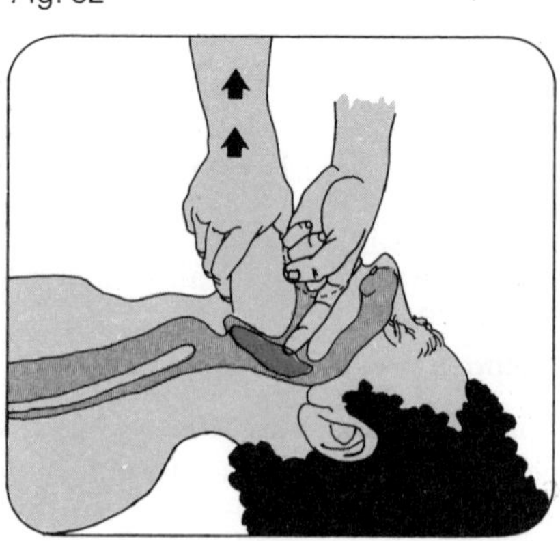

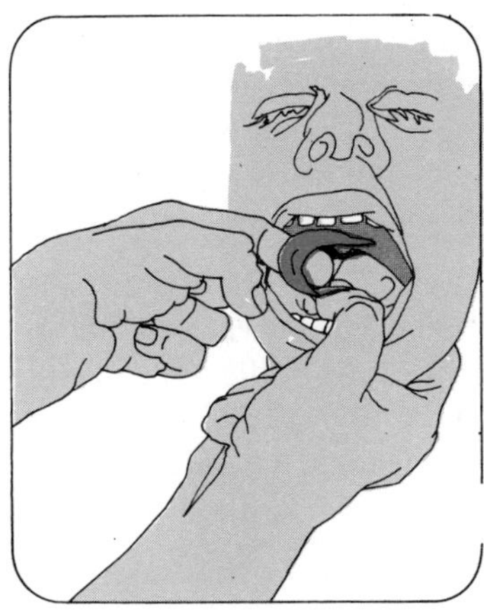

Fig. 83

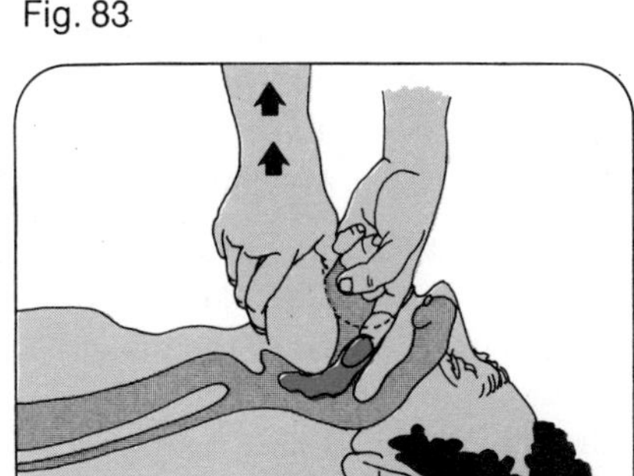

Remember the steps to follow for resuscitation of the unconscious victim:

1. Attempt to ventilate
2. Back blows
3. Manual thrusts
4. Finger sweep
5. Attempt to ventilate
6. Back blows
7. Manual thrusts

Foreign Bodies in the Skin

When a small splinter of wood or a glass fragment becomes embedded in the skin, or just beneath the surface of the skin, it should be removed to prevent infection.

If the object is close to the surface of the skin, use tweezers sterilized over a flame or in boiling water to pull out the object. If it is just beneath the skin, lift it out with the tip of a needle that has been sterilized in the heat of a flame. If it is embedded deeper in the tissues, only a health professional should remove it.

Foreign Bodies in the Ear

Seeds, beads, pebbles, or other small objects may be pushed into the ear by small children. Sometimes an insect crawls into an ear. Any object in the ear requires the attention of a health professional. An untrained person may push the object farther into the canal of the ear, perhaps causing injury to the eardrum and making the object more difficult to remove. Never use cotton swabs, hairpins, or other such devices to remove objects from the ear. Do not delay medical attention, particularly if the foreign body is a dried seed that may absorb moisture and swell, making it harder to remove.

If an insect has entered someone's ear, turn the victim onto his side and drip warm olive oil or baby oil into the affected ear canal. This will stop the buzzing (the insect usually drowns in the oil) and will cause the insect to float out. Then drain the oil by tilting the head to the other side. If this treatment is not effective, consult a health professional.

Foreign Bodies in the Nose

Blowing the nose hard is not an advisable method of removing a foreign body from the nose. Young children, particularly, should avoid doing this, because they may sniff instead, lodging the object more deeply or even inhaling it into the lungs. If an object is not easily removed, take the patient to a health professional.

Heat Exhaustion, Heat Cramps, and Heat Stroke

The body may suffer a number of reactions when exposed to excessive heat. The elderly, the very young, chronic invalids, alcoholics, and overweight persons are likely to have heat reactions, especially during heat waves in areas where moderate temperatures are normal.

Heat Exhaustion

In heat exhaustion, the body temperature is almost normal. In the body's effort to lose heat, blood pools in the capillaries of the skin, blocking circulation to vital organs and constricting the smaller veins. Symptoms of heat exhaustion include pale and clammy skin, tiredness, profuse sweating, dizziness, nausea (and perhaps vomiting), headache, and, in some cases, fainting (Fig. 84). First aid is as follows:

1. Move the victim to an air-cooled room but take care to avoid his becoming chilled.
2. Loosen any tight clothing.
3. Apply cool, wet cloths and fan the victim.

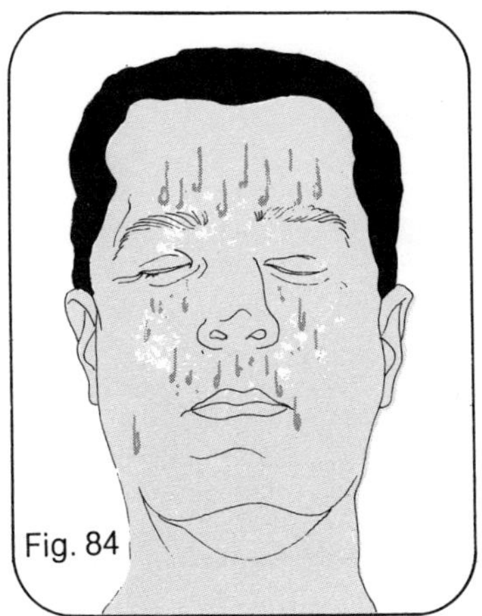
Fig. 84

4. Have the victim lie down with his feet elevated 8–12 inches (20.3–30.5 centimeters).
5. Give the victim sips of salt water (one teaspoon of salt per glass, half a glass every 15 minutes) for about 1 hour.
6. If vomiting occurs, stop giving the victim liquids and take him to a hospital.

The victim should make no attempt to resume activities for several days and should protect himself from exposure to unusually high temperatures.

Heat Cramps

Heat cramps involve muscular spasms and pain, generally in the muscles of the legs and abdomen. Cramps are caused by the loss of body salt and water (through profuse sweating), which is not replaced. Give first aid by replacing salt, giving salt water as described for heat exhaustion. Gentle massage is also helpful in relieving muscle spasms.

Heat Stroke

Heat stroke occurs when a person remains too long in great heat—usually the heat from the direct rays of the sun. Symptoms of heat stroke are very high body temperature—possibly 106°F (41.1°C) or higher—and complete absence of sweating. The skin is hot, red, and

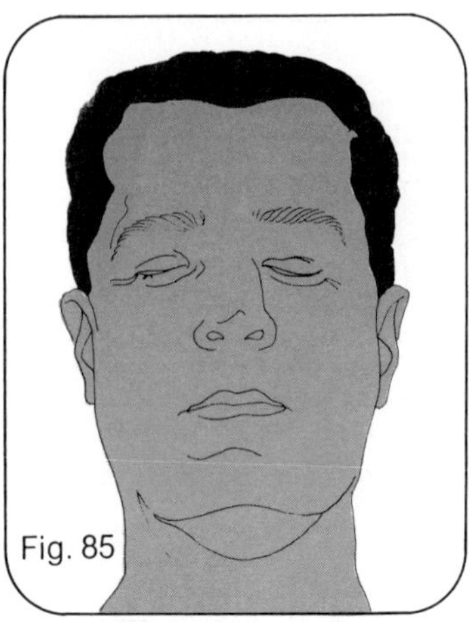
Fig. 85

dry (Fig. 85). Heat stroke, a life-threatening emergency, requires immediate medical attention. Call for medical help first, then take immediate steps to cool the victim's body quickly. Take care to avoid overchilling the patient once his temperature drops below 102°F (38.9°C). First aid is as follows:

1. Sponge the victim's bare skin with cool water or rubbing alcohol repeatedly OR apply cold packs continuously OR place the victim in a tub of cold water (do not add ice) until his temperature is lowered.
2. Turn on fans or air conditioners, if they are available, since drafts promote cooling.
3. If the patient's temperature starts to go up again, start the cooling process again.

Do not give the patient any stimulants (such as coffee or tea).

Frostbite and Exposure to Cold

Frostbite occurs when ice crystals form in the fluids and soft tissues of the skin. The effects are more severe if the injured area thaws and then refreezes. Usually the affected area is small: nose, cheeks, ears, fingers, and toes are the most commonly affected areas.

Just before frostbite occurs, the skin may be slightly flushed. When the skin turns white or grayish-yellow, frostbite has set in. Often there is no pain.

To treat frostbite, protect the affected area from further injury, warm it quickly, and maintain respiration. First aid procedures are as follows:

1. Bring the victim indoors as soon as possible and cover him with blankets or extra clothing.
2. Give the victim a warm, *nonalcoholic* drink.
3. Place the frostbitten area in warm (never hot) water. If warm water is not available or practical to use, wrap the affected area gently in a sheet or a warm blanket. Never apply a heat lamp or a hot water bottle.
4. Never rub affected areas.
5. Once the affected area is warm again, stop the warming process and have the patient exercise the area.
6. If the patient's feet are involved, do not allow him to walk after the affected part thaws.
7. If fingers or toes are involved, place dry, sterile gauze between them to keep them apart.
8. Elevate the frostbitten parts.
9. Give fluids—one level teaspoonful of salt and one half teaspoonful of baking soda to each quart (.95 liter) of lukewarm water, or mix two pinches of salt and one pinch of soda in one glass of water.
10. Obtain medical assistance as soon as possible.

Hypothermia

A person with hypothermia has an abnormally low body temperature 95°F (35°C) or lower. Hypothermia occurs when the body loses heat faster than it can produce it.

Hypothermia may occur on any person who is exposed to extremely cold temperature without adequate protection. Many elderly persons, however, develop hypothermia after exposure to relatively mild cold temperatures in the range of 60–65°F (15.6–18.3°C). The likeliest victims among the elderly include the very poor who cannot afford adequate heating, the very old, and persons whose body temperature control does not respond normally. Infants under 1 year of age sometimes get hypothermia, since their body temperature control may not be fully developed.

Prevention of Hypothermia

To protect against accidental hypothermia—

- Avoid prolonged exposure to cold without protection. (The elderly and infants should not be exposed to even mild cold.)
- If you are on medication, check with the doctor to make sure that the medicine does not change your body's response to cold. (Phenothiazines may do this.)
- Have someone stop in or call you periodically if you live alone and are elderly.
- Have adequate bed clothing.
- Eat heat-producing foods (fats and carbohydrates).
- Drink hot, sweet drinks. *Do not drink alcoholic beverages,* because they lower the body temperature.
- Add external heat as needed.
- If you are an older person, increase the room temperature to at least 70°F (21.1°C).
- Wear adequate clothing, protecting critical body areas such as the head, neck, sides of the chest, and groin. Several layers of clothing will keep the heat in better.
- Avoid using plastic rain gear without insulation. Make sure that down-filled items are fluffy and that the material can "breathe."
- Check cold-weather clothing and rain gear for leaks before wearing. (Rain gear may be tested in the shower.)
- Stay dry.
- Use body energy wisely. If it is extremely cold, do only those things that are absolutely necessary for survival.

Symptoms of Hypothermia

If the body temperature varies only one degree centigrade or two degrees Fahrenheit, the brain sends out signals to warn that problems are about to occur. It is important, then, to learn to recognize the symptoms of mild hypothermia:

- Shivering—usually the first sign.
- Cold hands or feet, or both, resulting from loss of the surface circulation required to maintain the body's normal temperature.
- Clumsiness. Muscle control is not responsive because surface circulation is reduced, and coordination is difficult.

NOTE. People with poor body temperature regulation may not

shiver, but their bodies may lose heat when they need to retain it. Under these circumstances, hypothermia is harder to detect.

More symptoms occur when body temperature drops to 92–96°F (33.3–35.6°C).

- Severe shivering (shaking or rigid muscles, or both, caused by bursts of body energy and changes in the body chemistry). This condition may occur in only one arm or leg.
- Skin discoloration—pale or an odd pink, and possibly a puffy appearance.
- Skin coolness.
- Drowsiness.
- Slow, *irregular* breathing.
- Low blood pressure.

The final stage occurs when the body no longer functions and the body temperature is 78–86°F (25.6–30°C).* The victim will experience—

- Collapse, because brain centers have failed, and organs are only partially functioning.
- Imminent death—Respiration and heart function stop and lungs may hemorrhage, causing frothing at the mouth.

It is still not too late to help the victim revive. Don't assume that death has occurred. Get the victim to medical help *immediately*, if possible.

First Aid for Hypothermia

While transporting the victim to facilities and equipment, if available—

- Provide the victim with protection and insulation from cold, wind, and water.
- Keep the victim's use of energy to a minumum but keep him awake if possible.
- Take immediate steps for rewarming the victim. The process should be gradual but rapid enough to cause the victim to adjust to the warmer environment.
- *Prevent after-drop* (further lowering of the body temperature after warming has begun), caused by the cool blood from the extrem-

*A regular clinical thermometer will not register this low. These temperature readings are used as an example of how cold the body may get before death occurs.

ities rushing back to the trunk, or center of the body. After-drop may stop the heartbeat and breathing and may kill the victim. Prevention of after-drop may be accomplished by carrying out the following steps:

First, rewarm the trunk in a bath.

Keep the victim's head out of the water. Start with a water temperature around 70°F (21.1°C), warm to the touch, and raise it to 110°F (43.3°C).

Apply cloths such as towels or blankets to the trunk *first.* Beware of causing superficial burns. Use insulated hot water bottles but wrap them to prevent a burn.

Retain the victim's exhaled air by covering his mouth and nose with a light cloth. Also, breathe into the victim's mouth as in mouth-to-mouth resuscitation (needed or not) to add warm air.

Use body heat. Strip the victim of all wet, cold clothing and place him on his side in a sleeping bag or blankets, between two stripped rescuers. Skin-to-skin contact on the front and back of the victim will provide body heat.

It is *very* important for all victims of hypothermia to be checked by a physician, since the effects of the cold may have caused other injuries—illness such as frostbite or pneumonia.

Sudden Illness

Fainting

When the supply of blood to the brain is reduced, a partial or complete loss of consciousness results, and fainting occurs. Recovery of consciousness almost always occurs when the victim is placed in a reclining position or when he falls as a result of the fainting. Since an injury may result from such a fall, other first aid assistance may be required.

A person who is about to faint is aware of certain symptoms. He becomes dizzy and somewhat nauseated, with possible accompanying numbness or tingling of the hands and feet, sweating, and possible disturbance of vision. His skin may be cold, moist, and extremely pale.

A person who feels that he may faint may be able to prevent a fainting attack by lying down or bending over with his head at the level of his knees.

If someone has fainted, first aid is as follows:

1. Keep the victim in a reclining position, loosen his clothing, and maintain an open airway.
2. If the victim has fallen, observe for signs of injury resulting from the fall and note suspected neck or back injuries.
3. If vomiting occurs, turn the victim on his side, or turn his head to the side, to allow for complete drainage and to prevent choking.
4. Do not give any liquid to the victim until he has revived.
5. Do not pour water on the victim's face; instead, bathe his face gently with a cloth wrung out in cool water.
6. Unless recovery is prompt, seek medical help. Observe the patient regularly, because fainting may be an indication of a developing illness.

Heart Attack

Heart attack usually occurs when one of the blood vessels supplying the heart becomes blocked. The victim usually experiences pain and shortness of breath. The pain is in the chest and often radiates to the left shoulder or arm. The victim may be very pale or may have a bluish discoloration of the lips, skin, and fingernail beds. As a rule, the victim is in shock. The heart attack may or may not be accompanied by loss of consciousness.

It is imperative to take *immediate* first aid action (1) when intense pressure, tightness, or squeezing in the center of the chest persists for 5 minutes or more, (2) when it spreads across the chest or to either the shoulder, the arm, the neck, or the jaw, and (3) when it is associated with sweating, nausea, vomiting, shortness of breath, or fainting.

First aid is as follows:

1. Place the victim in a comfortable position. Often, a sitting position is most comfortable.
2. If breathing stops, immediately begin artificial respiration.
3. Have someone call an ambulance or a rescue squad equipped with oxygen, and have the victim's physician notified.
4. Do not give liquids to an unconscious patient.
5. If the victim's heart stops beating, cardiopulmonary resuscitation (CPR, or heart-lung revival) must be given by someone who has had training in this technique. Most rescue squad and ambu-

lance workers have had this training. The American Red Cross and the American Heart Association offer CPR training through local chapters.

Seizures

Seizures (formerly called convulsions) are involuntary and are usually violent muscular spasms involving the entire body. During a seizure, the victim is unconscious. In infants and young children, seizures may accompany a period of high fever. Seizures that develop later in the course of a childhood disease are more serious and may indicate complications of the central nervous system. Seizures that occur in older children and adults may accompany, or be the result of, severe illness or a head injury or may be a form of epilepsy.

At the start of a seizure, the body muscles will be rigid for a few seconds. This phase is then followed by jerking movements and bluish color of the face and lips. Drooling or foaming at the mouth may occur. The patient may lose bowel and bladder control. After the seizure, the patient will be very tired and will sleep deeply.

First aid involves preventing the victim from hurting himself. Do not restrain him or try to stop his movements. Do not give any liquids. Do not place him in a tub of water. Give artificial respiration if it is indicated. If repeated seizures occur, consult the health professional and take the patient to the hospital. Report the length and characteristics of the seizure to the health professional.

Chapter 15

Being Prepared for Disaster

A disaster is an unfortunate event that may harm life or property, one that occurs more or less suddenly, and one over which people have little control. Disasters come in many forms and can occur at any place, at any time. Natural disasters include heavy rains, floods, hurricanes, tornadoes, blizzards, landslides, avalanches, earthquakes, lightning, and lightning-caused fires. Other disasters are associated with man: wars, transportation accidents, spilling of dangerous chemicals or radioactive materials, explosions, and fires. Some situations can either be the cause or the result of disaster, such as long-lasting power failures, collapsing buildings, epidemics, famines, and civil disorders.

Any person could become the victim of a disaster at some time or other. How well both the victim and his community manage the experience will determine the victim's chance for survival. Since most disaster situations develop quickly, the time to make a plan of action and to assign responsibility is *before* anything happens. Preparedness is the best defense against disaster—the best way to increase the chance of survival and to lessen the damage in any disaster situation.

NATURAL DISASTERS

Analyzing weather data and transmitting information about possible danger to the public is the responsibility of the National Weather Service (a branch of the National Oceanic and Atmospheric Administration of the U.S. Department of Commerce). Most major radio and television stations have direct wires from Weather Service offices and they interrupt their programs when there is important weather news. Local public safety, law enforcement, and civil defense officers are also informed when there is a forecast of severe weather. In recent years, great progress has been made both in forecasting severe storms and floods and in warning people in time to take shelter.

Every person should learn what system is used to warn the local community of potential disaster threats. For example, the signal may be one long blast on a fire or civil defense siren. Learn which radio and TV stations in your area can be depended on to provide weather warnings and keep tuned to those stations when conditions warrant doing so. In general, the terms "alert," "advisory," and "watch" mean that there is a possibility of severe weather or flooding, while "warning" means that there is actual danger for people in a specified area. Do not try to telephone radio or TV stations or a

Weather Service office for information during severe weather conditions. The telephone lines are sure to be busy. If you sight a tornado or know any other important information affecting public safety, report it to either the local law enforcement (police or sheriff) office, the nearest Weather Service office, or the local civil defense office.

Lightning

Lightning kills more people every year than hurricanes or tornadoes do. It is more common in some areas than others, but everyone, regardless of where they live, should know what do do during a thunder and lightning storm. During such a storm, stay indoors unless it is absolutely necessary to be outside, and stay away from plug-in electrical appliances, open doors and open windows, fireplaces, radiators, sinks, stoves, and metal pipes. Don't use plug-in electrical equipment, such as hair dryers, electric toothbrushes, or electric razors, during the storm. Also, don't use the telephone during the storm, since lightning may strike outside telephone lines.

If you are caught outdoors, avoid standing in an open area or standing under a tall or solitary tree or tower, since lightning will usually strike the tallest object in the area. If you are driving, stay in your car, which offers good lightning protection.

Given below are safety suggestions excerpted from the publication *Severe Local Storm Hazard in the United States: A Research Assessment,* by Waltraud A. R. Brinkmann and others.*

Don't take laundry off the clothesline.

Don't use metal objects like fishing rods and golf clubs. Golfers wearing cleated shoes are particularly good lightning rods.

Don't handle flammable materials in open containers.

Get out of the water and off small boats.

Seek shelter in buildings. If no buildings are available, your best protection is a cave, ditch, canyon, or under head-high clumps of trees in open forest glades.

When you feel the electrical charge—if your hair stands on end or your skin tingles—lightning may be about to strike you. Drop to the ground immediately.

Tornadoes

Although small in area affected and of short duration, tornadoes are the most violent of all storms. They have struck all 50 states and in every month of the year but they are most numerous over the central plains in the spring. They most often develop in the late afternoon or early evening hours.

A tornado *watch* alerts people to the possibility of tornado development and may cover an area as large as several states. It may stay in effect for several hours. During a watch, follow your normal routines while listening to the radio and observing the sky for unusual cloud conditions.

A tornado *warning* is issued only after a tornado has been sighted. It indicates the location of the tornado and the probable path of the storm during a certain time period, usually an hour or less. If a warning is given, people in the path of the storm should take immediate safety precautions.

The lowest floor of a sturdy building offers the greatest safety. In houses, the basement is the safest place to be. If there is no basement, take shelter in a small room in the center of the house, away from all windows. Taking shelter under a workbench or sturdy table or furniture may give additional protection. Keep some windows partly open on the side of the house away from the storm's approach. If time permits, secure items outside the home (garbage cans, lawn furniture, toys, signs, etc.). They should either be anchored securely to keep them from being blown away or should be brought indoors. Mobile homes are unsafe during windstorms, even when anchored with tie-downs. Occupants should take shelter in the nearest sturdy building or lie flat in a ditch or ravine.

If you are in a school, office, or factory building, stand in an interior hallway on the lowest floor, away from windows. Avoid large rooms with unsupported roofs.

If you are in a car and are caught in the storm's path, leave your car and lie flat in the nearest ditch or ravine. It may be possible to drive away from the storm's path by driving at a right angle from it, but don't try to outrun a tornado. (Tornadoes usually move from southwest to northeast.)

Hurricanes

Hurricanes form at sea and strike most often along the Atlantic and Gulf coasts, between June 1 and November 30. Strong winds, high tides, and giant waves damage coastal areas, while torrential rains and flooding follow the path of the storm as it moves inland. If the calm "eye" of the hurricane passes overhead, there may be a short period when the winds die down and the sky clears. The winds then begin again with great force, but from the opposite direction.

A hurricane or tropical storm *advisory* refers to information issued by the Weather Service as it tracks a tropical storm or hurricane. A *hurricane watch* means that a hurricane moving toward the coast may threaten a specific area within a specific time period. During a watch, follow normal routines but keep listening to radio or TV. Check your supplies of flashlight and radio batteries, water, nonperishable foods, first aid items, and prescription medicines. Make certain your car's gas tank is filled. Have tools and boards on hand for emergency repairs and for boarding up windows against the storm.

A *hurricane warning* means that the storm is expected to strike a specific section of the coast within 24 hours or less. If a hurricane warning has been issued, persons in the threatened area should take immediate action:

- If evacuation is advised (as in low-lying coastal areas, which may be flooded by rising tides, or in other areas that may be cut off or flooded by swelling streams), begin procedures for evacuation immediately.
- Stay indoors during the storm if evacuation is not advised.
- Store drinking water in clean bottles and jugs. Store water for other purposes in the bathtub.
- Protect windows with storm shutters, boards, or tape.
- Secure outdoor objects such as garbage cans and lawn furniture, or store them indoors.
- Have tools and boards on hand for emergency repairs. Quick repairs can sometimes be made while the hurricane's "eye" passes over.
- Keep your car fueled, since service stations may not operate for some time after the storm.

Floods

In the usual slow-rising flood, there is time to warn and evacuate people from the threatened area. However, in a flash flood caused by sudden heavy rains or the breaking of a dam, there may be no time for evacuation. In that case, try to move to higher ground, such as up a hill or mountainside. *Never* try to drive out of a flash flood area. If you cannot get to higher ground, stay where you are and wait for rescue.

Do not try to travel after the water rises. The current may be very strong. Bridges may be washed out, and flooding across roads may be much deeper than it appears.

Earthquakes

The chief danger in an earthquake is from collapsing buildings. If you can get outdoors, stand in an open area, away from buildings, and wait for the tremors to stop. If you can't get outside, stand in a doorway. Be very cautious about reentering structures that may have been damaged.

If possible, turn off electricity and gas, and be alert for possible fires. Report broken water mains, downed power lines, and gas leaks to the local police or fire department.

MAN-MADE DISASTERS

Fire

All families are under the risk of fire. This risk can be reduced by heeding recommendations about open flames and electrical wiring and by the use of smoke and heat detectors in appropriate locations. All family members should be aware of procedures and priorities for dealing with fire:

- Plan at least two escape routes from every room in the house. If halls and stairways are filled with smoke or flames, it may be necessary to escape through bedroom windows. Make sure that children know how to unfasten screens or storm windows. If bedrooms are upstairs, consider installing an escape ladder (usually rope) or have the children sleep in rooms with easy rooftop access, or consider cutting extra doors through closets so that the children can get to a room with rooftop access.
- Sleep with bedroom doors closed so that heat, flames, and poisonous smoke or fumes will be held back and you will be given time for escape. As a fire precaution, instruct each person to feel his

bedroom door before opening it. If the door feels hot or if there is smoke leaking in around the edges, the door should not be opened. The emergency escape route should be used.

- Hold periodic home fire drills and agree on an outside meeting place so that you can check to see if everyone is safe.
- Use special stickers on the windows or follow the suggestions of local fire authorities for other ways in which to identify sleeping rooms of children, the elderly, or the handicapped.
- Place and maintain smoke and heat detectors as recommended by fire authorities and the manufacturer.
- Keep a fire extinguisher in the kitchen, and possibly others in the garage and basement. Know how to use them and follow directions for their maintenance. Check consumer reports for information on kinds of fire extinguishers that offer maximum protection.
- Make sure that every telephone has the fire department's telephone number glued to it, or know how to contact the fire department through the telephone operator.
- See that every family member understands the important priorities when a fire is first discovered.
  (1) Inform the others and get everyone out of the house. Do not take time to get dressed or collect valuables. Close windows and doors to help slow the spread of fire and give extra time for escape.
  (2) Call the fire department from a neighbor's house, the nearest pay phone, or a street alarm box.

Every family member should thoroughly understand the following rules for dealing with fire:

- Call the fire department, then try to fight the fire only if it is still small. Use a fire extinguisher or try to smother the flames with a heavy coat, rug, or blanket. If the fire is contained in a wastebasket or cooking pot, cover it with a metal lid to shut off the air supply. If the fire is in the oven or clothes dryer, leave the door shut and turn off the appliance.

- If a person's clothing catches fire, he should lie down and roll to smother the flames. A rug, blanket, or coat can be wrapped around the victim to help smother the fire. He should remain lying down, since the flames are less likely to reach his face.

- If you are trapped in a burning building, remember that the safest air for breathing is always low, near the floor, since smoke and heat rise. The smoke is as deadly as flame, since it contains poisonous gases such as carbon monoxide. Holding a wet cloth over your mouth and nose will help to prevent inhaling the smoke but will not provide protection from poisonous gas.
- Close windows and doors to help slow the spread of fire.

Nuclear Disaster

It is as important today as ever to be informed about and prepared for nuclear disaster resulting from an enemy attack or an industrial accident. Saving life and lowering the risks of body damage are the key tasks in relation to nuclear disaster, as they are in all types of disaster. Radiation fallout, which may result in death or radiation sickness, is the major threat of nuclear disaster.

When there is a nuclear explosion, large amounts of soil and debris are drawn up into the highly radioactive (mushroom) cloud, where the radioactive products of the detonation condense on and into the debris, producing radioactive fallout particles. Within a short time, these particles fall back to earth. On the way down, and after they reach the ground, the radioactive particles give off gamma rays (like X-rays), too much of which can kill or injure people. Also, radioactive material may leak into the air as the result of an accident. The particles give off most of their radiation quickly, making the first few hours or days the most serious. Exact fallout patterns cannot be predicted. Fallout from a single explosion might cover several hundred miles downwind, a few miles upwind, and dozens of miles crosswind. Gamma rays are very penetrating and can pass through solid material (such as wood or cement) to damage or destroy body tissue. Over a period of time, the body is able to repair most of the injury. But when the body has been exposed to large amounts of radiation in a very short period of time, death may be caused.

Radiation sickness results from accumulated exposure to radiation. The effect of radiation may be very slight symptoms, or death may occur, depending on the total amount absorbed by the body, the length of time during which the dose was accumulated, and the amount of the body exposed to the radiation. A very large dose received in a short period of time (a few days) may result in death, while the same large dose over a long period of time (up to a year) may cause no serious illness, although the long-term effects are known.

In order to be prepared for nuclear disaster, you should—

- Know your local emergency action plan
- Understand nuclear attack hazards in your area
- Know the attack warning signal
- Know the locations of fallout shelters
- Improvise protection if no shelter is available
- Prepare emergency supplies
- *Follow official instructions*
- Check with your local civil defense agency for more specific instructions

INDIVIDUAL AND FAMILY PREPAREDNESS

Individuals and families should be prepared for all types of disaster—man-made and natural—and particularly for the kinds of disasters most likely to strike where they live. Every family should have a preparedness plan for any emergency situation in which either the family or the community (or both) is likely to be involved. Education for emergencies is the first step for every family member, and this chapter presents the basic concepts in preparing for and coping with disaster situations.

Learning basic skills for meeting emergencies increases the individual's capacity not only to help himself but also to contribute to the welfare of the family and the community. Examples of emergency preparedness courses offered by the Red Cross are those in first aid, cardiopulmonary resuscitation (CPR), home nursing, and foreign body obstruction of the airway.

Home Supplies for a Community Disaster

A family can best survive a community disaster by staying in the home until the danger passes. For such a situation, the family should have on hand and ready for use at all times the following items:

- A battery-powered radio and extra batteries. (The radio may become the family's only link with the outside world after a disaster, and the information and instructions it provides may save lives. The radio is not just for entertainment.)
- Flashlights and extra batteries. (Although candles and lanterns can be used for emergency lighting during a power failure or dis-

aster situation, they greatly increase the danger of fire at a time when people cannot count on help from the local fire department. Telephone lines may be down, streets may be blocked with debris, the firemen may be busy with rescue work elsewhere, etc. If you do not have a flashlight, it is safer to sit in the dark.)

- First aid supplies (see chapter 14).
- An emergency supply of canned foods and fruit juices, water in jugs or plastic containers, instant beverages, and sealed boxes of crackers and other foods that don't need cooking or refrigeration. (Include paper plates and paper cups and premoistened disposable washcloths for an emergency cleanup. A camp stove or charcoal grill can be used for emergency cooking, but only *outside the house.* In addition to the risk of fire, indoor use can cause death from carbon monoxide poisoning. Also, a camp stove that is not in good working condition may leak gas.)

Emergency Evacuation of the Home

In some disaster situations, you may have to leave your home. *Always* follow official instructions for evacuation of homes in specific areas. Think now about what you would need to take with you if you were forced to evacuate your home and go to a shelter. Such items might include—

- Eyeglasses, dentures, hearing aids, special foods such as formula for an infant, and prescription drugs needed on a regular basis by any member of the family
- Sturdy shoes and clothes appropriate to the weather, such as raincoats and waterproof boots
- For a small child, a favorite toy or blanket that the child is used to sleeping with, to give comfort in strange surroundings
- Cash, checkbook, credit cards, driver's license, and any other important papers
- Blankets, if possible
- Extra clothing

To remove large amounts of clothing or personal belongings from your house in a hurry, use large plastic garbage bags, or spread a blanket on the floor, pile wanted items on it, pick up the four corners, and drag it out. Since the easiest way to transport extra clothing is to wear it, pull on an extra pair of slacks and sweater. If flooding is a threat and time permits, you might move some valuables to a second or third floor or to nearby higher ground.

Before leaving the house, turn off the electricity at the main switch, turn off the water faucets tightly, and unplug all appliances. If there is time, seal electric wall outlets with waterproof tape.

What To Do After a Disaster

Some guidelines for individual and family behavior after a disaster will be useful:

- Do not try to travel until there is official word that roads are clear and bridges are intact. If you are not in danger, stay where you are.
- Stay away from the disaster area unless you are qualified to help and are willing to work. Sightseers block emergency traffic and get in the way, adding to the problems faced by rescue workers.
- Stay off the telephone in order to keep lines free for emergency telephone calls. Use the telephone only to report to the police if there are downed power lines, broken water lines, or blocked streets. After the major disaster has passed, contact relatives or close friends to notify them of your safety.

If you are not sure about the safety of your water supply, purify water by *one* of the following methods:

- Boil the water vigorously for 10 minutes.
- Add 12 drops of tincture of iodine per gallon, mix, and let stand 30 minutes.
- Add 8 drops of chlorine laundry bleach per gallon, mix, and let stand for 30 minutes.
- Use water-purifying tablets, following directions on the package.

If your house is badly damaged, be cautious about reentering. Wear sturdy shoes at all times. Wear thick gloves when attempting any salvage or rescue work. Broken glass, torn metal, splintered wood, and exposed fiberglass insulation are all hazards to hands and feet. Be sure that the electricity is turned off and that major appliances are unplugged. If appliances have been exposed to the weather, do not use them again until they have been checked by a repairman. Be alert for escaping gas. Turn off the gas, if possible. Prevent fires: be alert for spontaneous combustion in wet materials such as hay, rags, or clothing (which may suddenly burst into flame as late as 2 weeks after the disaster).

HELPING OTHERS

Most disasters affect more than one family. Lives are disrupted, and individuals and families need help. People must help each other to meet the immediate demands of the disaster situation. Although each disaster situation is different from every other, both in details and in extent of damage, the following problems are nearly always present:

- Many persons, injured or sick, will need help at the same time.
- Deaths may occur.
- Some persons may be isolated and may need to be rescued.
- Families may be separated.
- Homes may be destroyed or may become unsafe.
- Communication, transportation, and utility services may be disrupted.
- Possessions may be lost that represent the savings of a lifetime.

There is always immediate need for medical care, food, clothing, and shelter for disaster victims. In addition, there is a danger of communicable disease because of contaminated water supplies, inadequate toilet facilities, and crowding.

Assisting Individuals

Helping in a disaster situation begins with being aware of your own reactions to the disaster. Different people respond in different ways to disaster. Most people respond in ways different from their usual behavior. People who have had the opportunity to prepare for what happens are more likely to proceed calmly. Most people are able to do what is expected of them at the time of the disaster.

It is helpful to know that normal responses to a disaster may include anxiety, trembling, pounding heart, rapid breathing, perspiration, muscular tension, urinary frequency, mild diarrhea, and nausea. Knowing this should help prevent concern that physical illness is occurring also. Less severe symptoms are often helped by engaging in group activity; more severe symptoms need to be brought to the attention of trained personnel.

Neighborliness is most helpful to those affected by disaster. In addition to keeping calm yourself, specific, helpful actions that you might engage in include—

- Reassuring and sympathizing with others.
- Helping to carry out directions of trained persons.
- Providing food and preparing food for meals.
- Sharing blankets, clothing, and supplies with other disaster victims.

- Providing companionship and distracting activities for children, disabled persons, and others who are upset.
- Volunteering to help with specific jobs that are within your competence, such as making or answering telephone calls or assisting with transportation.

Assisting Through the Red Cross

The American Red Cross is a voluntary agency designated by the United States Congress to render assistance when disaster occurs. It provides—

- Health services for the ill and injured
- Food for disaster victims and volunteer workers
- Temporary shelter for persons evacuated from their homes
- Clothing for disaster victims, if needed
- Assistance in meeting other needs of disaster victims

All people can help the Red Cross to help disaster victims, whether the victims are in one's own community or elsewhere. Volunteers for such help should call their local chapter, which coordinates the efforts of the helping agencies and individuals. Contributions can be made, through the chapter, in volunteer time, money, or any material items being asked for.

Volunteers with skills gained from Red Cross first aid or home nursing courses may be put to work assisting doctors, nurses, or professional Red Cross workers in first aid stations or shelters, where they will help to care for the injured, sick, or emotionally upset. Volunteers without medical or nursing skills may be assigned in a variety of other capacities, such as—

- Working in a rescue center or shelter
- Serving food at shelters or from mobile canteens
- Working at a clothing distribution center
- Keeping records and doing other clerical work and answering telephone inquiries
- Babysitting
- Providing transportation

Volunteers with other skills can increase their ability to help themselves and others through taking other Red Cross preparedness courses.

Disaster workers who volunteer to help with disaster relief must be prepared to work under conditions of chaos and confusion. They must learn to recognize their own limitations—to do what they can and then stop to rest. If they collapse from fatigue or allow themselves to become too upset with the problems they see around them, their usefulness is ended.

Disaster victims must be cared for with warmth, understanding, and honest reassurance. They have been subjected to unusual emotional as well as physical stress. Reassurance that they are not alone in their trouble, and that they and their families will be helped, is very important. The volunteer who listens carefully and sympathetically while an upset person talks out his fears and tensions is being very helpful.

COMMUNITY PLANNING

Planning for a mass disaster involves many elements of the community. On the national level, disaster plans are made by the U.S. government together with the American Red Cross. On the community level, government, civil defense, emergency service agencies, public health officials, and police and fire departments coordinate their disaster plans with Red Cross chapters and other volunteer groups. In a disaster situation, local government agencies are responsible for—

- Issuing official warning and designating hazardous areas
- Evacuating all persons from hazardous areas
- Maintaining emergency communications and transportation services
- Providing police and fire protection for the disaster area

After a disaster, government agencies are responsible for cleaning debris from public property and for repairing streets, water and sewage systems, and public buildings. The government also helps some people through existing community welfare services. For example, food stamps or donated commodities may be made available to disaster victims. If the area is proclaimed a major disaster area, other help may be made available from the federal government. This assistance may include unemployment insurance, temporary housing, individual grants, and low-cost loans for rebuilding homes and businesses.

During and after a disaster, the Red Cross offers additional emergency help to individuals and families. The information it keeps on all disaster victims who were given medical aid, were hospitalized, or were assigned to shelters goes into a central Red Cross disaster headquarters in the disaster area, where it helps to reunite families and answer the inquiries of worried friends and relatives. In the clean-up and rehabilitation period that follows a disaster, the Red Cross issues emergency orders that can be used like cash at local stores to buy food, clothing, essential household furnishings, occupational supplies and equipment, and material for temporary repairs.

Chapter 16

Philosophy and Principles of Home Nursing

The philosophy of home nursing is tied closely to the dynamic nature of the American Red Cross. From its beginning, the Red Cross has worked to prevent illness, to relieve suffering, and to promote the fullest possible enjoyment of life by people. In the early 1900s, Red Cross societies throughout the world recognized that many people, especially volunteers, were interested in receiving instruction in practical home nursing skills. Following the reorganization of the American Red Cross in 1905, Mabel Boardman, the national leader, promoted the ideas that knowledge of good health care for mothers and babies could prevent diseases and that nursing skills could be valuable in times of epidemics. Jane Delano, the first director of what is now the American Red Cross Nursing and Health Services, was the person responsible for putting these ideas into practice. Classes in Home Hygiene and Care of the Sick were conducted in the District of Columbia branch of the American Red Cross as early as 1908. When the National Committee on Red Cross Nursing Service was established the following year, one of its aims was to form classes in home nursing throughout the country. In 1913, the first Red Cross textbook on home nursing was published, *Elementary Hygiene and Home Care of the Sick,* by Jane A. Delano and Isabel McIsaac. Since that time, home nursing instruction has been one of the most active programs in Red Cross chapters.

The American Red Cross in 1912 was one of the early pioneers in training nurses to provide care of the sick in rural homes. In 1913, the service became known as the Town and Country Nursing Service. The nurses taught hygiene, care of the teeth, nutrition, sanitation, prevention of disease, and many other matters related to health. As the country developed and rural living increased, the need for home nursing instruction grew. The service provided by the Red Cross nurses and their instruction of volunteers and family members gained much public attention, particularly during the influenza epidemic of 1918–1919. Persons who had learned the skills were able to help relieve the suffering of their families and neighbors.

Changes in society and changes in health care since the early 1900s have resulted in the hospitals becoming the primary place for care of the ill and injured. Even so, people have continued to seek Red Cross instruction in home nursing and care for mothers and babies. People seem to realize that families can better maintain their health and enjoy life more when they know more about nutrition, exercise, signs and symptoms of disease, and other matters affecting their health.

Now, with the increasingly higher cost of health care, interest in home nursing is again becoming widespread. With an increasing number of persons over 65, home health care is an attractive alternative to care in hospitals or nursing homes.

PHILOSOPHY OF HOME NURSING

Nursing is the art and science of giving care to others. It first involves care for the whole person—body, mind, and spirit—and requires attention as well to the person's environment.

Nurses recognize the basic human needs of all human beings:

To be well, healthy, and active
To have security
To love and be loved
To be accepted
To feel worthy
To be independent
To be successful
To be creative
To have a set of values
To have food, shelter, and clothing

Nursing is concerned with the physical care and emotional needs of a patient.

Home nursing is the care of the ill person in the home. It requires cooperation and careful planning between the patient and his family. Efforts must be made to provide safe care and to keep the patient comfortable while carrying out nursing measures that promote the highest possible level of wellness for both the patient and the family. The family and the patient (if he is able) need to plan activities that save time, energy, and money.

The Patient

The major goal of home nursing is to help the patient to be as independent as his condition permits. Some illnesses require the patient to use as little energy as possible and to get a great deal of rest, and in such a case the family should help the patient in every possible way. In many other illnesses, it is best for the patient's physical and mental health for him to be as active as possible, doing as much for himself as he can. In these situations, the family should encourage the patient to care for his own needs as much as possible. Elderly patients often need the chance and encouragement to do many things for themselves. Although it may take longer for an ill or elderly person to dress himself, his feeling of independence is important for his mental attitude and thus for his general state of health. The physical exercise he gets when doing things for himself also helps keep his muscles in good tone.

The patient's emotional state is as important as his physical condition. Illness brings limitations that many patients find difficult to accept. The need to depend on others can add to discouragement and depression. For this reason, it is very important for the family to involve the patient in his own care as much as possible. Even when he is physically unable to help himself, allow the patient to make decisions concerning his care. When the patient is asked for his opinion, the person providing care and the sick person together can often find the most satisfactory way to carry out a procedure such as a bed bath. When the patient has some control over his care, his mental outlook is likely to improve, and he may recover faster. Children, also, will benefit by being involved in their own care when they are ill at home.

The Home Nurse

The home nurse may be either a parent, husband, wife, child, relative, or friend. The patient himself may serve as home nurse to the extent that he can provide his own care. The role of the home nurse may shift from one family member to another, and friends may help too. In order to avoid confusion, it is generally a good idea for one person to have the major responsibility for the patient's care. This role includes communicating with the health professional and other sources of services for the patient, planning activities, and keeping schedules for necessary treatments and medications. Written schedules and records of important observations regarding the patient's physical and emotional condition are often advisable.

BASIC PRINCIPLES OF HOME NURSING

Nursing care should be planned around the needs of the patient. Since each patient's physical and emotional needs are different, the duties of the home nurse will vary from one type of illness to another and from one household to another. There are, however, several basic principles of home nursing to be considered in the care of any ill person. These include—

Hygiene

Attitude and personal appearance

Safety

Comfort

Economy

Effectiveness

Common sense and good judgment form the basis of *all* nursing measures. It may be important to adjust living arrangements to meet the needs of both the ill person and the family. Often it is necessary to review household tasks to see whether some can be omitted or made easier. Such planning adds time for the care of the patient and makes sure that no one person has too much to do. The home nurse who includes each family member in helping to keep the household on an even keel is practicing good management, and good psychology as well.

Hygiene

The home nurse should take several actions to protect both patient and nurse from injury and infection. Handwashing is one of the most important of these actions. Its purposes are—

To protect the patient from bacteria on the home nurse's hands

To protect the home nurse from infections from the patient

To protect other people who might come in contact with the home nurse or with things that the nurse touches

To promote personal cleanliness

The home nurse should wash both *before* and *after* giving care to the patient, and before handling supplies that will touch the patient. When the home nurse is giving care to more than one patient, the nurse's hands should also be washed *between* caring for patients.

Use warm running water for handwashing when possible. When running water is not available, pour water for both soaping and rinsing over the hands from a pitcher or a can into a basin. If water for handwashing is unavailable, as in a disaster situation, use a commercial, premoistened, disposable small towel; or rub liquid detergent or an alcohol solution over your hands. Then wipe your hands clean with tissues or paper towels.

Handwashing for a home nurse involves more attention to hygiene than does normal handwashing. The correct procedure is as follows:

1. Assemble necessary equipment: soap, water (if running water is not available), clean towel, container for soiled towels.
2. Roll up long sleeves if necessary. Remove your wristwatch or push it well up on your arm. Remove any jewelry that might be harmful to the patient or that might collect dirt.
3. Wet and soap your hands thoroughly, using friction to work up a good lather. Wash the entire surface of your hands, between the fingers, around and under the nails, and well above the wrist. A nail brush may be helpful for removing dirt and particles from under your nails.
4. Rinse the bar of soap so that it will be clean for the next use. This helps prevent the growth of bacteria on the soap. Place the soap in a well-drained soap dish.
5. Rinse with hands lowered to allow the soap, dirt, and soiled water to drain off your hands into the sink or basin.
6. Repeat the last three steps (to remove dirt and oil).
7. Dry your hands by using a paper towel or a clean cloth towel, or by shaking your hands in the air. The occasional use of hand cream or lotion helps avoid chapping, which is not only uncomfortable but also can cause breaks in the skin that can admit infection.
8. Place soiled towels in the laundry or in a waste container. Rinse and dry the washbasin, if one was used.

The home nurse should also keep fingernails trimmed and clean, to avoid scratching the patient and, of course, for hygienic purposes.

The use of a coverall apron is recommended when someone is caring for an ill person: it keeps the home nurse's clothing clean and may prevent the spread of disease to or from the patient. The side of the coverall that touched the patient should be folded together after use, and the coverall should be hung near the door, inside the sickroom, ready for use again.

Attitude and Personal Appearance

The general attitude of others around him will certainly affect the patient's outlook. In addition, the home nurse's behavior can greatly affect the patient's physical and emotional condition. An attitude of cheerfulness offers the patient support and encouragement, gains his cooperation, and promotes a positive outlook, which may speed his recovery.

Most people do not like to be sick and dependent on others for help. If you are the home nurse, it might be helpful if you were to imagine how you might feel if you had the patient's illness. It might also be good to encourage the patient to express his feelings about receiving help. Listening is one of the best ways to show a real interest in the patient's feelings. In this way, the home nurse comes to a greater understanding of what the patient is experiencing. The home nurse can then be sympathetic and tolerant when the patient seems demanding, uncooperative, or ungrateful.

Being flexible and giving the patient an opportunity to make some of the decisions regarding his care is also helpful. The home nurse might say, "Would you like to rest now and walk later?" or "Would you like to sit up for dinner or stay in bed?" (In giving the patient choices, the home nurse must be prepared to accept his decisions.) When changes in the patient's condition or treatment schedule occur, the home nurse should be able to adjust to the changes with calmness and resourcefulness.

Personal appearance is also important. The home nurse should be clean and dressed neatly but comfortably.

It will help the patient to relax if the home nurse keeps the sickroom clean and neatly organized. When the home nurse has everything under control, the patient will be able to rest better, knowing that he can depend on the home nurse for proper care.

Safety

Safety in caring for an ill person involves prevention of the spread of illness, proper use of drugs and proper giving of treatments, and prevention of accidents. Knowing how to handle soiled articles, how to dispose of discharges from the nose and throat, and when and how to wash the hands properly provides protection both for the patient and for the people around him. The necessity for storing drugs safely, administering any drug in the correct way, and carrying out treatments as prescribed are of extreme importance.

The prevention of accidents is important for the home nurse, the patient, and the family. Any accident that occurs could disrupt the routine of the entire family. Preventing accidents involves identifying safety hazards and eliminating them.

Comfort of the Patient and the Home Nurse

The comfort of the patient is one of the goals of home nursing because it promotes the patient's recovery and a feeling of well-being. The comfort of the home nurse is also very important. Through good posture and body mechanics, the home nurse avoids back and muscle strain while caring for the patient.

A dry, clean, well-made bed and the use of pillows for support contribute to the patient's comfort and are essential to good rest and sleep. (Comfort that encourages the patient to remain in one position for too long, however, can be harmful. The sick person should move about in bed unless the health professional tells him not to. Moving helps him to maintain muscle tone, get needed exercise, and avoid deformities to the joints.)

Good posture is important both for the patient and for the home nurse. For the patient, good posture means keeping the various body parts in proper line, whether sitting, lying, or moving. The home nurse, through good posture and the use of proper body mechanics, avoids strain on joints and muscles, avoids injury, and will be less fatigued. In this way, the home nurse also saves energy, is more comfortable, and is better able to help the patient.

Body mechanics is the way in which the body moves and maintains balance. Points for the home nurse to remember in using good body mechanics and in maintaining good posture are—

- Maintain normal spinal curves by keeping your chest up, holding your head erect, and tightening the muscles of your abdomen and buttocks.
- Stand with your feet comfortably apart, with one foot forward (to maintain a wide base of support).
- Wear comfortable shoes that provide support for your feet.
- Use the muscles of your arms and legs to provide power when moving or lifting an object. Do *not* lift with the back muscles, because doing so will result in strain and injury.
- Carry heavy objects close to your body to prevent strain and save energy.
- Stand close to the work area. When possible, raise the work area to a level that lessens the need to stoop and bend. When stooping is necessary, keep your back straight and flex your hips and knees.
- Move a patient or other heavy object by pushing, pulling, rolling,

turning, or sliding, since these methods require less effort than lifting.

- Alternate periods of rest and activity to help maintain good muscle tone and to prevent tiring yourself.

Economy

Economy in nursing care means the best and most efficient use of energy, time, money, and household equipment. The home nurse should save—

- Steps and time, by planning a work schedule and by collecting needed equipment before starting a task
- Energy, by making sure that instructions for nursing care are understood by all concerned
- Money, by improvising nursing equipment
- Money and time, by planning meals ahead of time and purchasing all needed items at one time
- Money, by comparing prices on prescription drugs
- Money and materials, by taking proper care of home appliances and household articles
- Energy, by using correct body mechanics

Home Nursing Effectiveness

As with most other tasks, there is more than one way to perform any nursing skill. The test of any method is its effectiveness. The home nurse should ask, "Does it work? Is there a better way that is safe for the patient and for me? Will it save time, money, or equipment?" Both the home nurse and the patient should feel free to try new ways of performing the necessary procedures. If there is any doubt about the safety or effectiveness of the proposed method, the home nurse should seek approval of the health professional.

Chapter 17

The Basics of Home Nursing

Nursing care at home should be planned around the needs of the patient and must be flexible so that it can be adjusted to meet changing circumstances that may occur. Factors such as age, sex, physical handicaps, and the patient's attitudes and feelings about his illness will affect the amount and kind of nursing care he needs.

Of primary concern in nursing care at home are the diagnosis and the severity of the illness as well as the general physical condition of the patient at the time he became ill. No two illnesses are exactly alike, and nursing care must be given differently in different situations.

Factors to consider in planning nursing care that apply in most situations include—

- Establishing a flexible routine and involving the patient in planning his care
- Organizing the patient's room
- Providing for bed and bedding
- Providing for personal hygiene
- Preventing the spread of disease
- Providing for special nutritional needs
- Providing rest and physical activity
- Preventing the side effects of limited activity
- Allowing and encouraging the patient to do as much for himself as possible
- Providing emotional support

More detailed instructions for carrying out some of these procedures are included in other chapters. Suggestions for ways in which to meet the patient's psychological needs are included throughout.

ESTABLISHING A FLEXIBLE ROUTINE

The routine of the patient's day will vary according to the nature and severity of the illness, but the nursing care will always include the providing of—

Meals
Medicine (if ordered)
Treatments (as ordered)
Grooming
Rest and exercise as necessary
Activities for passing time and for mental stimulation

The home nurse should plan the above routine so that the schedule is flexible enough to permit the patient to get the care he needs at the time he needs it. The patient himself should help to make the plan for his care, if at all possible.

The home nursing schedule should take into consideration the usual habits of the sick person. As long as these habits do not endanger the patient himself or anyone else, he should be allowed to continue them. For example, if the sick person has been accustomed to taking a bath at night before going to sleep, this practice should be continued. Also, many people eat a light meal at lunchtime and have the main meal of the day in the evening. Reversing this practice might be upsetting to the patient. The home nurse should not make an issue of a habit that is harmless and only requires that the nursing schedule be adjusted.

The needs and schedules of other family members are another consideration in establishing the routine. All members should take part in planning the patient's care so that the best possible schedule and division of tasks and responsibilities can be found. The plan should be reviewed every week or two to be sure that it is working well and that each family member is doing his part.

ORGANIZING THE PATIENT'S ROOM

The room selected for the patient confined to bed for a long period of time should meet both the patient's needs and the needs of those who will be giving the nursing care. The patient's room should be sunny and airy. It should be quiet, private, and near the bathroom. It should offer a convenient and uncluttered arrangement of personal belongings and furniture. The patient should be able to call, ring a bell, or signal in some other way and have the signal heard in other parts of the house so that he can get assistance when he needs it. A separate room is generally not necessary for the sick person, unless there is communicable disease or the sick person is easily disturbed by others.

An important consideration when selecting a room for the patient may be the nearness of the room to a bath, a toilet, or running water. If the patient is able to move about by himself, the closeness of the toilet may save him energy and make it easier if he has to get up at night. If the patient is confined to bed, it is much easier for the home nurse to carry water only a short distance. Sometimes the most suit-

Fig. 86

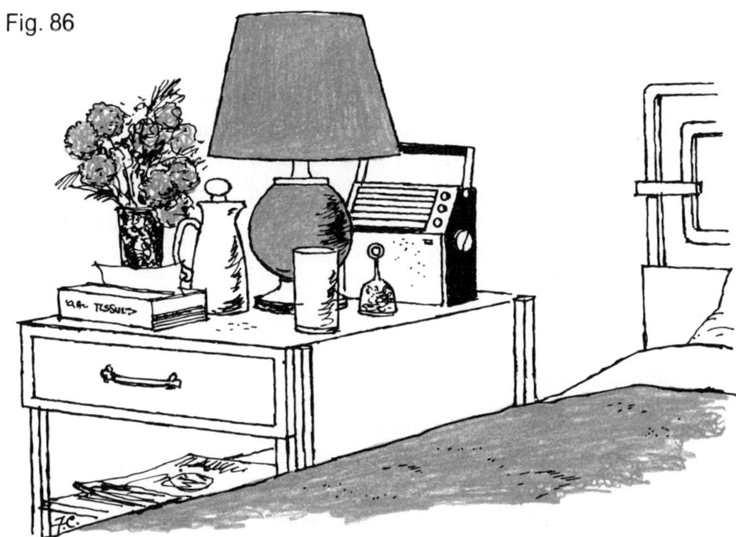

able room is not located near a toilet; in that event, a bedside commode may be improvised (see chapter 24), might be borrowed from a community agency, or might be available for rental from a hospital supply store.

A neat room can be an asset to both the patient and the home nurse. The furniture should be placed to make it easy for the home nurse to attend to the needs of the patient. There is no need to strip the room of the personal belongings and decorations that make it charming and attractive. Artwork of children may be an enjoyable addition to the room. A clock and calendar are helpful to the ill person for keeping track of time and date.

The temperature of the room should be warm enough to keep the patient comfortable and to prevent chilling when he is bathed or is uncovered for any reason. Adequate ventilation should be provided at all times.

Light should not shine directly into the patient's eyes. The bed should be placed so that light from a window comes from the side or the back of the bed; if neither is possible, the shades should be lowered or a screen placed so that glare can be avoided. Light from a bedside lamp should come over the patient's shoulder and should be bright enough to prevent strain and tiring of the eyes during reading. When a night light is needed, a small light may be plugged into a wall outlet, or a flashlight may be made available.

Providing a comfortable chair in the room will encourage family members and guests to sit down and talk with the patient, keeping him in touch with family activities and helping him to feel that he is important to them. A plant, an aquarium, or a household pet, if it is permitted and wanted, can be a source of great pleasure to the patient, whether he is young or old. A radio, a record player, or a television set can provide recreation for the patient who has to be alone much of the time. A telephone may allow the sick person to keep in touch with other family members and friends. (If the patient is hard of hearing, most telephone companies can install a device on the telephone to increase the volume.)

Cleanliness and order in the sickroom are important to the welfare and comfort of the patient, and order in the room is a real time-saver for the home nurse. Cleanliness involves keeping the patient and his bedding clean, promptly removing all soiled articles from the room, and keeping the room clean and free from dust. Careful washing of hands before and after giving nursing care is a basic precaution against the spread of infection.

Noise may be upsetting to the sick person, and small noises are often more disturbing than loud, unusual sounds. Sounds that recur often, such as those made by creaking doors, rattling windows, flapping shades, and dripping faucets, are often very disturbing. Talking or whispering outside the patient's room may also be disturbing.

PROVIDING FOR BED AND BEDDING

The quality of the mattress and bedding and the type and placement of the bed are especially important when the patient has a long-term illness that confines him to bed for a major part of the day and night. Good bed planning for nursing care includes such factors as the height of the bed, a firm mattress, protection for the mattress and bedding, and blankets that are ample and warm.

The Bed

The bed should be placed so that there is easy access on all sides, or it should be easy to move. When a patient must remain in bed for a long period of time, it will be much easier for the home nurse if the bed is of a convenient height that allows care for the patient without undue strain on the home nurse's back and shoulder muscles. However, if the patient is able to be in and out of bed daily, an elevated bed should not be used, because it increases the likelihood of accidents. It is possible to raise a regular bed by the use of blocks made at home (see chapter 24). If blocks are used, the casters should be removed to make the bed more stable.

In many communities it is possible to rent or borrow a hospital bed. (The health professional, the health department, or the local hospital can usually give advice on how to obtain a hospital bed.) Hospital beds have several advantages in addition to their height: they can be operated mechanically to provide a backrest and other support for the patient, they make it easier to change the patient's position, and side rails can be put in place to keep the patient from falling out of bed.

The Mattress

A good, firm mattress is essential to the comfort of the patient. Although modern mattresses are built to give extra support for the heaviest parts of the body, it may be necessary to use a bed board to make the mattress firm and level and to prevent the patient's body from sagging. A bed board of heavy cardboard or ¾-inch (2-centimeter) plywood that fits the length and width of the mattress may be placed between the springs and the mattress to provide support. (A door removed from a closet may work well also.) If the mattress is too rigid, it will not conform to the natural body curves. A foam rubber pad placed on top of the mattress will provide a softer surface.

The mattress will be more comfortable and will wear more evenly if it is turned regularly from end to end and from side to side. Exposure to sun and air for a few hours once a week, if possible, and regular, thorough brushing or use of a vacuum cleaner will keep the mattress clean and will help to avoid odors. The mattress should be enclosed in a washable cover for protection and cleanliness. If the patient is incontinent or is very ill, a waterproof mattress cover may be advisable. Any mattress cover used should fit tightly, without wrinkles.

A special air mattress may be recommended for the patient who has, or is likely to develop, pressure sores. An alternating pressure mattress, which is an electric device and quite expensive, might be bought or, in some communities, rented. A good substitute for such a mattress would be a sturdy camper's air mattress filled with water and placed on top of the regular mattress (see chapter 24 for details).

Sheets and Blankets

The most important factors in choosing sheets and blankets for the patient's bed are smooth fit, ease in laundering, and ample size, to insure sufficient tuck-in while keeping the patient warm and the blankets clean.

The bottom sheet must provide a tight, smooth surface. Flat sheets have to be anchored by being tucked under the mattress, and they tend to loosen with movement of the patient. Fitted sheets have the advantage of remaining almost free from wrinkles and will remain in place without adjustment.

The length of sheets and blankets is important, both for comfort and for cleanliness. Use of sheets 104 to 108 inches (264.2 to 274.3 centimeters) long insures having an ample amount to tuck in under the mattress and also allows for folding a wide area of the top sheet over the blankets to help keep the blankets clean. An extra-long blanket has the advantage of reaching high enough to keep the patient's shoulders warm and still being long enough to tuck in at the lower end of the mattress.

The fabric content of sheets and blankets is a matter of personal choice. Sheets of cotton and synthetics combined are easy to wash and dry, but some people find them too warm or difficult to maintain free of stains. Cotton blankets wash well and are suitable for use in mild weather. Woolen blankets and those made from synthetic fibers are warmer than cotton blankets but need special care in washing (or may need to be dry cleaned). Whatever blankets are chosen, they should be clean, soft, light in weight, and warm enough for the patient's comfort. If an electric blanket is used, carefully follow the directions for use.

A draw sheet (see page 428) placed lengthwise across the center of the bed is an aid in moving the patient in bed and offers additional protection to the bedding. A draw sheet may not be necessary, however, if the patient is out of bed much of the day and is able to go to the bathroom or to use a commode. If additional protection is necessary for the bedding of an incontinent or very ill patient, a rubber or plastic sheet could be used under the draw sheet, or under a cotton blanket or small mattress pad. Consult the health professional regarding useful commercial supplies, especially for incontinent males.

If a bedspread is to be used, choose a lightweight cotton one that can be laundered easily. A bedspread does provide protection for the blankets; a flat sheet of an attractive printed fabric could be used for this purpose.

Pillows and Other Supports

Supplies that may be needed to provide support for the patient in bed include several pillows of varying sizes and degrees of softness (feather pillows fold better), a folded or tightly rolled blanket placed in a pillowcase, towels and washcloths, and a footboard or some substitute that provides needed support for the feet. Waterproof pillow protectors or plastic bags may be used under the regular pillowcases if the patient is incontinent or likely to vomit.

PROVIDING FOR PERSONAL HYGIENE

The home nurse should see that the patient's needs for cleanliness, grooming, and elimination are met.

If the patient is able to get up and go to the bathroom, it may be enough to offer a steadying hand to him as he walks to and from the bathroom. There should be good lighting in the bathroom. The floor should be free from loose rugs or mats, pools of water, pieces of soap, toys, and other hazards. Handrails installed next to the toilet and in the bathtub and shower are helpful.

Even when the patient is able to get up and go to the bathroom, there are times when it is more convenient for him to wash his hands before meals in the sickroom. It is always useful to have a basin for washing hands and face or for soaking feet and perhaps to have another smaller basin for caring for the teeth and mouth. (See chapter 24 for suggestions about basins.) When the patient is helpless, the home nurse will, of course, have to assist him in this activity. (See chapter 21 for procedures to follow for giving a bed bath and similar care.)

Mouth Care

When the patient is able to care for his own teeth and mouth, the main responsibility of the home nurse is to provide him with the necessary equipment. The patient who brushes and flosses his teeth while in bed will need a toothbrush, toothpaste, dental floss, a glass of water, and a bowl or basin in which to spit out the toothpaste. He may also need a towel to protect his nightclothes. The patient who wears dentures and is confined to bed will need a container in which to soak and clean his dentures, as well as a toothbrush and dentrifice. Many patients find the use of a mouthwash refreshing. (The procedures for regular toothbrushing, flossing, and care of dentures are given in chapter 2.)

How often mouth care is carried out depends on the patient's habits, preference, and physical condition. Certain illnesses and medications can cause the mouth to taste bad or to feel dry and uncomfortable. Mouth care may be required more often during periods of illness. Some severely ill or unconscious patients may need mouth care as often as every 2 hours.

Some illnesses cause the patient to breathe through his mouth more than usual. If the mouth becomes dry or the lips become chapped and cracked, a substance to prevent drying should be used. The mouth can be rinsed with a mixture of half glycerine and half lemon juice. For the lips, use a thin layer of mineral oil, petroleum jelly, the glycerine and lemon juice mixture, or a commercial lip balm. In any event, use only small amounts of these materials.

Cleanliness and Grooming

Attention to appearance and grooming are important for the personal comfort, cleanliness, and morale of the patient. The patient will feel better if he is wearing clean and attractive clothing and if his hair is combed and brushed. Women should be encouraged to continue to use cosmetics. Cleanliness for the patient involves his taking at least the following measures:

- Washing hands after toileting and before meals
- Taking a daily bath or shower, or at least washing the face and genital area daily
- Attending to mouth care in the morning on awakening, after meals, and before going to sleep
- Putting on clean clothing daily, or as needed
- Applying powder, if desired, to the body (particularly to the genital area and under the breasts of women)
- Applying cream or lotion to dry areas—elbows and feet particularly
- Soaking hands and feet weekly and giving appropriate care to nails and calluses

Elimination

Special provision for elimination must be made if the patient is confined to his bed. A bedpan may be necessary. Using a commode or putting a bedpan on a straight chair may be more natural and comfortable for the patient. (See chapter 20 for the use of a bedpan or bedside commode.)

Constipation may be a problem of the sick person. Causes of constipation include the illness itself, inactivity, drugs, changes in the amount and kind of food eaten, or, perhaps, the slowing down of all body processes. Constipation may become more likely if the patient has difficulty in using a bedpan or experiences delays in getting to use the bedpan or toilet. (Information in chapter 2 can be helpful in dealing with the problem of constipation.)

PREVENTING THE SPREAD OF DISEASE

There are three points to remember in preventing the spread of infection:

- Maintain good hygiene when the patient is confined to bed.
- Prevent the spread of communicable illness from the ill person to others.
- Prevent the spread of communicable illness from others to the already ill person.

In most instances, the entire family has already been exposed to the communicable disease before a diagnosis is made. For this reason, isolation (separation from others) of the patient is of limited value. This fact is especially true of the acute communicable diseases, which are of relatively short duration and are usually most infectious during the onset of illness and before the symptoms are easily recognizable.

The method of preventing the spread of communicable disease depends upon the type of disease involved. In general, communicable diseases are transmitted by discharges from the nose and throat, from the intestinal tract, and from open sores or wounds on the skin. Chapter 12 describes several communicable diseases and ways in which those diseases are spread. The greatest sources of danger are through direct contact with discharges from the patient and through air droplets. Covering one's mouth when coughing or sneezing and safely handling and disposing of all body discharges are of primary importance in preventing the spread of the disease. Follow the general precautions listed in chapter 12 as well as the specific precautions given by the health professional.

A patient who is already sick will often have lower resistance to infectious diseases than will a healthy person. The sick person is much more likely to become ill after exposure to infected persons. For this reason, only persons who are in good health should be allowed to visit the very ill patient. Keep anyone, especially small children, with a cold and runny nose away from the very sick person.

Good hygiene practices with respect to body wastes may be difficult to carry out when the patient is confined to bed. The patient, his bedding, and particularly the bedpan, must be kept clean (see chapters 20 and 21 for procedures). The use of disposable pads under the buttocks of the patient may be helpful. Cleanliness prevents the likelihood of infection of the skin, the urinary tract, or the digestive tract.

PROVIDING FOR SPECIAL NUTRITIONAL NEEDS

During illness accompanied by fever, the body has a greater than normal need for protein, vitamins, minerals, fluids, and calories in general. This need results from increased activity in the chemical processes of the body. Protein, vitamins, and minerals are used up faster than usual, and the body's need for fuel is also increased. A diet that contains more carbohydrates and protein than usual may be ordered or advised in order to supply the body's need for extra fuel and body-building material. In addition, the diet should contain more liquids than usual, since much body water may be lost through sweating.

To meet the higher energy requirements, increase carbohydrate intake by adding starchy foods such as cooked breakfast cereals, potatoes, pasta, or bread or rice served with butter or margarine. Sugar in the form of jellies, jams, syrups, or honey may also be increased, but a large intake of these foods may dull the appetite and furnish only calories with only a few vitamins or minerals. Acutely or chronically ill patients may be fed with specially prepared diets that include extra vitamins, minerals, and protein. Although meats are a good source of protein, the patient's appetite for meat may be so poor that other sources, such as milk and other dairy products, must be increased. To increase protein without adding bulk, dried skim milk may be added to many foods.

During illness, adequate fluid intake is especially important. Fluids are necessary to prevent the dehydration (drying out) of the tissues, which may occur due to fever, vomiting, or diarrhea. Fluids regulate body processes and help prevent constipation. They also help to keep secretions of the nose and respiratory tract moist and less thick, and thus easier to expel. Unless the doctor orders otherwise, offer the patient water and juices often. Fruit juice frozen in an ice cube tray may appeal to sick children and others who like such foods.

If the patient has had a severe illness, he may tolerate only small amounts of food at a time, and he may need especially nourishing food. Small feedings at frequent intervals are usually better for the patient than over-feeding at regular mealtimes. Nourishment at midmorning, midafternoon, and bedtime may be advisable in addition to regular meals. A high caloric diet, one that offers especially nourishing foods, may be ordered for a patient who is very weak or who has lost a lot of weight that he needs to regain. (Be aware, however, that high caloric foods that are rich in fat or sugar can be upsetting to the patient's digestive system.)

The amount and nutritional quality of food eaten by the sick person, as well as the selection and preparation of the food, may be a very important part of his treatment and progress. Appetite is often poor during illness. Foods served to the patient should therefore be those that he likes, if his diet allows them. Care should be taken to make sure that each food is well (but only moderately) seasoned, tastes and smells good, and is as appetizing and attractive as possible. Fresh, colorful foods should be selected, and vegetables should be cooked in as small an amount of water as possible and served at once. Liquids served hot must be only pleasantly hot so as not to burn the lips and tongue. Foods that are not highly seasoned or spicy are usually easier to digest.

Special Diets

Many patients are on special diets prescribed by their physician. All persons, including sick persons, need a well-balanced diet (see chapter 2). The health professional should be specific about what kind of diet the patient should have.

A *liquid diet* (Fig. 87) is often ordered for the patient who is acutely ill, who is suffering from some digestive condition, who has had surgery, or who, for some reason, is unable to swallow solid food. Offer frequent feedings to the patient on a liquid diet, in order to satisfy nutritional requirements of the body.

Fruit juices, tea, or coffee, some carbonated drinks, strained soups, milk, eggnog, thin custards, and ice cream are included in the *full* liquid diets. Because sugar is a good source of energy, the doctor may

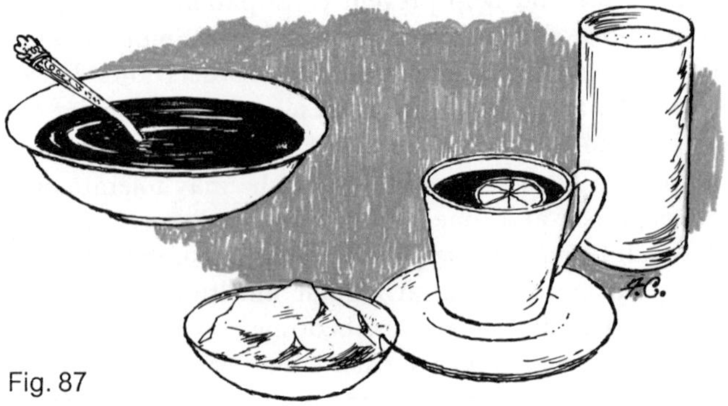

Fig. 87

request that certain drinks be sweetened. Gruel can be made by cooking cereal (such as oatmeal) thoroughly, then straining it and diluting it with water or milk to make it easy to drink. Salt and butter or margarine may be added to make it more flavorful, if the patient prefers. Flavorings such as vanilla and nutmeg are often added to milk or eggnog to make them more appetizing. Patients experiencing nausea and vomiting or who are acutely ill may be restricted to *clear* liquids. The clear liquid diet includes gelatin, tea, broth, and some carbonated beverages. It is not possible to provide nutrients necessary for maintenance of body functions through a liquid diet; therefore, the health professional should be consulted regarding nutrients if it becomes necessary for the patient to be on a liquid diet for very long. (See Charts I and II, on pages 370 and 373, for sample menus.)

As the patient progresses toward recovery, the health professional may offer a *soft diet,* which will include buttered toast, breakfast cereals (except bran), soft-cooked eggs, strained or pureed vegetables, and baked or mashed potatoes. (See Charts I and II for sample menus.)

When the patient is allowed to have a light or full diet, he probably can eat many of the same foods that are prepared for the family (general diet). Preparing identical menus for the patient and the family eliminates additional work for the home nurse.

A *low sodium diet* may be prescribed for some patients. Since sodium is a principal ingredient of salt, this diet usually involves reducing salt intake. Sodium causes the body to retain fluids, and its use may need to be restricted in patients with hypertension, cardiovascular disease, and diseases of the kidney or liver. In a *strict* low sodium diet, *all* salt must be omitted from cooking and as seasoning. (Fortunately, a salt substitute is usually permissible.) Foods with natural sodium must also be omitted from the diet, including pork, lunch meats, seafood, and canned meats. (There are foods available prepared especially for persons who must restrict sodium intake. In some areas, the sodium content in drinking water may be high, and the person may need to use distilled water. Check with the local health department for information.) Persons on a low sodium diet should follow the health professional's diet instructions and should be alert to signs such as nausea, muscle weakness, and dizziness; if these signs occur, the individual should contact the health professional at once, because the sodium level in the body may be too low. The American Heart Association has booklets that may be helpful to persons who need to follow a low sodium diet.

The cooperation of the patient is essential if he is on a special diet. He should understand the importance of the benefits to be gained by restricting certain foods and the damage that these foods might cause to his body. This is particularly true for the patient on a sodium-restricted diet or a diet for diabetes.

CHART I
FOODS ALLOWED ON FULL LIQUID, SOFT, AND GENERAL DIETS

Type of Food	Full Liquid Diet	Soft Diet	General Diet
Fruits	Fruit juices Strained fruits	Fruit juices Cooked and canned fruits (without seeds, coarse skins, or fibers) Bananas	All cooked and canned fruits Citrus fruits All other fruits
Cereals and cereal products	Gruel, strained Infant cereals with milk	Cereals, dry or well cooked Spaghetti and macaroni, not highly seasoned	All
Breads	None	Enriched white and whole wheat bread Soda crackers	All
Soups and broths	Broth Soups Strained cream	Broth Soups Strained cream	All
Eggs	Eggnogs	Soft-cooked eggs	Eggs cooked all ways

CHART I (cont'd)

Type of Food	Full Liquid Diet	Soft Diet	General Diet
Dairy products	Milk—sweet and buttermilk Cream Milkshakes Butter and margarine	Milk—sweet and buttermilk Cream Butter and margarine Cottage cheese Cream cheese Cheddar cheese used in cooking	Milk—sweet and buttermilk Cream Butter and margarine Cheese, all kinds
Vegetables	Strained vegetables Vegetable-beef soup Blended vegetable juices Creamed vegetable soups Tomato juice	Cooked: asparagus, peas, string beans, spinach, carrots, beets, squash Potatoes—boiled, mashed, creamed, scalloped, baked Salads: none	All, including salads
Nonfruit desserts	Ices Ice cream Plain gelatin Junkets Thin custard	Ices Ice cream Cereal pudding Custard Gelatin Simple cake Plain cookies	All

CHART I (cont'd)

Type of Food	Full Liquid Diet	Soft Diet	General Diet
Beverages	Tea, coffee, cocoa Coffee substitutes Milk and milk beverages Some carbonated beverages	Same as liquid diet	All
Sweets	Honey Syrup Sugar, dissolved	Same as liquid diet	All

CHART II
SAMPLE MENU FOR 1 DAY

Sample Family Menu for a Day	For Adult on Full Liquid Diet	For Small Child on Full Liquid Diet	How To Modify for Full Liquid Diet	Soft Diet
Breakfast				
Sliced oranges	Orange juice	½ cup orange juice	Squeeze oranges; strain juices.	Orange
Oatmeal	Oatmeal gruel	½ cup oatmeal gruel	Strain oatmeal through sieve; add milk to thin; serve with 3 tbsp. cream or milk and ½ tbsp. sugar.	Oatmeal
Toast with jelly				Toast with jelly
Coffee	Coffee with cream and sugar			Coffee
Milk (for children)		Full glass of milk		Milk (for children)
10:00 a.m.	Frosted milkshake	Frosted milkshake (1 cup, scant)		Frosted milkshake (if desired)

CHART II
SAMPLE MENU FOR 1 DAY (Continued)

Sample Family Menu for a Day	For Adult on Full Liquid Diet	For Small Child on Full Liquid Diet	How To Modify for Full Liquid Diet	Soft Diet
Lunch				
Potato soup	Potato soup	½ cup potato soup	Put cooked potato through sieve. Thin soup to desired consistency with stock, vegetable, water, or rich milk.	Potato soup
Peanut butter sandwich				Poached egg on toast
Coleslaw				
Fruit gelatin	Plain gelatin	½ cup plain gelatin	Omit fruit from gelatin mold.	Fruit gelatin
Milk	Milk	½ cup milk		
3:00 p.m.	Fresh fruit ade with ginger ale	Fresh fruit ade with ginger ale (1 cup, scant)		Fresh fruit ade with ginger ale (if desired)

CHART II
SAMPLE MENU FOR 1 DAY (continued)

Sample Family Menu for a Day	For Adult on Full Liquid Diet	For Small Child on Full Liquid Diet	How To Modify for Full Liquid Diet	Soft Diet
Dinner				
Tomato juice	Tomato juice	½ cup tomato juice		Tomato juice
Beef stew (with carrots, potatoes, tomatoes, celery, peas)	Strained beef broth	½ cup strained beef broth	Just before thickening stew, remove enough broth for patient; strain, reheat, and serve. Vegetables may be added if sieved or blended in blender.	Beef stew (carrots and potatoes only)
Salad—cottage cheese and canned peach on lettuce				Peach and cottage cheese—no lettuce
Bread with butter or margarine				Toast and butter or margarine
Soft or stirred custard; plain cookies	Soft or stirred custard	⅓ cup soft or stirred custard	(Soft custard is a cooked eggnog and is less firm than regular custard.)	Soft custard; plain cookies
Coffee	Coffee			Milk
8:00 p.m.	Hot cocoa	½ cup hot cocoa		Hot cocoa (if desired)

Mealtime Atmosphere

If the patient is not able to go to the table to eat, prepare his tray and give it to him before the family eats, while the food is hot and most appetizing. If a lap tray is not available, one can easily be made from a large box (see chapter 24 for instructions). Since its appearance may affect the patient's appetite favorably or unfavorably, make the tray and its contents pleasing to the eye:

Fig. 88

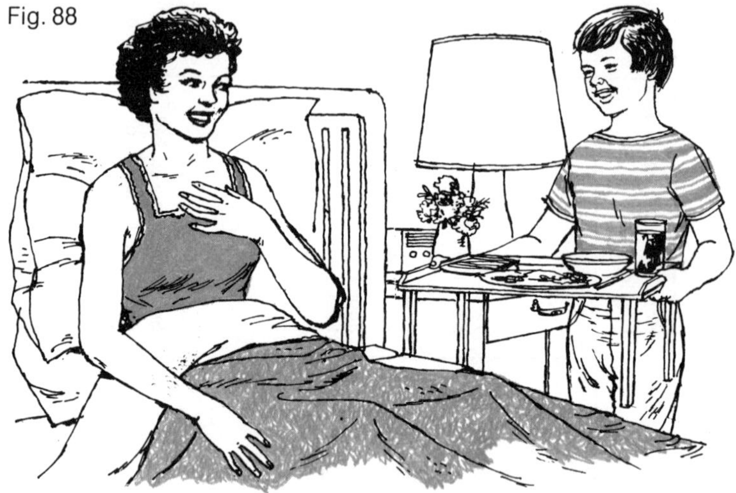

- Dishes should be attractive and in proportion to the size of the tray.
- The tray cover should be attractive and clean. Paper tray covers are convenient, inexpensive, and disposable.
- Different kinds of decorated or colored napkins can provide an element of interest and pleasure, both for adults and children.
- The practice of placing a fresh flower or a little surprise on the tray may help the patient to look forward to mealtime with pleasure.

Placing small portions of food on the plate may make it possible for the patient to eat all the food, giving him the satisfaction of "cleaning his plate."

Every effort should be made to see that the atmosphere at mealtime is most pleasant. The patient who is calm and relaxed will have less difficulty in digesting his food. Before the tray is brought into the sickroom, offer the patient the bedpan. Let him wash his hands and face with a wet washcloth so that he can be clean and refreshed for

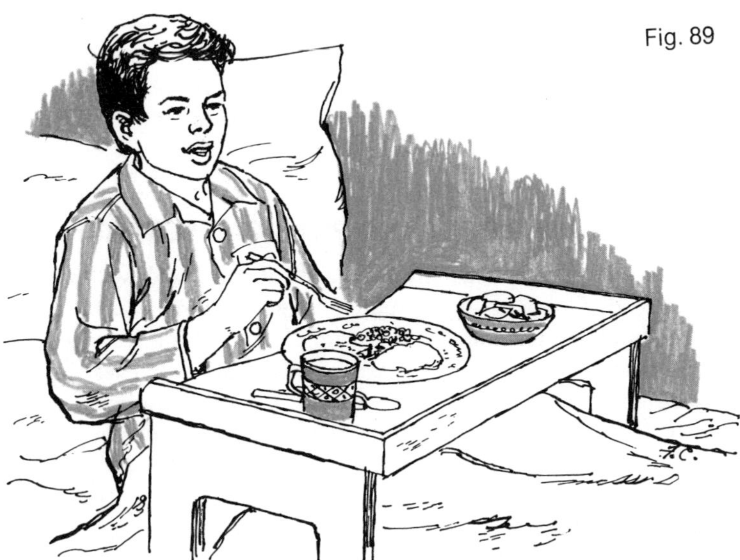

Fig. 89

his meal. Put the room and bed in good order and adjust the backrest or pillows to provide back support. Arrange the bed table comfortably and conveniently. If possible, the chronically ill patient should get out of bed into a chair at mealtimes; this will provide him with some activity and will aid his morale as well.

Eating when others are around is of great benefit for most people. Social contact can increase the patient's appetite and his desire to eat his food. If the patient is unable to come to the table for his meals, the home nurse or other family members should plan to sit and visit with him while he eats. If the patient is extremely lonely and needs more attention, he may refuse to feed himself and may insist that he be fed. In cases like this, it is important to try to see the reason for his behavior. If he merely wishes more attention, scheduling routine visiting periods might remedy the problem.

The average person prefers to feed himself, but helpless and weak patients or small children must be assisted (see chapter 20). The tray should be placed where the patient can see his food. When feeding the patient, give food in small bites, alternating various foods as he would do if feeding himself, or as he requests. Unless he is weak, let him hold his bread and butter and eat it when he wishes. Allow him to wipe his own mouth.

The kind and amount of food eaten should always be noted on the patient's record so that the health professional may determine whether the patient is taking enough nourishment. Changes in mental functioning, lack of energy, or skin breakdown (eruptions, dryness, cracking) should also be recorded, since these may be related to inadequate food and fluid intake.

PROVIDING REST AND PHYSICAL ACTIVITY

A person who is ill may feel tired and achy and probably will want to rest in bed. Going to bed usually means keeping warm, quiet, relaxed, and comfortable. This provides rest, builds resistance, and helps repair tissue damage caused by the illness. Bed rest is prescribed for the acutely ill. When the patient has an infectious disease, going to bed at the first appearance of illness will also help to prevent the spread of a communicable disease. A person with a fever, headache, nausea, sore throat, or runny nose should go to bed in a room by himself, or at least isolate himself from other family members until the health professional sees him or until he feels better.

Activity during an illness of relatively short duration should be encouraged. Such activity could include anything the patient is interested in that does not cause undue fatigue or emotional strain. A patient who is ill for a short time (less than 2 weeks) may be allowed to engage in exercises to maintain strength and normal range of joint motion. *All activity,* however, including the return to what is normal for the patient, should be carried out *gradually.* Sitting or getting out of bed for the first time should be done slowly, with adequate provision for support and assistance, because these activities may cause dizziness. Children are usually ready to do school assignments after their temperature has returned to normal or near normal.

Patients who have had surgery or who are returning home after hospitalization should follow their health professional's advice about exercises and the return to usual activities. Often they can exercise as much as they can tolerate. Sometimes special exercises to strengthen certain muscles are prescribed.

It is important that the patient keep interested in the world around him. Activating this interest may take more than conversation, diverting activity, and exercise. It could include reading to the patient and involving him in some recreation. Friends and family should not only provide company but should also keep the patient interested in relaxing projects or activities.

Because sleep helps restore the body, the home nurse should observe the length and quality of the patient's sleep. The number of hours during which a sick person sleeps should be observed and recorded as accurately as possible. Naps should also be noted, because the person who naps during the day may not sleep as long at night. The nature of the patient's sleep should also be observed: whether the patient is quiet or restless, whether he sleeps for short periods of time and wakes often, or whether he sleeps for several hours at a time. Information from the patient about his sleeping is not always reliable. When a person is ill, a short period of wakefulness may seem much longer than it really is, especially at night, when others in the household are asleep.

PREVENTING THE SIDE EFFECTS OF LIMITED ACTIVITY

The preceding principles of rest and activity, which apply to those who are ill for a short time, apply also to patients with long-term illness. When a person is immobile for long periods, however, special precautions must be taken to prevent complications. Adequate exercise should be a main concern.

When the health professional tells the patient to stay in bed, he is prescribing a form of treatment that often is as important as medicine. Without bed rest, medicine sometimes can do little good. As in a prescription, the health professional determines whether bed rest is to be partial or complete and for how long it should continue. With complete bed rest, there is a danger of rapid physical change: muscles lose their tone and become weak, and the patient may be unable to stand or to maintain his balance when he does get up. Complete bed rest is therefore prescribed only when it is absolutely necessary.

Exercise

Adequate exercise for the person confined to bed for long periods of time is very important. The health professional should advise on an exercise program for the patient. Active exercise maintains or restores muscle strength and tone and maintains the mobility of the joints. Sometimes the patient is so ill that there is little physical activity in his daily routine; in such a case, the home nurse should make a special effort to help him have some physical activity each day.

Letting the patient participate in his daily care, and giving him assistance in getting out of bed for meals and in walking around, will not only restore muscle strength but will also be a morale booster. Such activity insures that the patient who does not otherwise move about will maintain a full range of motion essential to keeping muscle strength and full use of his joints.

Planned range-of-motion exercises and correct body posture are extremely important in the prevention of contracture deformities. A contracture deformity occurs when a muscle tightens up from not being used, causing the joint to become stiff and the body part (such as an arm, wrist, knee, or hip) to become permanently bent or deformed. This condition is often seen in patients who find it more comfortable to stay in one position for long periods of time. It is much easier to prevent these deformities than to treat them once they appear.

To prevent contracture deformities, encourage the patient to keep his body in good position *and* to change his position as often as possible. (Chapter 20 provides guidelines for positioning and support of the patient in bed.) *Range-of-motion exercises* should be started early in the patient's illness and should be continued until he is moving about normally (see chapter 22). The home nurse may help the patient to do these exercises by moving the patient's body parts (arms, legs, joints, etc.) or may support the patient's efforts to do the exercises himself. When a patient has one-sided weakness and does not regain muscle strength in an arm or a leg, range-of-motion exercises should be continued at least twice a day. Sometimes several months of exercising the muscles is necessary before muscle strength returns and the limb becomes useful again.

The patient can aid in preventing contracture deformities by doing as much as he can for himself and by moving about in bed. When there is weakness or paralysis on one side, he can be taught to do range-of-motion exercises with the weak limbs by using the strong limbs.

Pressure Sores

Pressure sores, or bed sores (also known as "decubitus ulcers") are another hazard of bed rest. A pressure sore is an area on the skin that first becomes red and tender and then breaks down into a sore. Pressure sores result from lying in one position for a long period of time, thus causing loss of blood flow to the tissues, with resulting lack of nourishment to the tissues. Observation of the skin and of pressure areas is an important preventive measure.

Areas of the body most commonly affected with pressure sores include the skin areas over prominent bones such as the "tail bone," the shoulders, and the heels. A cast, splint, tight bandage, or even the bedding can create enough pressure to cause the skin to break down and develop sores that are difficult to heal. Wrinkles in the bottom sheet, crumbs, or anything that causes irritation or friction can also contribute to the formation of these sores. Improper placing and removing of the bedpan can cause irritation to the skin, which, if not cared for, will also cause a sore. Moisture, either from perspiration or from body discharges such as urine or stool, can also contribute to the development of pressure sores.

The prevention of pressure sores depends almost entirely on nursing care. Change the patient's position at least every 2 to 3 hours or as often as needed so that pressure is not maintained for a long period on any one body part. Turn the patient from side to side and from his back to his abdomen. Keep the skin clean and dry. Gently rub the pressure areas with a lotion to help stimulate circulation and bring needed nutrients to the skin. Baths and frequent back rubs are helpful in stimulating circulation. Good nutrition nourishes and strengthens body tissue, contributing to the prevention of pressure sores.

A firm mattress that provides for even distribution of body weight is desirable. Bedding that is free from wrinkles is also important. Large pieces of covered foam rubber placed under the body wherever there is pressure on bones will help to relieve pressure. An alternating pressure mattress may also be recommended to aid in the prevention of pressure sores (see "Providing for Bed and Bedding" section of this chapter).

Washable sheepskin or chamois skin placed under the affected part of the body, usually the buttocks, will help absorb moisture, relieve pressure, and protect the skin from irritation. If the sheepskin has fleece, the wooly side should be placed next to the patient's body. (If the patient is allergic to wool, synthetic sheepskin is also available and can be used.) A number of these pads will be needed so that the patient can always have a dry one. They may be washed and rinsed well by hand or in the washing machine, using lukewarm water and a mild soap. They must always be air dried, to keep the skins soft and supple.

Any redness at a pressure area should be reported immediately to the health professional so that he can recommend additional measures for the care of the patient. Treatment should begin at the first sign of redness, and observation for and prevention of further pressure sores should continue.

Chapter 18

Evaluating Your Patient

The home nurse should observe and evaluate the patient's mental and physical condition daily to determine whether it is improving or becoming worse. What the home nurse includes in the assessment depends on the nature of the patient's illness. The assessment may include information on temperature, pulse, respiration, blood pressure, amount of pain, whether a wound is healing, and other aspects of the patient's physical condition. Since the patient's mental state can also affect his rate of recovery, the home nurse will also notice whether the patient is happy, sad, bored, depressed, etc.

Changes in a person's health status can often be measured by certain body functions and states. For example, the internal temperature of most persons is about 98.6° Fahrenheit, or 37° centigrade. When the temperature is higher, the presence of an infection may be indicated.

The measurement of temperature, pulse, and respiration (referred to as vital signs) involves fairly simple procedures and can be done easily if the home nurse follows the instructions given. Taking the blood pressure (also a vital sign) and inspecting the throat can also be done by the home nurse with proper instruction. Each of these procedures is explained in this chapter.

TEMPERATURE

Normal Temperature

The healthy human body maintains an internal temperature that varies only slightly with the time of day or the amount of physical exercise. Therefore, a higher-than-normal temperature is often an indication of sickness. It is important to know what an individual's normal temperature is so that variations from the normal can be recognized when they occur.

Temperature can be taken by mouth (orally), in the rectum, or under the armpit (axilla). The most commonly used method of taking the temperature is by mouth. The normal mouth temperature of a well person is usually between 97.6° and 99.6° Fahrenheit, or 36.4° and 37.6° centigrade. When the temperature is taken rectally, it is generally 1 degree Fahrenheit or ½ degree centigrade higher than the oral temperature. When taken in the axilla, the temperature reading will be about 1 degree Fahrenheit or ½ degree centigrade lower than the oral reading. This variation in temperature is related to the closeness of the blood vessels to the surface next to the thermometer; the closer the blood vessels are to the surface (as in the rectum), the higher the normal reading will be. When you are reporting a temperature reading to the health professional, it is important to mention how the temperature was taken.

The Thermometer

Every home should have a clinical, or fever, thermometer. Clinical thermometers are inexpensive and are available with either Fahrenheit or centigrade scales. The family may choose whichever it prefers. (Braille thermometers are also available for use by the blind.) Another type of thermometer is an electronic device that shows a visual reading of the body temperature. Some electronic devices will show visual readings for temperature, pulse, and blood pressure. These devices, however, are much more expensive and are more likely to be found in a hospital setting.

The clinical thermometer is a glass tube filled with mercury, with a bulb at one end. The thermometer operates on the principle that mercury expands when exposed to heat. When subjected to body heat, the mercury rises in the glass tube and remains at the highest point registered. The narrowing at the bulb end prevents the mercury from returning to the bulb until it is shaken down. Since the clinical thermometer is made of glass, it breaks easily. It should be handled with care and stored in a thermometer case or rigid box when not in use. Too much heat will also cause the thermometer to break by making the mercury expand too rapidly. The thermometer should be kept away from any source of heat (such as hot water, a stove, or a heater) and should be cleaned only with cool water.

There are two types of clinical thermometers: oral and rectal. Oral thermometers have a long, slender bulb; rectal thermometers have a blunt, stubby, or teardrop-shaped bulb. *Do not use an oral thermometer to take a rectal temperature,* because the slender (almost pointed) bulb is likely to damage the sensitive tissue of the rectum. The blunt end of the rectal thermometer is not likely to injure tissue when inserted into the rectum.

The stubby thermometer is sometimes referred to as the universal thermometer because it can be used to take either oral, rectal, or axillary temperature, while the oral thermometer can be used only for oral and axillary temperature. *A thermometer that has been used to take a rectal temperature should never to be used to take a temperature by mouth.* It is wise to have two thermometers that are clearly marked, one for rectal use and one for the mouth, especially if there are small children in the family. If the only thermometer that is available is the blunt end (rectal) type, and if you are not sure how it has been used, use it only for taking rectal temperatures.

How To Use and Care For the Thermometer

Where To Take the Temperature

Most people prefer to have their temperature taken orally. Taking the temperature rectally is advisable when the patient cannot hold the thermometer safely in his mouth for the required time. Examples are an infant or young child, an unconscious person, a person with a mouth injury or with poorly fitting dentures, a person with a stuffy nose or other nasal obstruction, or a person having convulsive seizures. Occasionally it is preferable to take the temperature in the armpit, although this method is considered less accurate than the oral or rectal temperature.

How To Obtain the Correct Temperature

Whichever method of taking the temperature is chosen, the following procedure should be followed when using a clinical thermometer:

1. Before taking the temperature, make sure the mercury is shaken down to 96°F, or 35.6°C, or below.

   When shaking down the mercury, stand away from hard surfaces to avoid breaking the thermometer by dropping it or striking it against an object. (It is a good idea to shake it over a bed or couch.)

   Hold the top end firmly between the thumb and the first two fingers.

   Shake with a loose wrist action, as if shaking water off the hand.
2. Have the patient sit or lie down.
3. When taking the temperature, allow sufficient time for the mercury to rise: at least 7 minutes for oral temperature, 2 to 4 minutes for rectal temperature, and 10 minutes for axillary temperature.
4. Check any great rise or fall in body temperature by taking the temperature again, using a different thermometer if possible.

5. Do not take the temperature immediately after the patient has had a very hot or cold bath. Do not take the oral temperature immediately after the patient has been smoking, or after he has been eating or drinking hot or cold liquids. Wait 10 minutes to take the temperature after these actions. If the patient has had an enema, wait at least 30 minutes before taking the temperature rectally.

How To Read the Thermometer

Fahrenheit thermometers are usually marked from 94° to 108°F, and the long lines on the scale indicate degrees. The short lines indicate two tenths (2/10) of a degree. Centigrade thermometers are marked from 34° to 42°C. The long lines indicate degrees, and the short lines indicate one tenth (1/10) of a degree. The small arrow indicates the average mouth temperature, which is 98.6°F or 37°C. The front of the thermometer magnifies the mercury column in the glass tube, and the back is made of frosted glass so that the mercury will be easier to see.

To determine the temperature, find where the end of the mercury column is located on the scale. One method is to hold the top of the thermometer (the end away from the bulb) in the right hand and, in a good light, turn the thermometer slowly until you see where the wide band of mercury stops between the scale markings on the top and the numbers on the bottom. Another method is to place the thermometer on a flat surface with the white edge down, in a good light. Stand directly over the thermometer, moving over it until you can see the mercury column.

Read the scale at the end of the mercury column to include the degree and the nearest two tenths of a degree. Record the temperature, shake the mercury column down, and clean the thermometer. If unable to read the thermometer soon after taking a temperature, clean it and store it in a cool place until someone else can read and record the temperature. (The mercury will stay at the same temperature until the thermometer is shaken.)

To convert a centigrade reading to a Fahrenheit reading, multiply the centigrade reading by 9, divide by 5, and add 32. To convert a Fahrenheit reading to a centigrade reading, subtract 32 from the Fahrenheit reading, multiply by 5, and divide by 9.

How To Clean the Thermometer

Always clean the thermometer after using it. If you are not sure that it is clean when you are ready to use it, clean it before using it. The cleaning procedure (Fig. 90) is as follows:

1. Moisten a wipe (tissue, cotton ball, gauze square) with cool water and soap it well.
2. Hold the thermometer by the top, with the bulb over a sink or waste container. Beginning at the top, wipe down with a firm, twisting motion, using friction to get well into the grooves of the tube and around the bulb. Discard the wipe.
3. Moisten a fresh wipe with cool water and rinse the thermometer, using the same downward, twisting motion. Discard the wipe.
4. Soap and rinse again.
5. Dry with a fresh wipe using the same motion.
6. Place the thermometer in its case or box, bulb end first, for safety and cleanliness.
7. Store the thermometer in a cool, dry area.

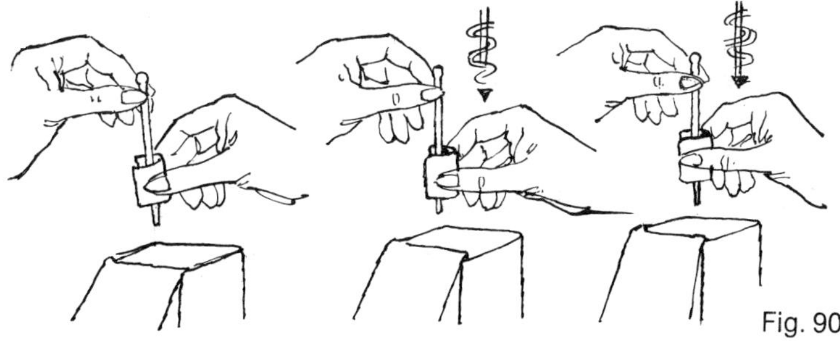
Fig. 90

Any time that one thermometer will be used to take the temperatures of two different persons within a short time, extra precautions should be taken to make sure that disease germs are not transferred from one person to the other. After cleaning the thermometer, let it stand in alcohol (90 percent ethyl or isopropyl, usually sold as "rubbing alcohol") for at least 10 minutes. After the soaking, rinse the thermometer well with water before using it again. It is a good idea to disinfect the thermometer in this way at the end of any illness, to make sure that it will be clean and safe to use when needed for the next illness. It should be remembered, however, that alcohol is not a substitute for washing, because it does not remove saliva or stool from the thermometer.

How To Take the Temperature

Oral Temperature

1. Assemble the necessary equipment: oral thermometer, equipment needed to clean the thermometer (wipes, cool water, soap), and waste container.
2. Wash your hands.
3. Make sure the mercury column is below 96°F (35.6°C).
4. Moisten the thermometer with cool water so that it does not stick to the patient's lips.
5. Place the bulb end well under the patient's tongue and a little to one side. Tell the patient to keep his lips closed, to breathe through his nose, and not to talk or bite down on the thermometer.
6. Leave the thermometer in place 7 minutes to insure an accurate measurement.
7. Remove the thermometer and with a tissue, wipe off the saliva, using a firm, twisting motion from the top downward over the bulb.
8. In a good light, read the thermometer and record the temperature.
9. Shake the mercury down. Clean the thermometer immediately.
10. Wash your hands.

Rectal Temperature

1. Assemble the necessary equipment: rectal thermometer, lubricant such as petroleum jelly, and equipment needed to clean the thermometer.
2. Wash your hands.

For an Adult

1. Explain to the patient the steps that will be taken and have him lie down on his side.
2. Make sure the mercury column is 96°F (35.6°C) or below.
3. Lubricate the bulb end of the thermometer so that it will slide easily into the rectum.
4. Gently slip the bulb about 1 inch (2.54 centimeters) into the anus (opening of the rectum) and hold it in place for 2 to 4 minutes. (If

the patient is able to do so, let him insert the thermometer himself and hold it in place.) Stay with the patient to be sure of safety and accuracy.

5. Remove the thermometer, wipe it, read it, and record the temperature.
6. Shake the mercury down. Clean the thermometer immediately.
7. Wash your hands (and the patient's, if he has helped).

For an Infant or Child

1. Explain to the child what is to be done.
2. Make sure the mercury column is below 96°F (35.6°C).
3. Lubricate the bulb end of the thermometer.
4. Position the child: have him lie on his side or abdomen so that his anus is visible. An infant or small child may lie face down on your lap with his legs hanging down at one side. An alternate position for an infant is on his back. Grasp his ankles with one hand and gently bend the child's knees to expose the anus.
5. Gently insert the bulb of the thermometer about 1 inch into the anus and hold it in place for 2 to 4 minutes. Hold the thermometer in place *at all times* by resting your hand against the child's buttocks so that your hand and the thermometer will move with the child. Help may be needed to hold a restless child.
6. Remove the thermometer by pulling it out in a straight line. Wipe it, read it, and record the temperature and the method used (R, for rectal).
7. Shake the mercury down. Clean the thermometer immediately.
8. Wash your hands.

Axillary Temperature

Temperature taken in the armpit may be called skin temperature. The average normal axillary temperature is 97.6°F, or 36.4°C, about 1 degree Fahrenheit (one half degree centigrade) lower than the mouth temperature. For this reason, the daily record should show that the temperature has been taken by the axillary method. The axillary method may be ordered for infants or when other methods are difficult to follow. In order for the axillary method (Fig. 91) to be reliable, the procedure given below must be followed carefully.

1. Assemble the equipment: clinical thermometer and equipment needed to clean the thermometer.

2. Wash your hands.
3. Make sure that the mercury is below 96°F (35.6°C).
4. Dry the area under the arm.
5. Place the dry bulb end of the thermometer carefully in the armpit and have the patient press his arm firmly against his body by grasping his opposite shoulder. Do not press the bulb sharply into the skin. It will be necessary to stay with an infant or child to make sure that the thermometer stays in place. The thermometer should remain in the armpit for 10 minutes.

Fig. 91

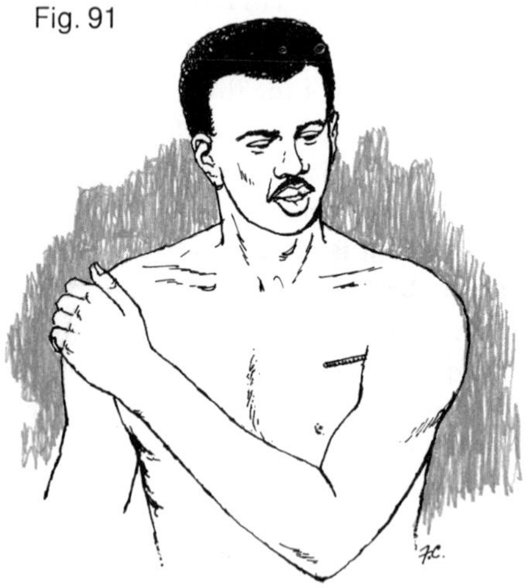

6. Remove the thermometer, wipe it, read it, and record the temperature and method used (A, for axillary).
7. Shake the mercury down and clean the thermometer immediately.

PULSE AND RESPIRATION RATES

The pulse is the throbbing of blood through the arteries, caused by the contractions of the heart as it forces blood through the vessels. Counting the pulse is one way to count the rate of the heartbeat. Respiration is the act of moving air in and out of the lungs—breathing. Each respiration is one full breath: one breathing in (inhalation) and one breathing out (exhalation), or one rising and falling of the chest.

Because both pulse and respiration rates generally increase as the temperature of the body rises, the count of pulse and respirations is an indicator of the patient's condition. A health professional may tell you how often to measure pulse and respiration. In general, if a patient is not feeling well, take temperature, pulse, and respiration (TPR) every 3 to 4 hours. If the pulse rate, respiration rate, and temperature of a child or adult are rising, you should take and record the TPR every hour. Report to the health professional if the patient's pulse rate is extremely rapid, extremely slow, or irregular. Also report shortness of breath, noisy respiration, or gasping for air.

Normal Pulse and Respiration

The pulse rate, volume, and rhythm will vary with age, sex, size, and physical and emotional condition. A pulse rate of between 70 and 90 beats per minute while at rest is normal for adults. The normal pulse at rest for babies and small children is somewhat faster than that of adults. The normal range of pulse for a baby or very small child is 100 to 130 beats a minute; for a newborn baby, it may be as high as 130 beats a minute. The normal pulse for a 3-year-old is about 110 beats a minute; and for a 12-year-old, about 80 beats a minute.

The respiration rate and quality vary with age and with physical and emotional condition. Normal, healthy adults breathe 14 to 20 times each minute. It is normal for a baby or a small child to breathe more quickly than an adult.

Since increased activity will increase the pulse and respiration rates, *pulse and respiration rates should be counted after the patient has been resting quietly for 10 minutes or more.*

How To Count Pulse and Respiration Rates

The pulse may be counted wherever there is a large artery near the surface of the body. Common places to take the pulse include the wrist (radial artery) and the neck (carotid artery).

The home nurse should consider the ease and comfort of the patient when choosing the site at which to count the pulse. The wrist is usually the easiest site. If the patient must stay in an unusual position, or if there is an emergency, it may be easier to find and check the pulse at the neck.

Both pulse and respiration rates may be counted while the temperature is being taken. *Respirations should be counted when the patient is unaware that it is being done,* since he is then less likely to change his rate of breathing (which he can control).

Following is the procedure for counting the pulse at the wrist and counting the respiration rate:

1. Have a watch or clock with a second hand placed so that it is clearly visible.
2. Have the patient sit or lie in a comfortable position.
3. Have the patient extend his hand in a relaxed position, supported on a chair arm, table, or bed, with the thumb up (Fig. 92). The arm may also be crossed over the chest so that respirations can be counted after the pulse is counted.

Fig. 92

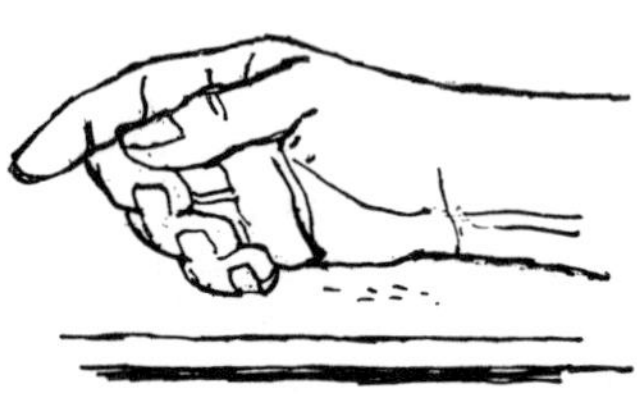
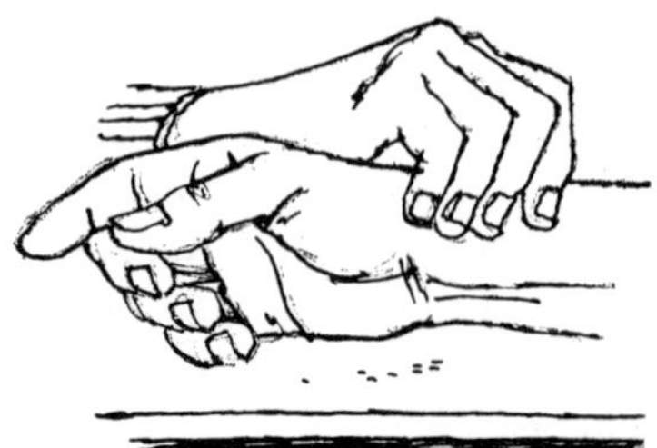

4. Locate the pulse by placing your fingers, *not your thumb,* on the thumb side of the patient's wrist, between the tendons and the wristbone (Fig 92). (The thumb has a pulse of its own, and it might be counted rather than the patient's.) Apply only enough pressure to feel the pulsing of the artery.
5. Count the pulse beats for one half a minute and multiply the number counted by two in order to calculate the rate per minute. If there is any doubt as to accuracy, count the beats for another half minute.
6. Count respirations while the fingers are still on the wrist, so that the patient will not notice that his breathing is being observed. Check the position of the second hand on the watch or clock; then count "one" when you see or feel the patient's chest rise as he breathes in. Count "two" the next time his chest rises, and continue counting for one half a minute. Multiply by two to get the rate per minute.

To count the pulse at the carotid artery, find the artery by first placing your fingertips on the person's Adam's apple, then sliding them down into the groove at the side of the neck (Fig. 93). Use only the fleshy pads of your fingers, not the very tips.

To check a baby's heartbeat, place the tips of your fingers on the

Fig. 93

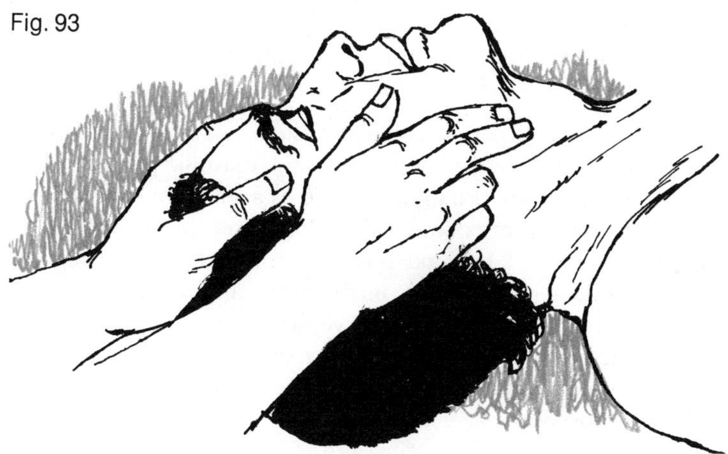

baby's chest, slightly below the line of the nipples and to the left of the breastbone.

Write on the patient's daily record the time, date, and rate per minute of the pulse and respirations.

BLOOD PRESSURE

Blood pressure is the force exerted against the blood vessels (arteries) when the heart pumps blood. It is one clue to the health of the heart and the blood vessels. Blood pressure measurements help health professionals tell if a person is suffering from high blood pressure (hypertension) or certain other conditions.

Occasionally it is important to keep a close watch on a patient's blood pressure. The health professional may request that the home nurse purchase the necessary equipment to monitor the blood pressure of a patient who has high blood pressure or disease of the heart or blood vessels. This procedure is more complicated than taking a temperature, since it requires coordination of eyes, ears, and hands. No one should expect to do it easily the first few times he tries. Persons who need to learn how to take blood pressure should contact their local Red Cross chapter for instructions.

The action, or "beating," of the heart has two parts:

- Contracting—when the heart pumps blood through the arteries to the parts of the body. The pressure in the arteries when the heart is contracting is called *systolic* (sis-TOL-ik) pressure; systolic pressure shows how hard the heart is pumping.

- Refilling—when the heart relaxes and fills with blood before the next contraction. The pressure in the arteries when the heart is relaxed and refilling for the next pumping action is called the *diastolic* (die-as-TOL-ik) pressure.

When you measure a person's blood pressure, you get two numbers: one for the systolic pressure and one for the diastolic pressure. The two measurements are usually expressed as a fraction: systolic over diastolic pressure. An example of a blood pressure for a healthy young adult is 120/80. Blood pressure is influenced by age, sex, emotional state at the moment, medications, and other factors. No two adults should be expected to have the same reading. Readings for the same adult may vary from day to day and hour to hour. Because so much variation is possible, care must be taken to follow the correct procedure.

Equipment

The home nurse will need two pieces of equipment to take blood pressure: a stethoscope (Fig. 94) and a blood pressure cuff (sphygmomanometer). The stethoscope merely picks up the sound of the

Fig. 94

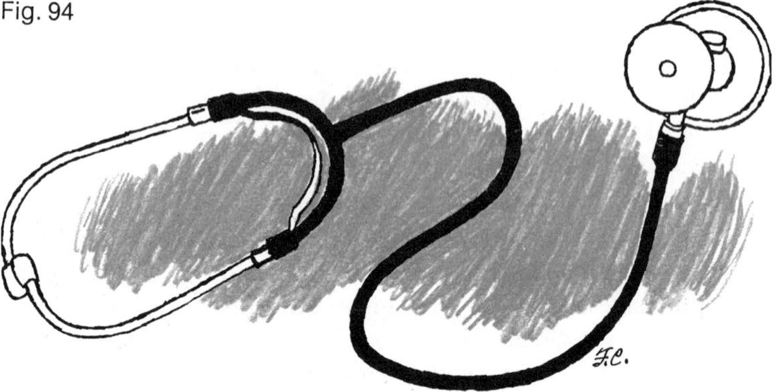

pulse and carries it to the ears of the listener. The blood pressure cuff has three parts:

An inflatable cuff, which is wrapped around the patient's arm.

A rubber bulb with a screw valve, which is twisted shut when air is to be pumped into the cuff and is opened when air is to be released from the cuff.

A gauge that registers air pressure in the cuff. There are two kinds of gauges: the aneroid type, which registers on a dial like a clock face, and the mercury type, which registers on a vertical column like a thermometer. Both are marked in millimeters from zero to 250 or 300.

The rubber bulb and pressure gauge are connected to the cuff by separate tubes.

This equipment is rather fragile and should be handled and cared for according to the recommendations of the manufacturer. It is also expensive. The health professional should be consulted before you make a purchase. Advice on the size of cuff to be purchased is particularly important. The standard cuff is designed for the arm of an average-size adult. If the patient has very large arms, a larger cuff will be needed. Smaller cuffs are available for children.

How To Take Blood Pressure

The following method is known as the palpatory-auscultatory (PAL-pa-to-ry–aus-CUL-ta-to-ry), or P-A, method of taking blood pressure. "Palpatory" refers to *feeling* the pulse. The first part of the P-A method is to estimate the systolic pressure while feeling the pulse. "Auscultatory" refers to *hearing* the pulse with a stethoscope. The actual blood pressure readings are determined by hearing the pulse, which is the second part of the P-A method.

1. Assemble the necessary equipment: stethoscope and blood pressure cuff.
2. Have the patient sit or lie comfortably with his arm extended, palm up (unless the health professional has ordered that the blood pressure should be taken while the patient is standing). If the patient is sitting, he should rest his elbow and lower arm on a table beside him. If in bed, he should lie flat with his arm extended, palm up, flat on the bed beside him in a relaxed position. The patient's sleeve should be rolled up so that the cuff can go directly on his arm.
3. Position the cuff on the patient's arm in such a way that the tube to the bulb is on the side of the patient's arm closest to his body. The bottom of the cuff should be about 1 inch (2.5 centimeters) above the bend of the elbow. Wrap the cuff snugly and smoothly. (If the cuff is so loose that it slides up and down on the arm when deflated, or if it is crooked so that the rubber air bladder bulges out, the measurement will not be accurate.)
4. Find the wrist pulse, close the valve, and squeeze the bulb

rapidly to inflate the cuff with air. As the cuff fills with air, it squeezes the arm, closing the artery and stopping the flow of blood.

5. When the blood is not flowing, you will no longer feel the pulse. *Read the gauge when the wrist pulse disappears.* This reading is the estimate of the systolic pressure.
6. As soon as you no longer feel the pulse and have read the gauge, open the valve and *quickly* let all the air out of the cuff.
7. Wait one or two minutes before you begin the auscultatory (hearing) phase of the P-A method.
8. Find the pulse in the brachial artery, close to the elbow and on the side of the arm nearer to the body. Place the bell of the stethoscope where you find the brachial pulse and hold it gently but firmly in place. Keep the tubes from moving, since the stethoscope will pick up sounds of the tubes touching things.
9. Inflate the cuff to a pressure 30 millimeters (mm) above the palpatory (feeling) estimate of systolic pressure. For example, if the estimate was 120, inflate the cuff to 150 millimeters. (When the pressure in the cuff is above the systolic pressure, no pulse sounds will be heard.)
10. Let air out of the cuff *slowly* and listen for a pulse sound in the arm. When the cuff pressure gets down to the person's systolic pressure, the pumping heart again forces blood to flow through the artery under the cuff. You can then hear the pulse through the stethoscope. The reading on the gauge when you first hear the pulse is the systolic pressure.
11. Keep letting air out of the cuff *slowly* (2 to 4 millimeters per second). Pulse sounds will continue and then disappear. The reading when the last pulse sound is heard is the diastolic pressure.
12. Open the valve completely and let the cuff deflate. Remove the cuff.
13. Record the two numbers as a fraction, systolic over diastolic.
14. Compare the reading to previous blood pressure readings. If either number is outside the expected range, repeat the procedure to check the accuracy of the measurement.

Points to remember:

- When you read the gauge, be sure that you are looking straight at it. If you are looking down at it or at an angle from the side, your reading may be incorrect.

- Air must be released slowly and gradually. The correct rate is 2 to 4 millimeters per heartbeat. If it is released too quickly, the pressure will drop 5 to 10 millimeters between heartbeats, and the reading is likely to be low.
- If air is released too slowly, the reading will be too high.

THROAT INSPECTION

The throat is one of the first areas of the body to signal illness. In many cases, a sore throat is an early symptom of a cold, but it may also be a symptom of an acute communicable disease. Early recognition and treatment of a sore throat are particularly important when the patient is among a large number of people, such as in a school.

Sore throats may cause some difficulty in swallowing, although small children seldom complain of this difficulty. Because infection is present, the lymph glands in the neck may become enlarged and tender. Another discomfort may be an earache, resulting from an inflammation caused by infection traveling through the Eustachian tube, which connects the throat to the ear.

Appearance of the Throat

The small flap hanging down from the top of the mouth is the uvula (YOO-vhuh-la), or soft palate. The tonsils are visible as flaps extending in and down from the sides (unless they have been removed by surgery). The arched opening at the back of the mouth is the throat. Normally, all parts of the mouth and throat are about the same pink color, and the lining of the throat looks smooth and shiny.

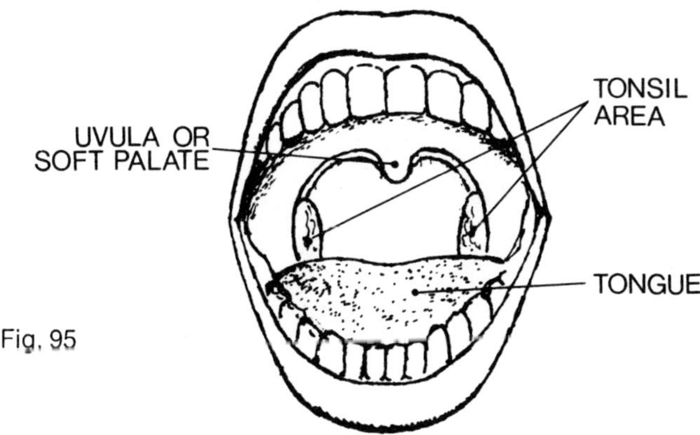

Fig. 95

How To Inspect the Throat

It is important to practice inspecting the throat when members of the family, particularly small children, are well. This gives the home nurse an opportunity to observe the normal appearance of each person's mouth and throat. It is also a good learning experience for a child; he will be more willing to cooperate when sick if he has had his throat inspected when well. If you are unable to see the back of the throat on the first attempt, let the patient rest before trying again.

When inspecting the throat, look for–

Bright red color. (Throat is redder than the inside of the mouth and different from its usual bright pink color.)

Swelling. (Throat seems full; tonsils seem enlarged and puffy.)

White, gray, or yellowish patches, usually on the tonsil area.

The inspection procedure is as follows:

1. Assemble the necessary equipment: wooden tongue depressor or spoon, tissues, flashlight.
2. Explain to the patient the steps that will be taken. Give the patient a tissue and instruct him to cover his mouth if he should need to cough. If a flashlight is not available, have the patient face a good light, near a window or a lamp.
3. Stand to one side to avoid being in the direct line of possible cough spray.
4. Support the patient's chin with one hand, and to help open the throat, ask him to say "ah."
5. Place the tongue depressor (or the handle of the spoon) about two thirds back on the tongue and use gentle pressure as necessary to bring the back of the throat into view. Ask the patient to say "ah."

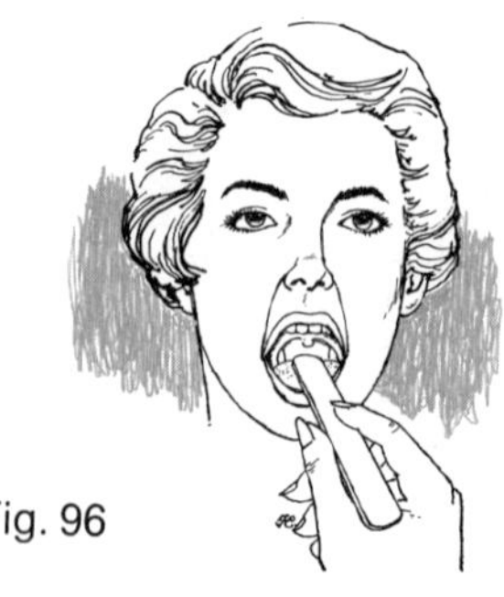

Fig. 96

6. Inspect the back and sides of the throat. Also note any unusual color and condition of the tongue and any unusual odor of the breath.
7. Discard the wooden tongue depressor. If a spoon was used, avoid touching the part that was in contact with the patient's mouth until the spoon has been washed well with hot water and soap.

If the throat is unusually red and swollen, or if white, gray, or yellowish patches are observed, encourage the patient to rest quietly and keep others away from him. Take his temperature, check for other signs of illness (for example, a rash, aching joints, productive cough, earache), and contact a health professional for instructions.

Chapter 19

Medications

Medicines are often needed to bring about a cure or provide relief for symptoms of specific illnesses. Medicines that can be sold only when prescribed by a doctor are called *prescription drugs.* Medicines that do not require a doctor's prescription are referred to as *over-the-counter* (OTC), or nonprescription, drugs. All medicines, however, should be used only on the advice of a health professional.

All medicines have the following common features:

- Potential benefit to the patient
- Potential for harm to the patient
- Limits in the amount that it is safe to use
- A generic name (which includes the names of the active ingredients)
- A brand name (the manufacturer's name for the drug)
- The possibility of becoming weaker under certain conditions (such as when stored for long periods of time before use, or when not taken as directed)
- Possible risk when taken in combination with alcohol or other drugs
- Variations in price

GENERAL PRINCIPLES REGARDING MEDICINES

Whatever symptoms a person may have, it is important that medicines be taken only on the advice of a health professional. The real cause of the symptoms must be known before the correct treatment can be started. Early diagnosis and treatment often makes cure more probable, and in a shorter period of time. In prescribing medicines, the health professional takes into consideration the person's condition, the active ingredient of the drug, the amount or dose of the drug, and how and when the drug is to be taken.

The health professional prescribes medicine for a specific condition of a specific person. Medicines have very specific actions. Some are made in such a way that they dissolve in the stomach; others are intended to dissolve in the small intestine or the large bowel. With some drugs, the active ingredients are released slowly over a period of hours, while others are made to release all of the active ingredient quickly. Some drugs go through the body slowly, while others are quickly excreted; some drugs tend to accumulate in the body after repeated doses. Some drugs must be taken right after a meal to avoid irritation to the stomach, while others must be taken on an empty stomach. Whichever way the drug works, it is prescribed with a planned action in mind. Medicine should be given only to the person for whom it was prescribed.

A combination of two or more drugs may change the action of the drugs. Sometimes a person may consult with or be cared for by more than one health professional. *It is very important that each health professional be informed of all medicines being used by the person,* including common OTC drugs such as aspirin.

Some persons cannot tolerate some medicines, and when these medications are taken, the response is an allergic reaction (an unexpected and sometimes serious set of symptoms). Penicillin is a good example of a drug to which some persons' bodies react badly. Whenever a person knows of any specific medicine that will cause an allergic reaction in his body, he *must* be certain to tell any health professional who may be prescribing medicines for him or giving or selling medicines to him.

THE PRESCRIPTION AND THE PHARMACIST

The health professional should prescribe the necessary drug or drugs by generic name. This allows the pharmacist to select the least expensive preparation when he fills the prescription. The federal government has set and enforces standards so that all drug preparations meet high standards for purity and content.

The Prescription

When the health professional writes a prescription, he usually includes the following information:

The name of the patient for whom it is written

The generic and sometimes the brand name of the drug

The form of medicine desired (capsule, tablet, or liquid)

The strength of the medicine

The amount or number of doses

The amount of medicine to be taken each time and the number of doses per day

Any special instructions such as whether the medicine should be taken before or after meals or only at bedtime

Whether the prescription can be refilled, and if so, how many times

The health professional's name

If a controlled substance such as a narcotic is ordered, the Drug Enforcement Administration (DEA) number of the prescriber

The Label

Pharmacists, physicians, and other health professionals work together to help patients have the facts they need in order to use medicines safely and so that the medicines will have the best effect. One method of giving facts is by putting them on the labels of medicine containers. The label should contain the following information:

The patient's name and the doctor's name

The name of the medicine

The amount of the medicine to be taken and the number of doses per day or the time of day the medicine is to be taken

Any special precautions or instructions

The name, telephone number, and address of the pharmacy

The prescription number

Information about refills

Some pharmacies use different-colored stick-on labels with special information such as "May cause drowsiness. Alcohol may intensify this effect," "Use care when operating a car or dangerous machinery," or "Caution: Federal law prohibits the transfer of this drug to any person other than the patient for whom it was prescribed." These precautions should be followed carefully. Check the label before leaving the pharmacy to be sure that all instructions are clear and understood, whether the medicine is for yourself or for someone else. Ask the pharmacist if there is any other information the patient should have about the medicine or the way in which it is to be taken.

The Container

For safety purposes, the government requires that medicine be given in containers that cannot be easily opened by children (called safety caps). These containers are often so hard to open that even adults, and many elderly and ill persons, may have difficulty in removing the safety caps. Regular screw-on caps can be requested and must be provided by the pharmacist if requested. However, the person may be asked to sign a form confirming that he made the request.

The Role of the Pharmacist

Many pharmacists are taking an active role in a national effort to increase the safety and appropriate use of medicines and to decrease the risk of ill effects and death. Some keep a record of all medicines prescribed for a patient (referred to as a "patient profile"). Some even remind patients to refill their prescriptions for medicines that are to be taken regularly over a long period of time (for example, drugs to control high blood pressure). Pharmacists are usually happy to discuss medicines, their use, and their expected effects with patients.

Costs and Services

Patients or their families are wise to compare prices and other services offered by pharmacies (drugstores) before having prescriptions filled. In the Washington, D.C., area, for example, prices have been shown to vary as much as 50 percent in different stores. Many pharmacies give a discount to persons over the age of 65. Some pharmacies are willing to deliver the medicines with no extra charge, and this saving may be an important consideration.

THE EFFECTS OF MEDICINES

Serious health conditions can arise from the use of specific medicines, from new or strong drugs used in treating complex health problems, from using two or more drugs within the same time period, and from attempts at self-treatment without the advice of a health professional. The tendency of persons to go to more than one physician and more than one pharmacy makes it more difficult to be sure that medicines are not used in dangerous combinations. The effect of a drug is often changed when it is used with another drug.

For all the above reasons, it is important that the patient, the family, and particularly the home nurse know what effects any medicine used is expected to have, and know what symptoms or side effects might indicate an allergy or other dangerous situation. If any of the following symptoms occur unexpectedly, they could be side effects of the medicine: nausea and vomiting, diarrhea, dizziness, skin rashes or hives, extreme restlessness, confusion, headache, and itching.

The patient and the home nurse should pay attention to swelling (particularly of the ankles and legs), changes in the size and color of skin lesions, significant weight changes, changes in behavior, and other things specifically mentioned by the health professional. It may be important to observe and record pulse and respiration rates, temperature, and blood pressure.

If any of these side effects or other unexpected symptoms do occur when taking medicines, the medicine should be stopped, and the health professional should be consulted at once.

STORING MEDICINES

All medicines should be clearly labeled and should be kept in a safe place away from children, preferably in a locked cabinet. Medicines should be kept separate from other bottles and jars. Medicines should be stored according to any special instructions on the container, such as "Keep refrigerated " or "Keep in a dark place." Liquid medicines should not be allowed to freeze.

Unused medicine should be promptly destroyed. Medicine in any container with no label, or with a label that cannot be read, should be properly disposed of. Active, dangerous drugs that are no longer used should be destroyed to prevent their doing harm to someone. Some drugs may become dangerous if stored too long.

Never simply throw unneeded medicine in the trash, because the medicine could be found by someone else and used improperly. Medicine may be flushed down the toilet; however, some medicines may discolor the porcelain. If medicine is to be put in the trash, wrap it in several layers of paper or mix it in with the other trash.

GIVING MEDICINES

In all cases when medicine is given, there are eight considerations with regard to the safety of the patient. These are known as the *Eight Rights*:

- The right medicine for...
- The right person...
- At the right time...
- In the right dosage form...
- In the right amount...
- By the right route...
- For the right response...
- With the right recording.

The health professional prescribes medicine for a specific condition of a specific person. Medicine should be given only to the person for whom it was prescribed. The instructions for its use are based on the diagnosis, the specific action of the specific drug in the specific size of the dose ordered. If medicines are to have the result intended, they must be taken *exactly* as ordered for as many days or weeks as ordered.

Some drugs may be taken several times a day or perhaps only once a day, depending on the drug used and the health professional's prescription. Often a person will have more than one medicine to take. It may be helpful to write out a schedule so that drugs and doses do not get mixed up.

Keeping written records of medications given and of the patient's reaction to the medication becomes extremely important when the patient's condition is serious or when his medication schedule is difficult to follow. It is then important to record such information as the date and the time given, the kind and amount of medicine given, and any effects observed. If the patient fails to take medication as ordered, this fact should be written down with the reason why it was not taken, such as "asleep," "refused," or "vomited the medicine."

If the health professional permits, medicine that has an unpleasant taste may be followed by a cookie, a cracker, fruit, or fruit juice. Persons on a special diet might not be allowed this choice. Care should be taken, however, not to overdo this practice with either adults or children, since they may associate the food with the medicine and come to dislike the food.

Giving Medicines by Mouth

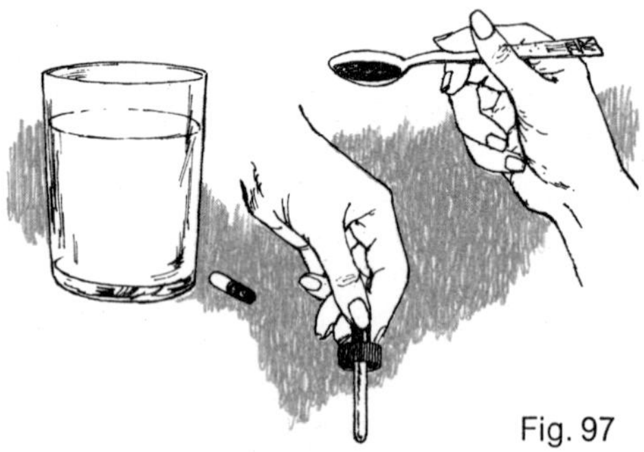

Fig. 97

When giving tablets, pills, or capsules—

1. *Read the label* when picking up the container and compare it with the doctor's order or the schedule for the patient.

2. *Read the label* again and pour the pill into the cap of the medicine bottle or into a spoon or a small glass.
3. Close the container and *read the label* again before putting the container back in its place.
4. If there is more than one medicine to give at the same time, prepare all tablets before giving any to the patient. (Read labels carefully.)
5. Give the medicine to the patient from the spoon or small glass.
6. Have the patient place the medicine on the back of his tongue, take a mouthful of water, tilt his head back, and swallow. (If the medicine is to be chewed by the patient, instructions should be followed.)
7. If the patient has difficulty in swallowing pills, try crushing the pill between two spoons. The medicine might then be mixed with applesauce or jelly and swallowed that way. *Capsules should not be opened* unless opening them is approved by the health professional.
8. Stay with the patient until you are sure he has swallowed the medicine.
9. Record on the patient's daily record the medicine taken, the time, and any other special information.

When giving liquid medicine—

1. *Read the label* when picking the bottle up and compare it with the doctor's order or the schedule for the patient.
2. Go to the patient before pouring the medicine.
3. If directed to do so, shake the bottle well.
4. *Read the label* and remove the bottle top. Keep the top clean by placing it upside down on the tray (if one is used).
5. Pour the medicine into the spoon or medicine glass, holding the bottle so that the label is toward the palm of the hand. This will prevent any dripping from making the label messy and unreadable.
6. If using a medicine glass, hold the glass so that the line for measuring the needed amount is at eye level. Pour the exact amount.
7. If using a dropper, hold it by the bulb with the point straight down, to keep the liquid from running into the bulb of the dropper. Count the number of drops out loud. If it is allowed, add a

small amount of water before giving the medicine to the patient.

8. *Read the label* again before giving the medicine to the patient.
9. Give the patient the medicine, making sure that he swallows it.
10. Record on the patient's daily record the medicine given, the time, and any other information.

After giving the medication, clean the glass, spoon, dropper, or any other equipment used. Put the medicine in a safe place according to the instructions on the label.

Rectal Suppositories

Suppositories are a form of medicine to be given by being placed in the rectum. They are often shaped like a small cone and are made with a cocoa butter base or other waxy material that melts at body temperature. There are different kinds of suppositories for different medicinal purposes. Some kinds of suppositories must be stored in the refrigerator to keep them firm until used and to make it easier to remove the wrapper and to insert the suppository into the rectum.

If the patient is able and wishes to insert his own suppository, he should be allowed to do so. Otherwise, the home nurse can do it for him. This is the procedure:

1. Explain to the patient the steps that will be taken.
2. Remove the medication from the refrigerator.
3. Help the patient get in a comfortable position (preferably lying on one side).
4. Unwrap the suppository.
5. Insert the suppository gently into the rectum, or let the patient insert it.
6. Hold the patient's buttocks together for a few moments until the urge to expel the suppository has ended.
7. Wash your hands, or provide for the patient to wash his hands if he has inserted the suppository.

Eye Medications

Eye drops or eye ointment may be ordered for a number of reasons: to soothe irritation, to cure infection, to relieve pain, or to dilate the pupils. The drops or ointment may be placed into the patient's eyes by a family member, or the patient may be able to do this for himself.

Eye Drops

Eye drops usually come in a small bottle with a top that has a dropper attached, or there may be a separate dropper. Eye drop solutions are also sold with a form of dispenser that fits over the bridge of the nose, thus making it easier to get the drops in the right place in the eye.

Pay attention to the expiration date on the bottle. Many types of eye drops are quickly outdated. Use *only* eye drops that are not outdated.

When instilling eye drops, be careful to see that both the dropper and the drops are kept clean. If the dropper touches the eye or any other object, it should be cleaned with soap and water and thoroughly rinsed before the dropper is put back in the bottle.

This is the procedure:

1. Wash your hands well before starting treatment.
2. Bring the medicine to the patient. *Read the label* to make sure that you have the right medicine and compare the instructions with the doctor's order or the schedule for the patient.
3. Explain to the patient the steps that will be taken.
4. Have the patient sit in a comfortable position or lie flat in bed, facing a good light, with his head tilted back if possible (Fig. 98).

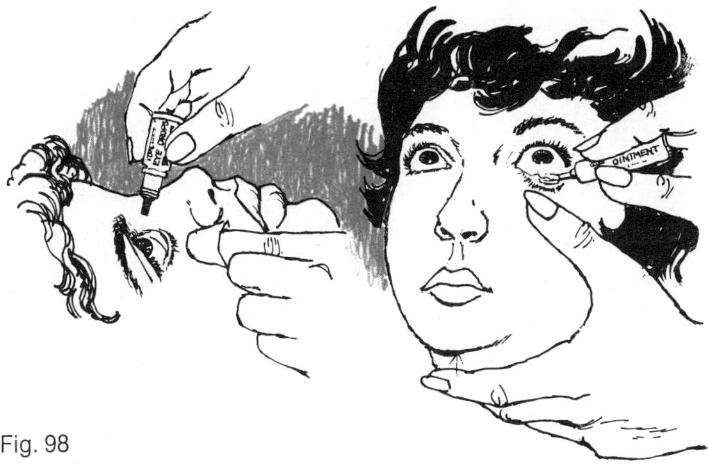

Fig. 98

5. *Read the label* on the container again.
6. Unscrew the cap and hold the dropper with the open end

straight down so that medicine does not go into the bulb. Draw up the amount of medicine needed. *Read the label* again.

7. Stand in back of or to the side of the patient. Draw down the lower lid of the patient's eye, using a tissue. Ask the patient to look up without moving his head.
8. Brace the hand holding the dropper against the patient's face to prevent injury to the eye if the patient should jerk his head while the drops are being given.
9. Hold the dropper above the lower lid so that the drops fall inside the lower lid, close to the nose. Squeeze out the number of drops ordered by the health professional. Do not let the dropper touch the eye.
10. Have the patient close his eye to distribute the drops, but he should not rub the eye.
11. Treat the other eye in the same way, if the health professional has ordered you to do so.
12. Dispose of any medicine remaining in the tube. Return the dropper to the bottle.
13. *Never* use the dropper for any other solution.
14. *Read the label* again before placing the container where it is usually kept.
15. Record the time when the drops were given, the condition of the eyes, and any reaction, immediate or delayed, on the part of the patient.

Occasionally there may be a slight stinging sensation and blurred vision immediately after the drops are put in the eye. The patient should be cautioned against squeezing his eyes tightly shut, using pressure with his fingers, or rubbing the lids forcefully.

If the patient administers the drops himself, he may do so in front of a mirror so that he can see what he is doing. Or he can lie flat without a pillow. In either case, the lower eyelid is pulled down, the eye dropper or dispenser is supported across the bridge of the nose, and the medicine is dropped on the inside of the lower lid.

Eye Ointments

Eye ointments are usually applied from a tube, and care must be taken to keep the tip of the tube and the ointment clean.

If the ointment is to be used on the inner surface of the eye, a small amount is squeezed from the tube onto the lower lid.

If the ointment is for treatment of the outer surfaces of the eyelid, any discharge or secretion on the outer surface of the lid should be rinsed away with clear water or solution ordered by the health professional before using the ointment. Then the ointment may be applied with a cotton-tipped swab or applicator.

Ear Medications

Ear drops placed in the ears may be needed to soften wax, to treat infection, or to relieve pain.

Have the patient lie on his side with the ear to be treated uppermost. Gently pull the earlobe back and upward. Drop into the ear canal the number of drops ordered by the health professional. The patient should continue to lie on his side for at least 30 minutes to allow the medication to enter the ear canal. (The health professional may specify a longer period of time.) If both ears are to be treated, wait the recommended time before instilling drops in the second ear.

Nose Medications

Nose drops or nasal sprays are frequently used to relieve nasal congestion. Nasal sprays, like all medicines, should be used only if recommended by the health professional. Over-the-counter nose medicines are not advised. If they are used, the manufacturer's instructions should be followed very carefully.

To instill nose drops, have the patient tilt his head back, then insert the tip of the dropper one-third inch (.84 centimeters) into the nose and release the specified number of drops (Fig. 99). Have the patient keep his head tilted back for several minutes to prevent the solution from escaping.

Fig. 99

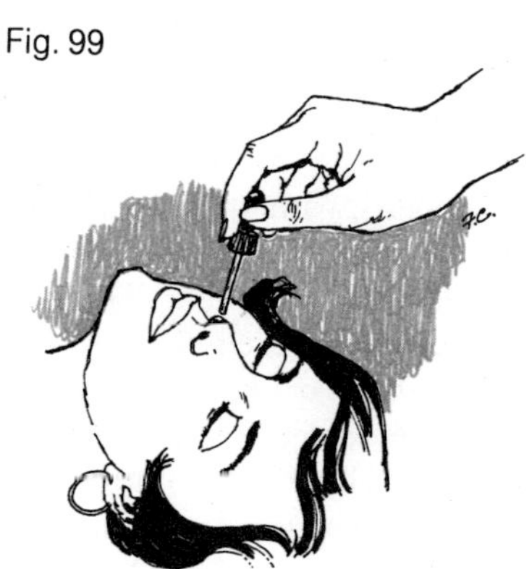

Nasal sprays are usually administered by the patient himself by breathing in as the spray is released.

Medicines Used on the Skin

Some medications are placed in creams or ointments that are to be used on the skin. Since some medicines used on the skin reach the bloodstream and can affect the whole body, it is important for any health professional who prescribes any new medication to know what skin medicines the patient is using.

As with any medications, follow the directions carefully when applying medicine to the skin. Be sure to wash the hands well first. Clean the area where the medication is to be applied before applying the medicine.

Inhalation Treatments and Oxygen

Some medicines that help the patient to breathe are made to be breathed in (inhaled). Some of these medicines are given by the use of humidifiers or vaporizers (see chapter 23). Some may be given from a hand-held sprayer or in an electric breathing machine. Sometimes oxygen is given as part of the treatment.

Hand-Held Sprayers

Medicines that are given in a hand-held sprayer are more common for home use. These medicines, like all others, should be used only according to the directions of the health professional. When the patient is using the sprayer, his lips should surround the opening that dispenses the medicine. The patient should breathe in very deeply through his mouth while at the same time spraying the medicine. Doing this provides needed relief as a fine mist enters the lungs.

Breathing Machines

Patients who have difficulty with their lungs and need frequent treatments over a long period of time may be advised to rent or purchase a machine to assist their breathing. These electric breathing machines and the medicines that are to be used with them must be used exactly as directed. Often, oxygen is used with this equipment. The health professional should demonstrate where and how to place the medicine to be dispensed by the machine. He should also set the controls of the machine so that the correct amount of air will be delivered at the right speed for the patient. The patient and his family should feel free to consult the health professional concerning any aspect of the treatment or the care of the equipment.

Oxygen

The usual purpose of oxygen is to ease the breathing of the patient, and it may be used in a number of ways. Oxygen may be given through a mask or a nasal tube or it may be given as part of treatment using a breathing machine.

However oxygen is dispensed, certain safety precautions must be taken to prevent fires or explosions. Each of these precautions is necessary to be sure of the safety of the patient and his family:

- Keep the room in which oxygen is to be used closed off from the rest of the house.
- Do not permit any smoking, lighting of matches, use of fire, or use of gas flame heaters in the room where oxygen is being used.
- Post "NO SMOKING" signs inside and outside the patient's room to remind the family and visitors not to smoke.
- Remove from the room any carpets (especially nylon) in which static electricity easily builds up. For clothing and bedding, use cotton or other nonstatic-producing materials instead of nylon. (A "static guard" substance might also be used.)
- Use a humidifier while oxygen is being used, to cut down the danger of sparks from static electricity. A humidifier will also help to prevent the drying effect that pure oxygen may have.
- Store oxygen tanks in a cool area, away from any source of heat.

Oral Medications for Children

Giving medicine to children requires special knowledge and skill. Almost all medicines ordered for children are ordered in smaller doses, usually on the basis of body weight. The "Eight Rights" in giving medication (see page 409) should be followed carefully in giving medicines to children.

Most toddlers and some older children will resist taking medicines to some extent. The home nurse or parents may need to persuade the child to take the medicine by mouth. The approach used should be positive, calm, and firm—but kind. The child should not, however, get the idea that he does not have to take the medicine. He should be helped to understand that the medicine is necessary to help him get well. If he asks, "Does it taste bad?" or "Is this the last time I have to take it?", he should be answered truthfully.

Some children are more willing to take medicine if they feel they are making the decision themselves. If the child wishes to hold the cup or glass himself, he should be allowed to do so. He may enjoy taking the medicine from a special small cup or glass such as a cup from a set of doll dishes.

It is a common practice to disguise the taste of some medicines in fruit juice or jelly. Every effort should be made to make the medicine as pleasant as possible.

If a child is not old enough to swallow a pill or capsule, the pill may be crushed. If it is allowed by the health professional, the capsule might be emptied into a spoon. The medicine will then dissolve if water is added. A drink of water or other liquid should follow the medicine.

Injections

Injections such as insulin can be given by family members or the patient himself after a health care professional gives instructions and supervises the procedure.

Chapter 20

Caring for the Patient Who Is in Bed

Bed rest is an essential part of the treatment for some illnesses. Whether the patient is temporarily weak and recovering from illness or whether he is unable to move his body (perhaps because of a stroke or paralysis), he will be greatly reassured if the home nurse knows how to care for him with skill and understanding. The patient will not only need to be made comfortable in bed through proper positioning and the use of pillows but will also need to have his position changed frequently to prevent pressure sores, shortening of muscles (contractures), and loss of muscle tone. Other important skills of the home nurse include serving attractive meals and perhaps helping the patient to eat them, and providing whatever help is necessary for elimination.

The patient should be encouraged to assist in his own care as much as is advisable, in order to provide some exercise for himself and to improve his morale. All lifting and moving of the patient should be done with careful attention to body mechanics to avoid strain and injury to either the patient or the home nurse. The home nurse who can help confidently, efficiently, and with understanding toward a person who is perhaps unaccustomed to being waited on "hand and foot" will do much for the patient's morale while at the same time insuring that he receives the best possible care during his illness.

POSITIONING THE PATIENT

For a patient confined to bed, good posture and frequent position changes are essential in order to prevent joint stiffness, deformities that may arise from prolonged inactivity, and pressure sores. Correct body position is the same whether a person is standing or lying down, and the patient's body may need special support to insure proper alignment of all parts of his body. Sick people have a tendency to curl up in bed with their backs, hips, and knees bent. They may lie in such a position to relieve pain or to keep warm. If a person remains in one position for long periods of time, it becomes more and more difficult for him to assume correct body position.

Basic to proper positioning is the proper equipment, including a firm mattress. Chapter 17 describes the bed and the bedding in detail.

The home nurse should keep the following points in mind with regard to positioning the patient in bed:

- Provide support for the back, maintaining the normal curves of the spine.

- Support the joints to prevent strain or deformity.
- Support the hands. If the patient tends to keep his hands closed, place hand rolls in his hands. A hand roll is made from one or two washcloths (or similar material), rolled tightly and taped.
- Position the patient's arms and legs carefully to prevent contractures (see page 424).
- Change the body position every 2 to 3 hours to promote circulation and to prevent pressure sores.
- Encourage movement to promote good muscle tone and to maintain the functioning of the joints.

Positioning the Patient on His Back

The patient will sometimes be lying flat on his back, using one pillow under his head and various other supporting pillows or materials. At other times, he will be raised to a sitting or half-sitting position, which can be achieved through the use of more pillows or backrests or by elevating the head of the bed in some fashion.

To position the patient using one pillow under the head—

1. Place the pillow under the patient's head so that it reaches under the shoulders.
2. Position the patient's arms comfortably at his side, with his hands open. If the patient tends to keep his hands closed, place a hand roll in each hand.
3. Place a small pillow or flat pad under the small of the patient's back, if it is comfortable for him.
4. Place small pillows or rolled bath towels alongside the hips to prevent the legs from turning outward.
5. Place a small pillow or pad under the patient's ankles to prevent pressure on the heels.
6. Support the feet by use of a vertical foot support so that the patient can brace his feet and keep them upright, unless the patient has a disease of the central nervous system. The support should extend about 2 inches (5.1 centimeters) above the toes to protect them from the weight of the bedding. This foot support prevents "foot drop." (For more information on foot supports, see chapter 24.)

To position the patient using three pillows—

1. Place two pillows lengthwise, crossed at the top and with the bottom corners together, so that they extend under the patient's shoulders.

2. Place one pillow crosswise at the top, under the head and reaching to the shoulders.
3. Place a small pillow or flat pad under the small of the back.
4. Place a pillow under each arm for support. Use hand rolls if needed.
5. If it is desired, place a flat pad or pillow under the knees *and* lower the legs to provide for a relaxing change of position. Do not place a pillow directly under the knees, since pressure at this point may cut off circulation.
6. Support the feet by use of a foot support. For more information on foot support, see chapter 24.

To position the patient using backrest and pillows—

1. Turn the patient onto his side using the procedures described on page 429.
2. Have the patient sit up or help him to sit up.
3. Place the backrest securely, with the slanting side toward the patient.
4. Place three pillows against the backrest as described above, crossed at the top and together at the bottom (Fig. 100).

Fig. 100

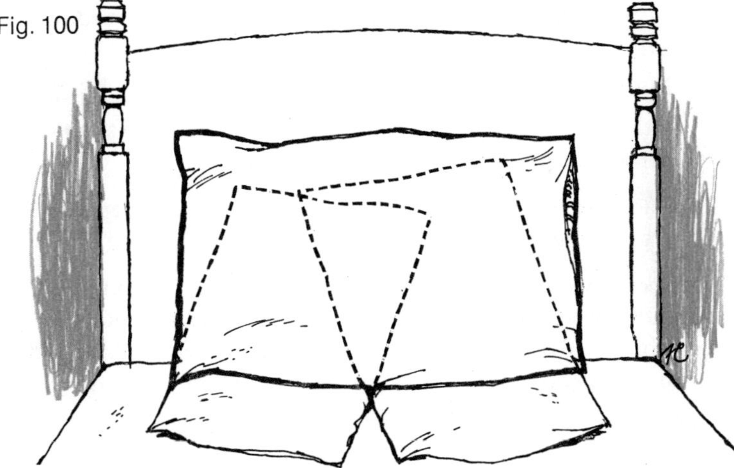

5. Have the patient move backward to a comfortable position.

Positioning the Patient on His Side

1. Turn the patient onto his side using the procedures described on page 429.

2. Place one pillow under the patient's head.
3. Place a pillow at the patient's back, lengthwise, and anchor it by pushing the edge of the pillowcase under the patient's back. Fold the outer side of the pillow under and tuck it in snugly against the patient to give more support, if it is needed.
4. Flex the hip and knee of the patient's upper leg, bringing the leg forward so that it does not rest on the lower leg. Position the lower leg comfortably.
5. Place a pillow lengthwise under the patient's upper leg to prevent skin surfaces from rubbing together and to provide correct support. The pillow should extend well under the foot so that the ankle and the foot do not drop and are kept level.
6. Make sure that the lower arm is in a comfortable position. The patient's upper arm and hand may be more comfortable if they are placed on a pillow, to provide support and prevent strain on the shoulder joint.
7. Use hand rolls if they are needed.

Positioning the Patient on His Abdomen

1. Turn the patient onto his abdomen using the procedure described on page 429.
2. Either position the patient to allow his toes to hang over the end of the mattress or place a pillow under his ankles to support his feet so that his toes do not touch the mattress.
3. Place a flat pillow under the patient's abdomen to keep the spine in good alignment and to help breathing.
4. Keep a woman patient more comfortable with a small pillow under her upper chest, to avoid pressure on her breasts. Foam rubber pads or small pillows may be placed under her shoulders to keep her from falling forward. If desired, place a large pillow under the abdomen and breasts.
5. Turn the patient's head to the side and place it on a small, flat pillow. Some people are more comfortable without a pillow.
6. Place the patient's arms at his sides, or raise them, depending on the patient's comfort and preference.
7. Use hand rolls if they are needed.

MOVING THE PATIENT

Having bed rest does not mean that the patient should never move. A person who is unable to move by himself should be helped to a new position every 2 to 3 hours. The purpose of changing the position of the bed patient is to relax him, to improve circulation, to prevent continued pressure on any part of his body over too long a time, to avoid strain on his joints, to prevent deformities, and to increase his level of comfort. Prolonged inactivity is damaging because the muscles lose their tone and may become shortened and resistant to stretching (a condition called contracture), and the joints may stiffen. If such inactivity continues for too long a period, the damage can become permanent.

The home nurse who cares for a patient who is in bed should both allow and encourage him to do as much for himself as possible. The patient should cooperate to the greatest extent of his strength. Doing things himself provides exercise for the patient and improves his morale—essential factors in his recovery. When assistance is needed, however, it should be provided. Before moving the patient, the home nurse should always explain to him the steps that will be taken, and the home nurse and the patient should coordinate their efforts, perhaps with a simple cue such as "one, two, three" or "ready."

The following are points to remember when moving a patient in bed:

- Explain to the patient the steps that will be taken, in order to gain his cooperation and to reduce any fear that he might feel.
- Encourage the patient to help as much as he can, since exercise will maintain muscle tone and help to prevent the complications of bed rest.
- Loosen the bed covers and remove pillows before moving or positioning the patient.
- Plan the move and signals to provide a smooth and coordinated move for the patient.
- Use the principles of body mechanics described on page 353 to prevent strain and injury to the back. Use a helper whenever it is necessary.
- Avoid breathing in the patient's face by keeping your head turned to the side when necessary.
- Change the patient's position every 2 to 3 hours or as advised by the health professional, to help prevent the development of pressure sores.

When the Patient Can Help

When moving the patient to the side of the bed—

1. Facing the side of the bed, place both your hands, palms up, under the patient's head or the pillow and shoulders. *On signal,* pull the patient's head and shoulders toward you.
2. Place your hands, palms up, all the way under the patient's hips and, *on signal,* pull his hips toward you. The patient can help by raising his hips and working with you.
3. Place your hands under the patient's knees and ankles and, *on signal,* pull his legs toward you.
4. Adjust the patient's body for proper alignment and comfort.

When helping the patient to sit up and lie down (Fig. 101)—

1. Help the patient to flex his knees.
2. Facing the head of the bed with your outer leg forward, lock arms with the patient by putting your near arm under the patient's near arm and your hand at his shoulder. Place your other arm around his shoulders to form a cradle, for support. The patient's head should rest on your near shoulder.
3. Adjust your posture for better leverage.
4. On signal, rock backward, pulling the patient to a sitting position. Continue to provide support if the patient feels dizzy. The patient can support himself in a sitting position by bracing his hands behind him on the bed.
5. Place pillows as needed.
6. To help the patient lie down, reverse the procedure.

When helping the patient to move up and down in bed—

1. If the patient will be moving toward the head of the bed, remove the backrest and pillows.
2. Have the patient flex his knees, and this will allow him to help push himself up.
3. If the patient is able, have him grasp the headboard of the bed with both hands. On signal, help the patient move up in bed as he pushes with his heels and pulls with his arms. If the patient needs more help to move up in bed—

   Explain to the patient the steps that will be taken.

   Facing the head of the bed, lock arms with the patient and cradle his head and shoulders as described in the procedure for sitting up.

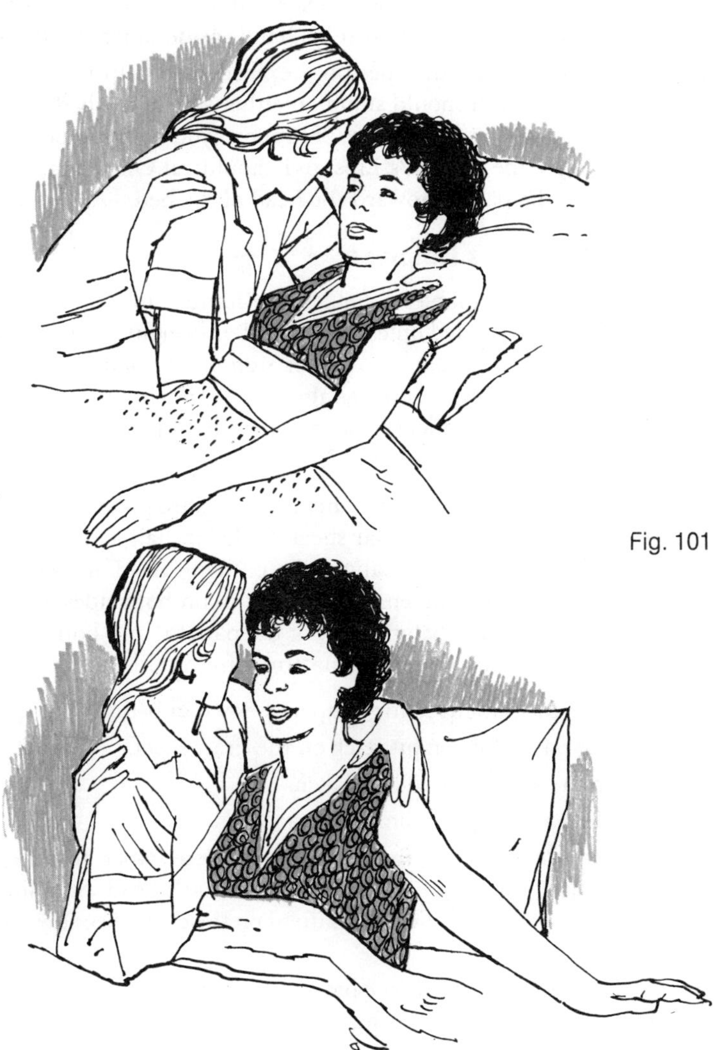

Fig. 101

Have the patient support himself by placing his hands behind him on the bed, keeping his arms as straight as is comfortable.

Place one hand low on the patient's back and the other hand, palm up, well under the thighs.

On signal, help the patient to move backward as he digs in and pushes with his heels.

4. If the patient will be moving toward the foot of the bed, repeat

the procedure described above, except that the patient digs in with his heels and pushes with his hands as he moves forward.

5. If both you and another person are needed to help move the patient, one of you should stand on either side of the bed, with knees flexed. Using a wide base of support, you both should join hands under the patient's hips and shoulders. On signal, you both move the patient toward the head of the bed.

When the Patient Is Helpless

When the patient is unable to help move himself in bed, two or more people will be needed unless he is very lightweight. The people helping should work in pairs on either side of the patient. They should plan the procedure and signals prior to moving the patient to provide an easy and smooth move. They should explain to the patient the steps that will be taken.

A draw sheet can be a great help in moving a helpless patient. It may be a sturdy crib sheet or a regular sheet, folded in half, end to end. The draw sheet should extend above the patient's head and below his hips and should be long enough to tuck in on both sides of the bed. It must be loosened before moving the patient, and both ends should be tucked neatly under the mattress after use.

When helping the patient to move up and down in bed—

1. Have the patient lie on his back on the draw sheet.
2. Explain the steps that will be taken.
3. Cross the patient's arms on his chest.
4. If one person is moving the patient up in bed, loosen the draw sheet, rolling the top of it close to the patient's head. Standing at the head of the bed, pull the patient on the draw sheet toward the head of the bed.
5. If two persons are moving the patient up in bed, gather the draw sheet into a loose roll on either side of the patient so that it can be grasped easily. Each person should face the foot of the bed with one foot forward and should grasp the rolled sheet firmly at the patient's head and hips. *On signal,* each should pull and lift slightly toward the head of the bed.
6. When moving the patient toward the foot of the bed using two people, have each person stand facing the head of the bed. Each should firmly grasp the rolled draw sheet at the patient's shoulders and hips and, *on signal,* pull toward the foot of the bed.

When turning the patient from the back to the side—

1. Explain to the patient the steps that will be taken.
2. Move the patient to the side of the bed, using the draw sheet, or using the method described on page 426.
3. Cross the patient's arms on his chest. Flex his knees for ease in turning, or cross his ankles so that the top foot is pointed in the direction of the turn.
4. Go to the far side of the bed so that the patient will be rolled *toward* you. Place one hand on the patient's far shoulder and your other hand on his hip.
5. Gently roll the patient, maintaining your grasp on his shoulder and hip. If using a draw sheet, roll the patient toward you by lifting the far side of the draw sheet.
6. Adjust the patient's shoulders and hips for good alignment, if necessary.
7. Place pillows for support as described on page 424.

When turning the patient from the side to the back—

1. Explain to the patient the steps that will be taken.
2. If the patient is large, move him, if necessary, to the side of the bed before turning him, to prevent his rolling too close to the edge.
3. Place the patient's knees and ankles together in a flexed position, supporting the joints from beneath.
4. Stand at the patient's back, facing the side of the bed, with one foot forward.
5. Place one hand on the patient's near hip and your other hand on his shoulder, palms down, and gently roll him onto his back.
6. Adjust the patient's shoulders and hips for good alignment if he is to remain in this position.
7. Place pillows for support as described on page 422.

When turning the patient from the back to the abdomen—

1. Explain to the patient the steps that will be taken.
2. Remove supporting pillows.
3. Gather the draw sheet into a loose roll at the patient's side. With the helper on the same side of the bed, together pull the rolled draw sheet and the patient close to the edge of the bed.
4. Place the patient's arms at his sides and put a flat pillow on his

abdomen. His hand closer to the center of the bed should be tucked well under his hip.

5. Support the patient's body while the helper goes quickly to the opposite side of the bed.
6. While you support the patient's head, have the helper grasp the rolled draw sheet on the far side of the bed at the patient's hips and shoulders and gently roll the patient toward the helper onto the patient's abdomen. The helper then releases the draw sheet.
7. Pull the patient to the center of the bed using the draw sheet.
8. Position the patient for good body alignment and comfort, with his face turned to one side. If necessary, move the patient toward the foot of the bed to allow his feet to hang over the bed, or use a pillow under his ankles.
9. Check and adjust the pad under the patient's abdomen for position and comfort. Adjust the patient's arms and legs, placing supports for comfort as described on page 424.

When turning the patient from the abdomen to the back—

1. Explain to the patient the steps that will be taken.
2. Remove the supports and loosen the draw sheet. Place the patient's arms at his sides. If his feet are hanging over the foot of the bed, pull him up in bed.
3. *With a helper,* pull the patient close to the edge of the bed by grasping the rolled draw sheet at the patient's shoulders and hips.
4. Move quickly to the far side of the bed while the helper tucks the patient's hand that is closer to the center of the bed well under the patient's hip.
5. While the helper supports the patient's head, grasp the far edge of the rolled draw sheet, gently rolling the patient onto his back.
6. Use the draw sheet to move the patient to the center of the bed, and then toward the head of the bed if necessary.
7. Adjust the patient's position, providing for good body alignment.
8. Place supports as described on page 424.

When lifting the patient to a sitting position—

1. Explain to the patient the steps that will be taken.
2. Have supports available.
3. With the patient lying on his back, stand facing the head of the bed with your outer foot forward.
4. Reach around the patient's neck and upper back with your near

arm. Your other arm should be pressed against the mattress next to the patient's shoulder to provide leverage.

5. To lift the patient, push against the mattress with one arm while bringing the patient to a sitting position with the other, shifting your weight from your forward leg to your back leg to help avoid back strain or injury. If the patient is heavy, two persons should be used to lift him, one on either side of the bed.
6. Support the patient while arranging the backrest and pillows to maintain a sitting or half-sitting position, as described on page 423.

FEEDING THE PATIENT

Every person, sick or well, has nutritional needs, and recovery from illness depends a great deal upon the diet. More information on the patient's diet is given in chapter 17.

If the patient is very weak or is unable to use his hands, he may have to be fed. If he is an adult who has always been accustomed to feeding himself, having to be fed by another person can be very upsetting for him. It is very important for the home nurse to understand the patient's reaction and to help him do all he can for himself. Mealtime should be a pleasant time. The home nurse or family member who helps the patient to eat can make him feel that it is a pleasure to share the time and experience. Sitting down, relaxing, and talking with the patient while he eats will help him to avoid feeling that his mealtime is a burden on others.

If the patient is blind, there are things you can do to make it easier for him to help himself and to enjoy his meal. If the blind person is feeding himself, describe where foods are placed on the plate by comparing them to the hours on a clock. For example, the meat is at 7 o'clock and the vegetable is at 5 o'clock.

If the patient is paralyzed or semiconscious, it is necessary to know before feeding him whether he is able to swallow. If the patient has trouble swallowing, consult the health professional before giving fluids or food. If the patient is paralyzed on one side, it is important to place the spoon on the side that is not weak.

Preparing for Mealtime

The patient should be offered the use of a bedpan before mealtime. Then the following preparations should be made:

1. Have the patient wash his hands or have them washed for him.

2. Raise the patient's head and shoulders if this is allowed by the health professional, using pillows or a backrest. The patient's head should recline in a comfortable position. Do not let the neck bend forward, because swallowing will be interfered with.
3. Depending on the patient's condition, allow him to have mouth care, such as the use of a mouthwash, before eating, to improve his appetite.
4. Protect the patient's clothing from possible spilling of food by placing a napkin or towel on the patient's chest, tucked into the neck of the nightgown or pajamas.
5. Place napkins or other protective coverings over the pillow and other bedding as needed.
6. Arrange the food attractively. Hot foods should be served hot, and cold foods cold.

Feeding a Helpless Patient

The most important things to remember in feeding a helpless patient are—

Be sure that the patient can swallow.

Give small amounts of food to avoid choking.

Obtain the patient's cooperation by avoiding any sign of haste.

Be sure that foods are not so hot that they burn the patient's mouth.

The procedure is as follows:

1. Wash your hands.
2. Sit beside the patient in a position that is comfortable and that allows ease in feeding him. Avoid hurrying.
3. Test the temperature of hot soup or coffee to make sure that it is not too hot. Pour a few drops of the hot liquid on the inside of your wrist (Fig. 102): it should sting but not redden the skin. (Some patients, particularly the elderly, may be less sensitive to pain and therefore may be more easily burned.)
4. For soft foods and liquids, fill the spoon two thirds full and remove any drip from the bottom of it by touching the bottom to the plate or bowl.
5. Touch the patient's lower lip with the side of the spoon, then tilt the spoon toward the lip, allowing the food to run into the mouth (Fig. 102). Allow the patient time to swallow.
6. Give liquids through a drinking tube or a straw (Fig. 102). Stir

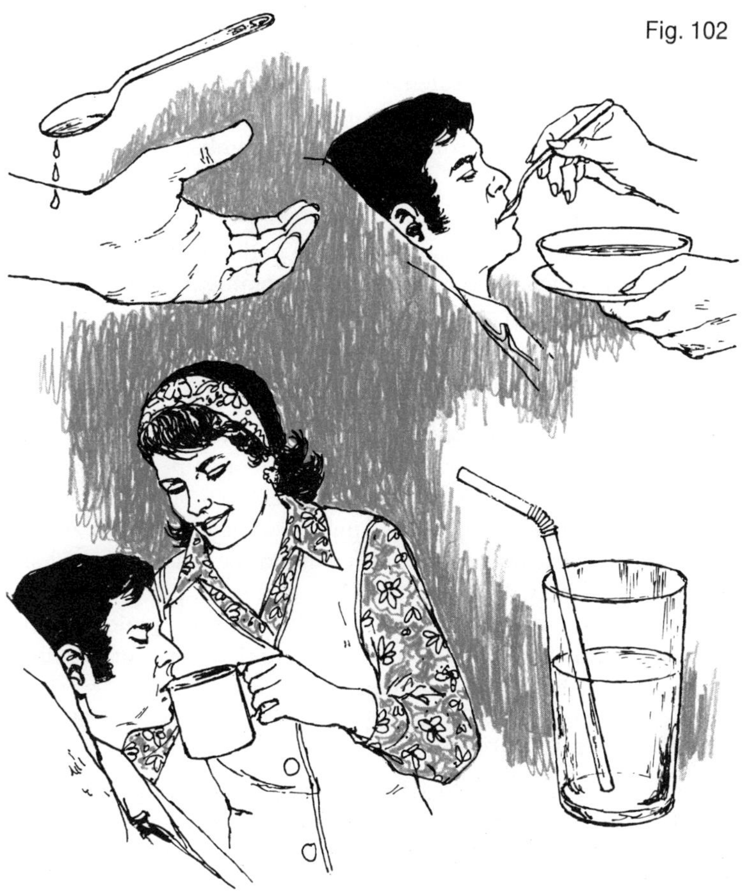
Fig. 102

the liquid first to distribute the heat evenly. Place one end of the straw in the side of the patient's mouth. Make sure the other end stays below the level of the liquid so that no air is swallowed. The patient can then suck the liquid through the straw and swallow at his own pace.

7. When liquids are given from a cup (Fig. 102), support the patient's head and raise it slightly by placing one of your arms under the pillow. Hold the cup with your other hand. Let the patient control the rate of flow by placing his hand under the cup.
8. If the patient can chew solid foods, offer them on a fork or a spoon, depending on the patient's ability and preference.

9. Allow plenty of time between mouthfuls. Alternate solid foods with liquids. If the patient cannot see the food clearly, tell him what you are giving him each time.
10. After the patient has eaten, help him wipe his mouth and allow him to wash his hands again if he wants to. Remove the tray and soiled dishes, brush away any crumbs, and straighten the bedding.
11. Provide for mouth and teeth care.
12. Record on the daily record what the patient ate, at what time, and how much. Record appropriate comments concerning his appetite and his enjoyment of the food.

PROVIDING FOR ELIMINATION

A patient who is unable to get to the bathroom will need a way to have bowel movements and to urinate (void, or empty, his bladder) in his own room, and perhaps without getting out of bed. A bedpan or a bedside commode serves this purpose. If the patient is able to get out of bed, he can use a bedside commode or can sit on a bedpan placed in a chair by the side of the bed. Since it is natural for persons to sit up to have a bowel movement and to urinate, the patient should be helped into a sitting position during elimination if sitting up is allowed by the health professional.

The Bedside Commode

When the patient is able to get into a chair but is unable to walk to the bathroom, a bedside commode can be provided. Using the commode rather than a bedpan is more satisfying to the patient and makes elimination easier. Getting in and out of bed to use the commode also provides important exercise for the patient.

The commode chair should be sturdy, comfortable, and of a height that makes it easy for the patient to get on and off. For comfort and safety, the commode chair should have arms. It may be easier to use if the arms are removable. A commode may be easily improvised by placing a bedpan on the seat of a sturdy wooden armchair. Although this arrangement raises the seat level, the few extra inches in height may be an advantage to the patient when he is getting on and off the chair. (See chapter 24 for improvisations.)

The procedure for getting onto a bedside commode is the same as the procedure for getting into a chair (see chapter 22). The patient should be allowed as much privacy as possible, but safety precautions must be maintained. If the patient is dizzy, however, someone should stay with him while he is using the commode.

In some communities, commode chairs may be available on a loan basis through such agencies as the American Cancer Society or the American Red Cross. It is also possible to rent or purchase commode chairs through dealers in hospital equipment and supplies. Check the yellow pages of the telephone book for information.

Any commode chair can be made to resemble a regular chair when not in use by the addition of washable cushions or slipcovers. The commode must be kept clean and free from odor at all times.

The Bedpan

If the patient is unable to get out of bed, he will need to use a bedpan in bed. If it is allowed, he should be in as close to a sitting position as possible to provide for more complete emptying of the bowels and bladder. Raising his head and shoulders by use of a backrest of pillows will help him to feel more comfortable and natural.

If the bedpan is to be used mainly in bed, it is wise to make up the bed with a waterproof pad or sheet under a cotton draw sheet in order to protect the middle part of the bed in case of spills. A disposable pad or improvised bedpan (see chapter 24) may also be used.

There are several measures that can be taken to add to the patient's comfort while he is using a bedpan. One is warming the bedpan before use, since a cold bedpan is very uncomfortable. Warm the bedpan by running warm water inside it and rotating the water around the sides of the pan, then pour the water out and dry the seat of the pan. Sprinkling the bedpan with powder will also add to the patient's comfort, particularly if the patient's skin is moist. For elderly or very thin patients, a soft pad placed between the patient's buttocks and the bedpan will increase comfort and help prevent skin irritation.

When the Patient Can Help

1. Assemble the necessary equipment: warm bedpan, bedpan cover, bell or other call system, toilet paper, equipment for hand-washing, bed protector, newspaper to protect the furniture.
2. Have the patient lie on his back with his knees flexed.
3. Place the bed protector under the patient's hips.

4. Place the bedpan on the bed beside the patient, with the open end toward the foot of the bed. Hold the pan at the side or the back to avoid handling the open end and thus soiling your hands.
5. Place one of your hands under the small of the patient's back. *On signal,* help the patient lift his hips. With your other hand, slip the pan under the hips and adjust it for comfort. If the patient has strength in his arms, he can help lift himself by using a trapeze bar above the bed (if one is available).
6. Raise the patient to a sitting position if the health professional permits, placing supports at his back.
7. Put the toilet paper where the patient can reach it. Leave the room to give him privacy unless he is too ill to remain alone. Make sure that the bell is within easy reach so that the patient can signal for you when he is finished.
8. If the patient is unable to clean himself, use the toilet tissue to clean him. Wipe female patients from front to back (to avoid bringing soil from the rectum to the vaginal area). Place the soiled tissue in the pan.
9. When the patient is finished, help him lift his hips so that the pan does not pull against his skin. (Place one hand under the lower part of the back to help him raise off the pan.) Remove the bedpan promptly.
10. Remove the bed protector, then cover the bedpan and take it to the bathroom.
11. Allow the patient to wash his hands and help him to get into a comfortable position in bed.
12. If ordered to do so by a health professional, and if only urine is present, measure the urine and record the amount.
13. Record the amount of bowel movement, the consistency, and the color.
14. If the contents of the bedpan are unusual, save them and report to the health professional. Otherwise, empty the bedpan into the toilet.

When the Patient Is Helpless

Generally, one person should not attempt to place a helpless patient on a bedpan. The home nurse should have someone assist at the opposite side of the bed. The procedure is as follows:

1. Assemble equipment as on page 435, as well as several covered pillows or folded blankets.

2. Turn the patient on his side, facing the helper.
3. Place a large pillow or two small ones lengthwise against the patient's back, from the shoulders to the upper buttocks.
4. Place a large pillow or two small ones lengthwise against the patient, from his thighs to his feet, building a platform on which he can be placed.
5. Protect the ends of the pillows and the bed between them with a waterproof bed pad (see chapter 24).
6. Place the bedpan on edge against the patient's buttocks, as close to the desired position as possible. Press downward with the bedpan on the mattress and hold it in place as the helper turns the patient onto the bedpan and the platform of pillows. Check to see that the bedpan is properly adjusted.
7. If it is permitted, raise the patient to a sitting or semisitting position, using pillows and backrests for support.
8. Allow the patient time to use the bedpan. Provide privacy if it is safe to leave him.
9. Cleanse the patient, using toilet paper or a warm, moist washcloth if the patient is unable to cleanse himself. This can be done while the patient is on the bedpan or after he is rolled onto his side. (Always wipe from front to back on female patients.)
10. Hold the bedpan flat on the bed to avoid spilling the contents, while the helper rolls the patient off the platform of pillows onto his side.
11. Remove and cover the bedpan. Set it aside on a protected surface.
12. Remove the pillows and wash the patient's hands.
13. Position the patient in good body alignment, using necessary supports.
14. Take the bedpan to the bathroom.

The Urinal

Male patients usually use a urinal when urinating. The urinal is a bottle-shaped container and can be improvised (Fig. 103) if a regular urinal is not available (see chapter 24). There is also available a special urinal designed for females. The procedure for using a urinal is as follows:

1. Help the patient place the urinal if he is unable to place it himself. Avoid exposing the patient.

Fig. 103

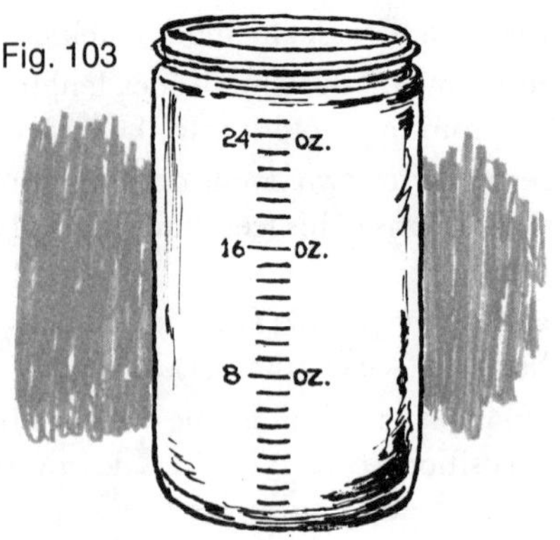

2. Remove the urinal promptly after use, cover it, and take it to the bathroom.
3. Allow the patient to wash his hands.
4. If ordered to do so by the health professional, record the amount of urine and note any unusual appearance.
5. If the appearance is unusual, save the contents and notify the health professional. Otherwise, empty the urinal into the toilet.

Cleaning the Bedpan or Urinal

1. Empty the contents of the bedpan or urinal into the toilet, unless the health professional has ordered otherwise.
2. Rinse the bedpan or urinal with cold water, loosening any remaining content from the sides.
3. Use hot, soapy water and a toilet brush to cleanse thoroughly.
4. Rinse well and dry.
5. Cover the bedpan and keep it out of sight when it is not in use.

The Incontinent Patient

Incontinence is the inability to control the escape of urine from the bladder or the escape of stool from the rectum. This condition may be only temporary, but with some types of disability or injury, and often in senility (a personality change that may occur in old age), it may be more or less permanent. A patient who has suffered a back injury that has caused paralysis of the lower part of the body may suffer permanent incontinence, while the patient who has had a stroke may have only temporary incontinence.

Incontinence can be extremely embarrassing for the patient. He should be reassured that he is loved and accepted despite his problem. Although in some cases the incontinent patient can be trained to regain control of his bladder or bowels, or both, the home nurse and the other members of the family will have to accept the problems that arise in caring for an incontinent patient. Every effort must be made to keep the patient clean, dry, and free from odor. In addition to having his daily bath, the patient needs to have his bed linen changed and his back, buttocks, and genitalia bathed and carefully dried each time he becomes wet, to keep him comfortable and to prevent skin irritation or breakdown. The skin should be thoroughly washed and carefully dried following each bowel movement as well.

A patient may be kept dry by use of a urinal, a special urine bag, waterproof protective pants over an absorbent pad, adult-sized diapers, or other special commercial supplies, particularly for males. However, the psychological effect of the use of diapers must be considered if this method of control is to be used. The home nurse may wish to talk with the health professional in deciding what is best for the patient. If the patient's condition indicates it, the health professional may order or insert a catheter (long, flexible rubber or plastic tube with small diameter) to help maintain dryness.

Special measures also should be taken to protect the bedding. A waterproof sheet may be used to completely cover the mattress and should be placed under the regular bottom sheet. A waterproof sheet should be placed under the cotton draw sheet. Either a disposable bedpan or an improvised pad may be placed under the patient's hips.

If there is no physical impairment or other apparent reason for the incontinence, the patient, unless he is senile, can usually be trained to regain control.

Training the Incontinent Patient

Neither the patient nor his family should accept incontinence as a problem that cannot be solved. Incontinence means that the body is not functioning correctly, and the health professional should give guidance to the home nurse in solving the problem.

Before any program for bowel or bladder training, or both, is started, a careful and thorough evaluation of the patient and his potential must be done by the health professional with the home nurse and the family (and the patient if he is able to participate). The patient's physical condition as well as other social and emotional factors that might affect the incontinence will be considered. A training program should not be started unless it has a good chance of success.

Special efforts must be made by the patient and the home nurse to restore control over the bladder or the bowels, or both. Regaining control over this aspect of body function is extremely important for increasing a patient's independence and self-confidence.

Bowel Training

The first step in bowel training is to determine what was normal bowel functioning for the patient before he became incontinent. He may have had bowel movements every day, every other day, or every third day. He may have had bowel movements after breakfast or after dinner. When the bowel training program is begun, a schedule should be planned to meet the patient's needs. It may be necessary to allow the patient to attempt a bowel movement two or three times a day. When a schedule is found that meets the patient's needs, *stick to it.* Make sure the patient's diet includes foods that help him have soft but firm stools that he can pass without undue straining.

Diet, which includes foods from the basic four food groups (see page 35), is very important for insuring normal bowel functioning. Some foods, such as prune juice, fresh fruits, and bran cereals, tend to stimulate bowel function. Certain other foods, such as vegetables, fruits, and salads, will make the stools softer and easier for bowel movements. Plenty of fluids (2–4 quarts, or 1.9–3.8 liters, per day) will also help.

Activity and exercise tend to increase bowel activity. It is therefore important for the patient to do as much for himself as possible.

A sitting position is more natural and allows better use of the muscles necessary to have a bowel movement. Whenever possible, therefore, the patient should use a toilet or a bedside commode. If the patient is bedridden, raise him to a sitting position on the bedpan if possible.

If the patient fails to have a bowel movement for a 3-day period, the health professional should be consulted. Stool that stays in the body too long becomes hard and difficult to pass. The health professional will determine the best way to stimulate a bowel movement —by using suppositories, laxatives, or enemas.

Bladder Training

Many things important to a bowel training program are also important to a bladder training program. A sitting position (on a toilet or a bedside commode) is very important for complete emptying of the bladder. Drinking plenty of fluids (2-3 quarts, or 1.9-2.8 liters, per day) is also important. Physical activity helps to stimulate the bladder to function. To help prevent incontinence during the night, fluids should not be given beyond midevening.

Find a schedule that includes normal times for urination. Most people need to empty their bladders when they first awaken in the morning. Many will urinate soon after drinking fluid. Note when the patient becomes wet—if, for example, he is usually wet at a certain time, such as 3:30 p.m. If the patient is incontinent only at night, plan two or three opportunities for him to urinate during the night by providing the urinal or helping him to the bathroom, depending on his condition. At first it may be necessary to provide opportunities to urinate as often as every 2 hours. These time intervals may gradually be lengthened as control is established.

Some patients may lose the usual sensations that indicate the need to urinate. This type of patient may be helped to recognize the need to urinate by noting sensations such as restlessness, sweating, chills, headache, or a feeling of fullness that occurs when the bladder is full.

Certain steps can be taken that stimulate urination and assist in helping to regulate the patient. The following measures can be taken while the patient is on the commode or the toilet: let water run from a faucet where the patient can hear it; run warm water over his hand; have him rock forward and backward; press gently on his lower abdomen with your hands; or pour warm water over his genital area.

Chapter 21

Keeping the Sick Person Clean and Comfortable

Depending on his condition, an ill person may be able to assist in his care or may need a considerable amount of help in maintaining personal cleanliness. The home nurse may need to assist the patient only by helping him to the bathroom, where he can wash himself, and by providing the necessary equipment. The patient who does as much for himself as he can will feel better and will also benefit from the exercise.

When it is necessary to provide extensive help for the patient in bathing, mouth care, washing hair, etc., it is a good idea for the home nurse to help put the patient at ease by using this time for conversation. Discuss the family and anything else on the patient's mind and encourage him to express his feelings about his illness.

This chapter covers practices and procedures for maintaining patient cleanliness and, therefore, comfort. It also includes information on giving back rubs and on changing the bed linens.

BATHING

Bathing cleans, refreshes, and stimulates circulation, all of which helps to maintain or improve a person's level of wellness. In addition, bathing is an activity that provides excellent exercise for the patient when he does all or any part of it for himself. While helping to bathe a patient, the home nurse should observe his general reactions, noting any changes in ability to move parts of the body and any changes in skin conditions.

When a patient is able to be out of bed, he may have a choice as to how he bathes. He might use a basin on a table beside his chair, or he can bathe at the bathroom sink, take a tub bath, or bathe in the shower. The type of bath the patient takes and the amount of help he requires will depend on his physical condition and strength. Points to remember about assisting a patient in bathing include those below:

- Have the room warm to prevent the patient from becoming chilled.
- Allow the patient to do as much for himself as he can.
- Allow plenty of time.
- Use good body mechanics when assisting a patient into or out of the bed, bathtub, or shower.
- Keep the patient covered (with a robe or a blanket).

- Observe and make note of the patient's skin and bony areas, checking for pressure sores.
- Report any unusual symptoms to the health professional.
- Provide the patient with as much personal privacy as possible.

Bathing at the Sink or From a Basin

When the patient is using a sink or a basin for bathing, provide him with the equipment he needs, such as soap, towels, and washcloths. Make sure that he has appropriate clean clothing to put on after the bath. The home nurse usually will need to provide only limited assistance, such as washing the patient's back, and therefore only needs to stay nearby to help when needed. If the patient is using a basin for his bath, the home nurse should assist by changing the water a few times to insure that it is clean and comfortably warm.

The Tub Bath

Tub baths are generally recommended as soon as the patient can walk, with assistance, as far as the bathroom. Before the patient takes his first bath, safety precautions against slipping and falling should be taken, and the use of certain helpful items should be considered.

Use of a nonskid rubber tub mat with suction cups or adhesive safety strips fastened to the inside of the tub is essential.

"Grab bars" on one or both sides of the tub are very helpful, giving the patient something to hold onto when getting into and out of the tub. One kind is permanently fastened to the wall. Another kind clamps onto the side of the tub and can be removed when no longer needed. Be certain, however, that the safety grip is completely immovable, or it will not be effective. To determine where a safety grip should be placed on the tub, get into and out of the tub yourself, and mark the spot that offers good leverage but does not interfere with getting into and out of the tub.

A low bench or a stool inside the tub is desirable if it is difficult for the patient to lower himself and get up again. A special bath stool can be purchased, but an old, sturdy wooden chair, with legs cut shorter and covered with rubber tips, will serve just as well and will also offer support for the patient's back.

Soap on a rope, a dish mop, or a sponge on a stick may be more useful than the standard washcloth for the patient who has limited use of his arms. A movable shower spray that fastens onto the tub faucet is helpful for rinsing arms, back, and shoulders.

The following is the procedure for preparing a weak or handicapped patient for a tub bath:

1. Make sure the bathroom is warm, so that the patient will not be chilled.
2. Fill the tub one third full of warm water (test the temperature with your wrist) before the patient gets in, and leave the water in the tub until after he gets out. (The water will help support the patient's weight, making it easier for the patient to lower and lift himself.)
3. Have towels, bath mat, clean nightgown or pajamas, and bathrobe on hand.
4. Help the patient to the bathroom. Have him sit down on a straight chair or in his wheelchair and remove his clothing. Help the patient *only* as much as is needed.
5. Place the straight chair or the wheelchair so that the patient faces the side of the tub, leaving him enough room to lift his legs onto the side of the tub. Steady the chair or lock the brakes on the wheelchair.
6. Have the patient lift one leg at a time, so that his *feet* are over the side of the tub. (Assist him if necessary.) Roll or push the chair close to the tub so that his *legs* are over the side of the tub. Again steady the chair or lock the brakes.
7. Have the patient hold the grab bars or sides of the tub and slide off the chair and onto the edge of the tub, placing both feet on the mat in the tub. If he needs help, support his body under his arms from behind (or use a draw sheet around his waist) and help him turn enough so that he can slide onto the bathtub seat or stool. If there is no seat or stool, help the patient to lower himself gradually into the tub.

(Whether you stay in the room with the patient or let him bathe alone will depend on his condition. If you leave, provide a way for the patient to call you. *Never leave a very young child, an elderly person, or a weak person alone in the tub. Stay near.* Assist the person with the bath if necessary, especially by washing his back.)

8. To get the patient out of the tub, support him under the arms (or use the draw sheet), helping him to a sitting position on the side of the tub. If the patient is able, have him hold the grab bars or

the two sides of the tub. (There is an alternate method for getting out of the tub, which is especially useful for persons who have difficulty in getting up from a sitting position: With the nonskid rubber mat in place, have the patient turn over onto his hands and knees. Have him place one hand on each side of the tub, push himself up, and rise to a standing position, holding onto the safety grip.)

9. Steady the chair or the wheelchair and have the patient slide backward onto the chair, then lift his legs out of the tub. Then turn the chair sideways. If a wheelchair is being used, release the brakes after the patient is in the chair.
10. Help the patient to dry himself thoroughly. Allow him to do as much as possible for himself.
11. Give assistance as needed in dressing. If the patient will be returning to bed, have him get into a clean nightgown or pajamas. The patient may wish to remain out of bed if permitted to do so by the health professional. He will probably need to rest for a while after the activity.

After the patient is comfortable, clean the tub and tidy up the bathroom. Put soiled clothing in a laundry hamper or a closed container. (Wet washcloths and towels, however, should dry before being placed in a hamper.)

Bathing in the Shower

Patients who have difficulty in getting into or out of a bathtub may find it easier to bathe in the shower while sitting on a bench or an old wooden chair. Some patients prefer a shower over a tub bath, regardless of their disability. There should be nonskid strips or a rubber mat with suction grips on the floor of the shower (be sure it does not cover the drain), and grab bars should be available for the patient. A shower cap should be available if desired.

When the patient is going to take a shower, start the water and adjust the temperature before he gets in, to make sure it is not too hot or too cold. Remember that the older patient may have lost skin sensitivity and may be burned without knowing it.

The Bed Bath

In situations when the patient is unable to bathe in the tub, in the shower, or at the sink, a bed bath is indicated. Only the acutely ill or helpless person will need to be bathed by someone else.

As soon as the patient's condition permits, he should be encouraged to do as much as possible for himself. Although it may take more time when the patient helps to bathe himself, the important consideration is that the patient is getting exercise and is caring for himself as much as possible. If he can do no more than wash his face and hands, he should be allowed to do so.

How often a patient needs to be bathed depends upon the patient. If he is elderly, he may not require a daily bath, since the skin of an older person tends to be drier. If the patient has a fever, the need for bathing is greater because of the greater amount of perspiration. The home nurse's common sense as well as the patient's wishes will determine how often, or at what time of day, a bath should be given.

Mouth care, necessary treatments, and changing of the bed linens can all be done at bath time, so that the patient need not be disturbed after his bath. Before beginning the bed bath, be sure that the room is comfortably warm, is free from drafts, and is arranged so that the patient will have privacy. The patient should be offered the opportunity to use the bedpan before the bath. All equipment needed for the bath should be collected and made ready to use. Needed items might be kept on a special tray or in a large basin. A lightweight, washable blanket for use as a bath blanket is needed to provide warmth and privacy for the patient (see chapter 24 for information on improvising a bath blanket).

Points To Remember

- Avoid chilling or tiring the patient.
- Encourage the patient to do as much for himself as he can.
- Protect the patient's privacy as much as possible.
- Change the bath water whenever it is soiled or soapy. Add hot water as needed.
- Give the bath from one side of the bed if it is comfortable for the patient. This is more efficient and saves the home nurse's energy.
- Observe and report to the health professional unusual conditions such as changes in the color of the skin or in bony areas.

Procedure

The following procedure is suggested as one method of giving a bed bath. Each home nurse will develop a pattern that is most comfortable for both patient and nurse and that will save the energy of both.

1. Set up a table or bedside stand. It should be of a comfortable height for the home nurse and should be protected by newspaper or plastic.
2. Assemble the necessary equipment:

   A large basin of warm water and a container or supply of hot water

   Two bath towels and one washcloth

   A cotton bath blanket for warmth and privacy

   Soap in a dish

   Skin lotion, body powder, or cornstarch

   A tray with toilet articles: hairbrush, comb, nail file, toothbrush, dental floss, mouthwash, toothpaste or powder or salt and soda

   Clean pajamas or nightgown, preferably with openings in the front for ease in putting on

   Clean bed linen

   A waste container and a pail for discarding used bath water if the bed bath is not given near a sink
3. Remove any unneeded pillows.
4. Lay the bath blanket over the regular blanket, then remove the regular blanket and the top sheet by sliding them from under the bath blanket. (If the top sheet will be used as a bottom sheet when the bed is remade, fold it and place it over a chair. When the bed is remade, a clean top sheet will be used.)
5. Remove the patient's pajamas or nightgown.

Wash the patient's face and ears as follows:

1. Place a bath towel under the patient's head to protect the pillow.
2. Wet the washcloth and wring it enough to keep it from dripping. If desired, make a bath mitt of the washcloth by wrapping it around your palm and fingers, holding it securely with the thumb and tucking in the ends at the palm so that the corners will not drag.
3. Wash the area around the patient's eyes gently with clear water, from the outer corner of the eyes toward the nose, using a separate corner of the washcloth for each eye to prevent the spreading of any infection that might be present.
4. Wash the rest of the face, with soap if desired, from the center of the face outward, using firm but gentle strokes. Rinse the face

carefully to remove all soap, since soap has a drying effect on the skin.

5. Dry the patient's face with a towel wrapped around your hand, holding the corners with the other hand to avoid dragging them across the patient's face.
6. Wash, rinse, and dry the patient's ears. *Do not use cotton applicator swabs in the ears,* because they may damage the eardrums.
7. Remove the bath towel from under the patient's head.

Wash the patient's arms and hands as follows:

1. Place a bath towel under the patient's arm and shoulder to protect the bedding.
2. Soap, rinse, and dry the arm, including the armpits, supporting the arm and using long, firm strokes from the wrist toward the shoulder (to increase blood flow in the patient's veins).
3. Place the basin on the towel at the patient's side and wash and rinse the patient's hand in the basin. If desired, allow the patient to soak his hand in the warm water for a few minutes. (For the arthritic or stroke patient, this is a good time for passive exercises. See chapter 22 for instructions.)
4. Remove the basin.
5. Dry the patient's hands and fingers well. Gently push back the cuticles with the towel and clean under the fingernails as needed. Apply skin lotion.
6. Remove the towel.

Wash the patient's neck, chest, and abdomen as follows:

1. Use clean water.
2. Cover the patient's chest with a towel. Pull the bath blanket down to the patient's abdomen. Hold the towel up with one hand while washing the chest with the other hand.
3. Soap, rinse, and dry the front of the neck, the chest, and the sides of the chest, using long, firm, gentle strokes. Wash and dry well under a woman's breasts. Observe the condition of the skin.
4. Leaving the towel over the chest, put a second towel over the abdomen. Pull the bath blanket down to the thighs.
5. Soap, rinse, and dry the abdomen, the sides of the trunk, and the upper surfaces of the thighs and the pubic area, using long, smooth strokes to avoid pressure and tickling. (The genitals are washed in a separate step later.)

6. Clean the navel carefully, using the corner of the washcloth or a cotton swab.
7. Pull up the bath blanket and remove the towels.

Wash the patient's legs and feet as follows:

1. Use clean water.
2. Fit the bath blanket snugly around one thigh at the groin, keeping the other leg covered. Help the patient flex his knee if possible.
3. Place a towel under the patient's leg and foot. Waterproof material might be helpful to further protect the bed.
4. Wash, rinse, and dry the leg, supporting the knee and using long, firm strokes from the foot toward the body. Examine the skin carefully for reddened or rough areas.
5. Place the bath basin on the towel and carefully lift the foot into the basin, supporting the knee and ankle with one hand.
6. Wash and rinse the foot well, especially between the toes. Lift the foot, then place it on the towel after removing the basin. Pat the foot dry, being sure to dry between the toes to prevent irritation and possible infection.
7. Clean the toenails if necessary. If the patient's skin is dry, apply lotion to the foot, the ankle, and the leg, as needed. Cover the leg with the bath blanket.
8. Follow the same procedure for the other leg and foot, changing the water as necessary.

Wash the back of the patient's neck, the back, and the buttocks as follows:

1. Use fresh, clean, comfortably warm water.
2. Position the patient comfortably so that his back is toward you.
3. Fold the blanket back to uncover the patient's back and buttocks.
4. Place a towel over the bottom sheet and the pillow. Tuck the sheet in under the patient's shoulder and back to keep the bed dry.
5. Soap, rinse, and dry the back of the patient's neck, the back, and the buttocks, using long, firm strokes. Examine the patient's skin carefully for reddened pressure areas or any breaks in the skin.

6. Give a back rub with lotion at this time or after the bath has been completed.

Wash the external genitals as follows:

1. Place a towel under the patient's buttocks to protect the bed.
2. Place a bath basin, soap, and towel within the patient's reach if he is able to help himself.
3. Allow the patient to wash and dry his genitals (for females, from front to back). If the patient is unable to wash himself, do it for him. (A female patient may also be washed by having her sit on a bedpan and pouring warm, sudsy water over her vaginal area, then rinsing with clean water and drying.
4. Cover the patient with the bath blanket.

After the bath—

1. Allow the patient to apply deodorant under each arm. (Soda bicarbonate may be used as a deodorant.)
2. Help the patient put on nightgown or pajamas.
3. See that the patient's hair is combed and arranged comfortably, and give assistance if necessary.
4. If a male patient wishes to shave, assist him if necessary.
5. Encourage a female patient to put on makeup.
6. Make the bed, using clean linen as needed (see page 460).
7. Remove the bath equipment and arrange the bedside table conveniently for the patient.
8. Make a note of any changes or unusual conditions observed during the bath, such as reddened areas resulting from pressure, any rash, swelling, lumps, sores, breaks in the skin, or a greater tendency to tire easily. Such conditions should be reported to the health professional.

THE BACK RUB

The purpose of the back rub is to refresh and relax the patient, to stimulate circulation, and to help prevent bed sores. The use of a lotion that will help to keep the skin soft and smooth is generally preferable to rubbing with alcohol, since alcohol is drying to the skin. The lotion should be applied to the home nurse's hands, rather than directly onto the patient's skin, to insure the patient's comfort.

Reddened areas should be given special care, because they indicate poor circulation in an area where pressure occurs. Slightly reddened areas should be massaged carefully. If the skin is very red and seems in danger of being broken, massage *around,* rather than *on,* the reddened area to stimulate circulation and to prevent breaking of the skin. (Make efforts to relieve pressure on any reddened areas by turning the patient more often or by using positions that avoid pressure on the affected area.)

A back rub can be given at the time of the bath, at bedtime, and whenever the patient's position is changed from a back-lying position, if he wishes.

The procedure for giving a back rub is as follows:

1. Assemble equipment: lotion or hand cream.
2. Lubricate your hands with lotion.
3. Face the head of the bed, with your outer foot forward and your knees slightly bent.
4. Apply pressure to the patient's entire back, including the shoulders, back of the neck, and buttocks. Keeping your hands flat and fingers together, use long, sweeping, firm but gentle strokes, starting low at the back and moving upward toward the neck.
5. Remember to keep lubricating your hands so that they glide comfortably over the patient's skin.
6. Observe the condition of the skin, paying special attention to bony areas and pressure areas. Give additional rubbing around any reddened areas. If the skin breaks open, contact the health professional.
7. Assist the patient into a comfortable position after the back rub.

CARE OF THE TEETH AND MOUTH

Mouth care is especially important during illness. How often mouth care is given depends on the patient's need. The patient's mouth should always be cleaned after he has eaten, and as often as needed for comfort. Some patients may need mouth care as often as every 2 hours. The health professional can give guidance concerning frequency. When the patient is unable to care for his own teeth, the home nurse will have to do it for him.

Points To Remember in Caring for a Patient's Mouth

- If it is necessary to hold the patient's mouth open, wrap soft material around the tongue blade or a spoon handle. *Never hold the patient's mouth open by placing your fingers in his mouth.* A human bite can be very dangerous.

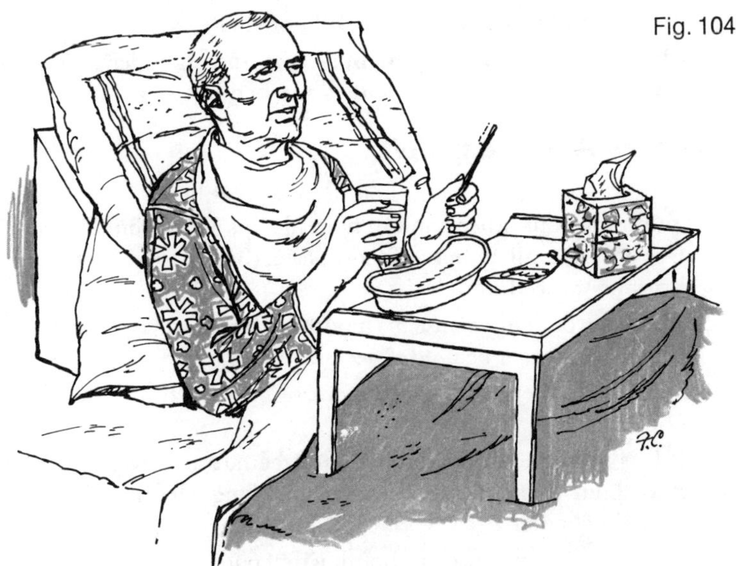

Fig. 104

- Use a child's toothbrush with soft bristles or a well-padded applicator to avoid damage to the gums and soft tissue.
- Observe the mouth, teeth, and gums for changes such as sores, bleeding, or very bad breath.

Mouth Care for the Helpless Patient

1. Assemble equipment:

   Toothbrush.

   Toothpaste (or substitute).

   Dental floss.

   Mouthwash. (A glass of warm water containing a half teaspoon of salt and a half teaspoon of baking soda can be used.)

   A glass of cool water.

   A towel.

   A small basin or container.

   Large-sized cotton-tipped applicator swabs.

   A waste container or paper bag.

2. Tell the patient what steps will be taken.
3. Position the patient. If it is permissible or possible, position him

in a sitting or half-sitting position. If he is unable to sit up, turn his head to one side so that he will not choke.

4. Place a towel over the patient's chest and shoulders, well up under the chin, to protect clothes and bedding.

When the Patient Can Spit

1. Brush the patient's teeth, holding the toothbrush in one hand and using your other hand to hold his lips away from his teeth. Use only a small amount of toothpaste. (See chapter 2 for toothbrushing procedure.)
2. Allow the patient to rinse his mouth with cool water. A drinking tube or straw can be used if necessary.
3. Have the patient spit the contents of his mouth into the basin or container.
4. If it is possible to floss the patient's teeth, use a strip of dental floss about 18 inches (45.7 centimeters) long. Use the technique given in chapter 2.
5. Have the patient rinse his mouth with cool water and empty his mouth into the container.
6. If the patient's mouth is dry, apply a glycerine and lemon juice mixture (four parts glycerine and one part lemon juice) to all surfaces of the mouth and tongue, using a large cotton-tipped applicator swab.
7. To prevent chapping of the lips, apply a thin layer of petroleum jelly, mineral oil, or glycerine and lemon juice mixture, or a commercial lip balm.
8. Take the equipment to the bathroom to clean it.

When the Patient Is Unable To Spit

1. Tell the patient what steps will be taken.
2. Use a moist toothbrush to clean the teeth. Take care to avoid damage to the gums.
3. If brushing is not possible, apply a solution of half water and half hydrogen peroxide with a cotton applicator swab. (This solution causes bubbles to form, which help clean the teeth.)
4. Moisten an applicator swab in mouthwash and press out the excess liquid against the side of a glass. (Instead of mouthwash, you can use a mixture of hydrogen peroxide or a mixture of glycerine and lemon juice.)

5. Steady the patient's chin with one of your hands and gently clean the inner surfaces of the mouth, the gums, and the tongue. Clean one section of the patient's mouth at a time, using a clean applicator for each section. Discard the applicator in a waste container or paper bag. Repeat the process with clean applicators until the entire mouth is clean.
6. "Rinse" the patient's entire mouth, using fresh applicators dipped in clear water.
7. Dry the mouth and chin with a towel.
8. If the patient's lips are dry, use an ointment or a lubricant on them.
9. Take the equipment to the bathroom to clean it.

Care of Dentures During Illness

A patient who wears dentures will frequently wish to keep his dentures in his mouth when he is ill. It is best if the person can wear his dentures most of the time, because it makes him look and feel better, helps him to eat, and slows the process of change in the shape of his gums, which can cause the dentures to fit poorly. However, it is not advisable for an unconscious patient to have his dentures in his mouth.

Dentures should be removed and cleaned at least once a day, and more frequently if needed. They may be cleaned according to the guidelines given in chapter 2. If the patient is unable to clean his own dentures, clean them for him. Your hands should be washed both *before and after* handling the dentures. Take great care to avoid dropping or breaking the dentures.

The dentures may be stored in water in an appropriate container in a safe place or may be returned to the patient's mouth. Mouth care should be given before the dentures are replaced in the patient's mouth.

CARING FOR THE HAIR

All patients should have their hair brushed and cared for daily to remove loose surface dirt and dandruff, to stimulate circulation of the blood in the scalp, and to make the patient as comfortable as possible. Cleanliness and grooming help to maintain the health of the hair, to improve the patient's appearance and morale, and to encourage the patient to take an interest in his personal hygiene.

Hair should be shampooed whenever it becomes oily or dirty. In some cases, a dry shampoo preparation, either spray or powder, may be preferred, depending on the patient's condition. At other times, a regular wet shampoo may be indicated. If the patient is able to be up and around, he may shampoo his hair himself in his customary manner. If he is unable to shampoo his own hair, the home nurse may do it for him. If the patient is allowed out of bed, the home nurse may wash his hair at the sink, in the shower, or in the tub. However the hair is washed, cotton can be used to plug the patient's ears to keep water out.

The procedure for washing the hair of a bed patient is as follows:

1. Assemble equipment: shampoo, a rinse if desired, a pitcher of warm water, several bath towels, waterproof protection for the bed, a shampoo pan or other improvisation for carrying water away from the patient's head (see chapter 24), a waste pail, a chair, or a low table.
2. Tell the patient what steps will be taken.
3. Have the room warm and free of drafts, to prevent chilling.
4. Raise the bed to a comfortable working height, if possible.
5. Position the patient on his back at the head of the bed in such a way that his head is over the edge of the bed. A pillow or rolled towel may be placed under the shoulders to make his head lower than his shoulders. (If the patient can sit up, he might lean over a table and have his hair washed in a basin.)
6. Place a waterproof sheet under the patient's shoulders and head and place a towel around his shoulders.
7. Place the waste pail on a chair or low table under the patient's head. Place one end of the shampoo pan under the patient's head and the lower end into the waste pail.
8. Wet the patient's hair by pouring water from the pitcher through the hair into the waste pail. (If there are two people to help, one pours while the other supports the patient's head and directs the stream of water through the hair.)
9. Work the shampoo through the hair and then rinse, repeating as necessary and working as quickly as possible to avoid tiring and chilling the patient.
10. Wrap a towel around the patient's hair while you remove the waterproof sheet and other equipment. Change sheets and nightgown or pajamas if they have become wet.

11. Use towels or a hair dryer to dry the patient's hair as quickly as possible.
12. Arrange the hair as desired.

Patients with longer hair who are in bed most of the time need special attention to their hair, since it is more likely to become tangled and matted. Many patients with long hair find that having braids is comfortable and helps to prevent tangles. (If braids are kept off to the side, it is easier to lie on the back.)

SHAVING

Many male patients prefer to be shaved each day, unless they regularly wear a beard. A man should be allowed to shave himself if he is able. Although he may not do a very good job, and it may take a long time, it is important to his sense of pride and gives moderate exercise if he can do it for himself. If he is unable to shave himself, the home nurse should make the shaving activity a part of the patient's daily care.

When shaving someone else's face, it is easiest to use an electric razor. A safety razor may be used when an electric razor is not desired or available.

If you are using a safety razor, use the type of lather preparation that the patient prefers. Take care to avoid cuts or nicks in the skin. After the face is lathered and shaved, use a warm, wet washcloth or towel to remove the remaining lather.

Some men like to use a shaving preparation before using an electric razor. Some men find an after-shaving preparation refreshing. If any nicks in the skin occur, a styptic pencil is useful in stopping bleeding.

Some women regularly shave their legs and under their arms. Even while sick, they may like to keep these areas shaved. The patient will usually let the home nurse know whether these areas need to be shaved and what method is usually used.

CARING FOR THE FEET

Proper care of the feet is important for all persons. Staying in bed for long periods of time decreases blood circulation to the feet, especially in old age, and when a person has certain types of disease such as diabetes, special care should be taken. (The advice of a health professional may be needed on how to care for the feet of a diabetic.) The following foot care procedure may be helpful:

1. Soak the feet in warm water to soften the skin and nails.
2. Pat the feet dry, especially between the toes, to prevent irritation and infection.
3. Rub the heels and soles of the feet to remove dead skin. A pumice stone is helpful in removing dead skin and can be purchased from most drugstores.
4. When necessary to cut the toenails, cut them straight across, leaving the corners square. Nail clippers are usually more efficient than scissors for this purpose. Check with the health professional when caring for a person with diabetes.
5. If the feet have a tendency to perspire between the toes, separate the toes with a thin layer of cotton and apply foot powder.
6. If the skin is dry, apply lotion.
7. Report any abnormalities (such as very thick toenails that resist cutting) to the health professional.

CHANGING THE BED LINEN

Clean, fresh linen on the bed, particularly after a bath, provides a patient with a feeling of comfort. Although the way the bed is made will vary somewhat, depending on the kind of bed and bedding needed, the home nurse should remember the following points when making the bed of a sick person:

- Top covers should be lightweight but warm and should be tucked in securely so that the patient remains covered.
- Toe space should be provided by making a pleat in the top sheet and blanket at the foot of the bed.
- When changing the linen, keep soiled linens away from your face and avoid shaking them excessively, in order to prevent the spread of infection.

Making an Empty Bed

1. Assemble equipment:

   Clean linen. (The top sheet that was on the bed may be used for the bottom sheet or for a draw sheet.)

   A draw sheet (an extra sheet or crib sheet).

   A waterproof pad for the mattress, if needed.

   A laundry bag for soiled linen (or newspaper to put soiled linen on).

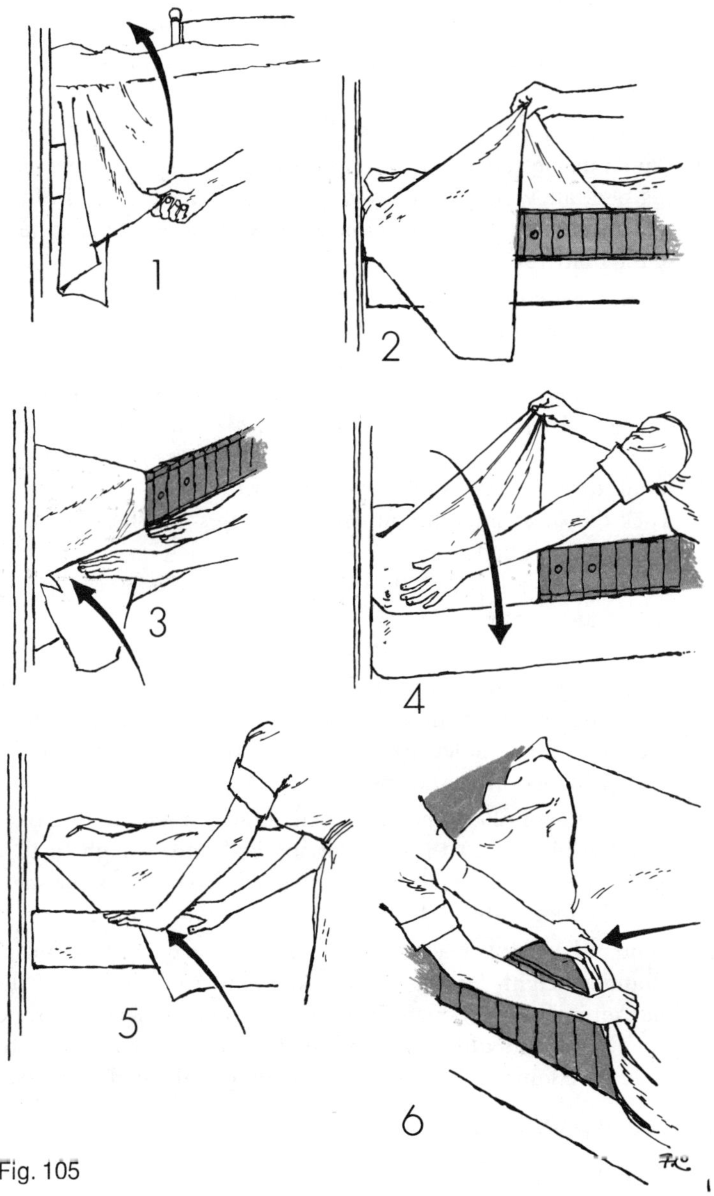

Fig. 105

2. Remove the bedspread, blankets, pillows, linen, and mattress pad, holding the bedding away from your face and clothing to

avoid contact. Remove pillowcases by turning them inside out to avoid touching the soiled side (see illustration). Place soiled linen in a laundry bag, in one of the pillowcases, or on newspapers on the floor. Fold any linen to be reused and place it over a chair.

3. If necessary, turn the mattress. Replace the mattress pad.
4. Put on the bottom sheet. If you are using a flat sheet, center it on the bed, allowing 18 inches for tucking under the head of the mattress to hold it firmly in place. Tuck the sheet in at the head of the mattress.
5. To make a corner at the head of the bed, grasp the selvaged (woven) edge of the sheet about 18 inches (45.7 centimeters) from the head of the bed. Raise it until it forms a straight line against the mattress, then let it fall back on the bed to form a triangle. Tuck the hanging part smoothly under the mattress. Then with one hand on the side of the mattress, use the other hand to bring the triangle forward over the side of the mattress. Tuck the sheet smoothly under the mattress all the way down the side of the bed.
6. Place a rubber or plastic sheet across the mattress before putting on a draw sheet if additional protection is needed.
7. Make a draw sheet by folding a regular sheet end to end. The folded edge should be at the top. Place the draw sheet across the center of the bed, with the folded edge positioned high enough to come under the pillow. Tuck the hanging part under the near side of the mattress.
8. Center the top sheet across the bed. Allow enough to fold back over the blanket at the head of the bed and enough to tuck under the mattress at the foot of the bed. Do not tuck the sheet in at the foot of the bed until after the blanket is in place.
9. Center the blanket across the bed and place the top end at shoulder height, leaving it loose at the foot of the bed. If the blanket is short, two may be used: place one blanket as desired to cover the shoulders and place the other so that it can be tucked well under the mattress at the foot of the bed.
10. Go to the other side of the bed.
11. Bring the lower sheet over across the bed and tuck it well under the head of the mattress. Anchor it by making a corner.
12. Gather the sheet in both hands along the upper edge of the

mattress, and with the backs of your hands uppermost and close together, pull the sheet diagonally, beginning at the head of the bed, and tuck it tightly and smoothly under the mattress all the way down the side of the bed (see illustration).

13. Pull the draw sheet smooth and tuck it under the mattress.
14. Provide toe space by making a pleat lengthwise at the foot of the bed, holding the sheet and blanket together (see illustration). Hold the pleat in place and tuck the remainder of the sheet and blanket under the mattress, making loose corners. (Another way of providing adequate toe space is to pull the bedding up over the toes, still allowing enough to tuck in at the foot of the mattress.)
15. Put on the pillowcase, keeping the pillow away from your face because it has been near the patient's nose and throat discharges. Place both hands in the clean pillowcase to free the corners. Grasp the center of the end seam with one hand outside the case and turn the case back over the hand. Grasp the pillow through the case at the center of one end (Fig. 106). Maintain your grasp until the corners of the pillow are adjusted in the corners of the pillowcase. Adjust and shape the pillow inside the case.

Fig. 106

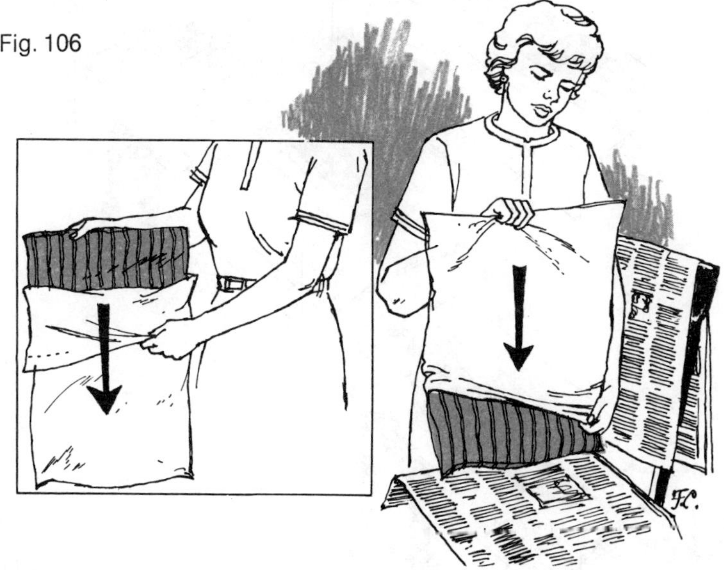

16. Fold the top sheet, the blanket, and the bedspread (if one is

used) in thirds toward the foot of the bed in such a way that the patient may easily grasp the top and pull up the covers.

17. Remove the soiled linen from the room with care, to prevent the spread of infection.

Making a Bed With the Patient in It

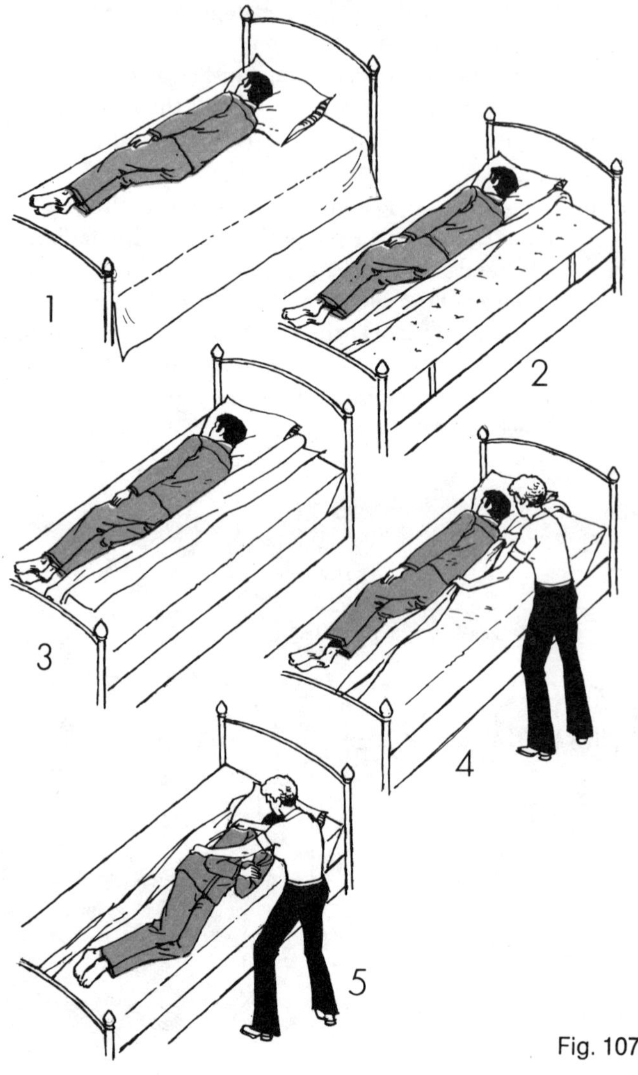

Fig. 107

A good time to make the bed is immediately after the bath. The procedure is as follows:

1. Assemble equipment: clean linen, an extra sheet for a draw sheet, a waterproof pad for the mattress if needed, a laundry bag or newspaper for the soiled linen.
2. Remove the bedspread, if any. Fold it and place it in a clean area.
3. Loosen the bedding on the side where you are working.
4. Loosen the top sheet at the foot of the bed.
5. Slide the top sheet down under the blanket and remove it. You might ask the patient to hold the top edge of the blanket while this is being done, or you might tuck the blanket under his shoulder to hold it in place. If the top sheet is to be used on the bottom or as a draw sheet, fold it and place it over the back of a chair.
6. Remove all pillows, or all but one for the patient's head.
7. Roll the patient (or have him roll) toward the home nurse. He should then be lying on his side (Fig. 107-1). (See chapter 20 for procedures for turning a patient in bed.)
8. Fold the blanket back close to the patient so that it will be out of the way.
9. Gather the bottom sheet lengthwise in a flat roll and push it close to the patient (Fig. 107-2). Gently pull the mattress pad smooth under the patient.
10. Change the bottom sheet:

    If using a flat sheet, fold it in half lengthwise. Place the fold of the clean sheet along the center of the bed lengthwise, allowing at least 18 inches (45.7 centimeters) at the head of the bed for tucking under the mattress. Unfold the sheet, allowing the top half to rest against the patient. Tuck the lower half of the sheet well under the mattress at the head of the bed. After making a corner, tuck the sheet well under the mattress all along the side of the bed (Fig. 107-3).

    If using a fitted sheet, place the corners of the sheet on the corners of the mattress at the head and foot on one side of the bed.
11. Tuck the remaining half of the sheet in a flat roll well under the soiled sheet, against the patient's back (Fig. 107-4). If the used sheet is wet or quite soiled, place a bath towel between it and the clean one.

12. Place the draw sheet across the center of the bed with the folded edge under the pillow area. Tuck the draw sheet under the mattress on the near side of the bed. Push the remaining half of the draw sheet under the soiled sheet, against the patient's back.
13. On signal, roll the patient from one side to the other onto the clean sheet. Support him on his side as you pull the bunched sheets out from under him (Fig. 107-5).
14. Roll the patient onto his back.
15. Go to the other side of the bed.
16. Loosen the bedding and remove the soiled bottom sheet and draw sheet, with the exposed (patient's) side of the sheet folded together, and place them with the soiled linen.
17. Smooth the mattress pad. Pull the edges of the clean bottom sheet to remove any wrinkles. If a *flat* sheet is used, tuck it well under the mattress at the head of the bed, make a corner, and tuck the sheet tightly and securely under the mattress all the way down the side of the bed. If a *fitted* sheet is used, place the corner of the sheet over the corner of the mattress at the head of the bed, then lift the mattress at the bottom of the bed to tuck in the remaining corner of the sheet.
18. Pull the draw sheet tight and tuck it securely under the mattress.
19. Remove the soiled pillowcases and place them with the other soiled linen. Put clean pillowcases on the pillows, taking care to keep the pillow away from your face. Adjust and shape the pillows inside the pillowcases.
20. Place pillows as necessary to provide comfort and proper body alignment for the patient (see chapter 20 for procedures).
21. Place a clean top sheet over the blanket, then remove the blanket and replace it on top of the sheet. Allowing room for the toes, tuck the top covers under the mattress at the bottom of the bed. Add the bedspread.
22. Remove the soiled linen from the room with care, to prevent the spread of infection.

Chapter 22

Exercise and Mobility of the Patient

THE IMPORTANCE OF EXERCISE

Exercise includes any use or movement of the body or any of its parts. It can be done in two major ways, active and passive. When the patient uses his muscles to move on his own, he is performing *active* exercise. When someone else moves parts of the patient's body while the patient relaxes, the patient is receiving *passive* exercise. In general, any type of exercise is good for the patient and helps him maintain or regain strength and muscle tone. However, there are certain conditions under which some exercises could be harmful, and it is of great importance when using exercise for a particular problem to have direction as to the most important exercises. This direction should be provided by a physician or a physical therapist. Consult the health professional regarding the type and amount of exercise for a specific patient.

Exercise has many good effects:

- It prevents muscle weakness and loss of muscle tone.
- It prevents deformities due to joint stiffness and shortening of the muscles and tendons.
- It improves circulation, which helps to speed the healing of wounds, to prevent pressure sores over bony parts of the body, to increase mental alertness, and to prevent dizziness.
- It helps to maintain strong bones and to prevent the development of kidney stones.
- It helps to improve the patient's appetite and to promote elimination of body wastes.
- It helps the patient to do things for himself, thus improving his mental outlook and helping him to get well faster.
- It helps to prevent the general discomfort associated with prolonged bed rest or immobility.

The patient should be encouraged to continue his daily activities of living, such as bathing, combing or brushing his hair, and feeding himself. Although it may take the patient longer than usual to do these activities, the benefits from them are many. One major benefit, in addition to that of providing valuable exercise, is that such activities help the patient keep or regain his ability to do things for himself.

This chapter includes discussions on range-of-motion exercises, on the process of getting out of bed and walking, and on special considerations for the patient with weakness of one side of his body.

RANGE-OF-MOTION EXERCISES

Each joint in the body has a normal range of motion; that is, the parts will move in specific directions and will do so when a person is normally active. So that joints can be kept flexible, they must move or be moved through all of the normal directions of movement for each joint. These exercises are known as range-of-motion exercises.

The major purpose of range-of-motion exercises is to maintain the flexibility of body joints, which might become stiff if not used. Range-of-motion exercises should be started very early in the patient's illness or disability. The exercises may be done when the patient is in bed, in a chair, or standing. Where and how they are done depends on the patient's condition and on the body parts needing special exercise.

The health professional should recommend whether active or passive exercises should be done. *Passive* range-of-motion exercises should be done for any body part that the patient is unable to move himself. During passive exercise, the patient relaxes while the home nurse moves the different parts of his body for him. If only one side is weak, as after a stroke, the patient may be taught to use the strong arm and leg to move and exercise the affected arm and leg. *Active* range-of-motion exercises are carried out by the patient. Active exercise includes three levels:

- *Assistive*—When the patient is assisted by the home nurse or by other means such as the use of weights to initiate or complete the movement.
- *Resistive*—When the exercise is made more difficult by the use of resistance from the home nurse or by the use of weights.
- *Free*—When the exercise is carried out by the patient himself. Active range-of-motion exercises provide an additional benefit: they help to increase muscle tone and to improve circulation.

The doctor, nurse, or physical therapist may demonstrate the exercise to the patient and his family and should advise on which parts of the body should be exercised, on the type and length of exercise, and on the number of times per day that the exercises should be done.

Each exercise should be repeated from two to five times at each session and at least once or twice a day (unless the patient is otherwise advised). In some cases, the exercises may be recommended three or four times daily. It may save time to combine an exercise session with the bed bath: the home nurse washes and dries one arm and then puts that arm through its range-of-motion exercises, and so on with each part of the body. Clothing and bedding should be arranged so that the patient is appropriately covered, but there must be freedom of movement for the exercise.

Points to remember about range-of-motion exercises are as follows:

- Consult a health professional such as a physician or physical therapist to determine the type of exercise (active or passive) that is best for the patient and the specific area to care for.
- Always explain to the patient the steps that will be taken and what he should do.
- Where appropriate, support body parts above and below the joint to be moved while the joint is in motion.
- Make the movements in a smooth and steady manner.
- Make each movement as complete as possible, while avoiding excessive pain for the patient. *If pain continues, consult your physician or physical therapist.*
- Observe the principles of good body mechanics (see chapter 16) to avoid back strain. Move the patient near the edge of the bed, so that he can be reached without your bending. Place the patient in correct alignment for passive exercises.

Directions for the major range-of-motion exercises are given here for use by or with the patient. These exercises can be done either by the patient or with the assistance of a physical therapist or public health nurse. If the home nurse is to assist, the instructions for the nurse's support to the body parts *above and below* the joint are given in italics. If they are to be carried out by the patient, the physical therapist or public health nurse can describe each step and teach the patient to do each exercise.

Exercise for the Neck

1. *Cup your hands over the patient's ears, grasping his head firmly.* Do not force his head into limited ranges.
2. Move the head slowly forward (as if looking down) and back (as if looking up).
3. Move the head slowly to one side and then the other (moving the ear toward the shoulder).

Exercise for the Shoulder

1. *Grasp the patient's arm by placing one hand just above his elbow, and with the other hand, support his wrist and hand.*
2. Move the arm forward and upward along the side of the head, so that the arm points over the head.
3. Return the arm downward to the side.
4. Move the arm sideways, away from the body to above the head, and return it to the side.
5. With the arm extending out from the shoulder, the upper arm resting on the bed and the elbow bent to 90 degrees, turn the lower arm down (palm toward mattress and then up—back of head toward pillow). Do not force the arm when movement is painful.

Exercise for the Elbow

1. *Grasp the patient's arm by placing one hand above the elbow, and with your other hand, support the patient's wrist and hand.*
2. Move the forearm, by movement at the elbow, toward the shoulder and then return the arm to the starting position.

Exercise for the Forearm

1. *With the patient's upper arm resting on the bed, the elbow bent and the hand in the air, grasp the patient's wrist with one hand and his hand with your other hand.*
2. Twist the hand so that the palm is pointing up, and then reverse the movement to have the palm point downward.

Exercise for the Wrist

1. *Grasp the patient's forearm and wrist with one hand and use the fingers of your other hand to carry out the exercise.*
2. Move the hand forward and backward and then from side to side.

Exercise for the Fingers

1. *Support the patient's forearm and wrist with one hand and use the fingers of your other hand to carry out the exercise.*
2. Bend the fingers and then straighten them.
3. Spread the fingers apart and then bring them together.

Exercise for the Thumb

1. *Support the patient's hand and fingers with one hand and grasp his thumb with the other hand.*
2. Move the thumb across the palm and then straighten it out.
3. Move the thumb in a wide, circular motion.

Exercise for the Hip and Leg

1. *Support the patient's leg by placing his ankle on your upper arm or shoulder, holding his knee in extension with one hand.*
2. Bend the hip by moving the leg upward as far as possible with the leg straight, and then bend the leg at the knee.
3. *Support the patient's leg by placing one hand under the ankle and the other hand just under the knee.*
4. Move the leg outward from the body as far as possible. Keep the leg level with the pelvis.
5. Return the leg and then move it across the other leg as far as possible.
6. *With the patient's leg resting on the bed, place one hand on top of the knee and the other on top of the ankle—or with both the patient's hip and knee flexed, place one hand under the knee and with the other, grasp the ankle.*
7. Twist the leg inward (toe toward center), then outward (toe toward edge of bed).
8. Lying on the side or the stomach, move the entire leg back as far as possible.

Exercise for the Knee

1. *Bend the patient's leg at the hip, raising the leg high, and support the leg by placing one hand just under the knee, then grasp the patient's ankle with your other hand.*
2. Bend the leg at the knee, then straighten the leg.

Exercise for the Ankle

1. *With the patient's leg resting flat on the bed, place one hand just above the ankle and grasp the heel in the palm of your other hand, with the sole of the foot resting against your forearm.*
2. Move the foot up and toward the leg.
3. Move the foot down and away from the leg.
4. Turn the foot so that the sole faces away from the body and then in toward the body. Do not allow the knee to turn.

Exercise for the Toes

1. *Hold the patient's foot with one hand and use your other hand to carry out the exercise.*
2. Bend the toes down toward the ball of the foot, then up and back.

GETTING FROM BED TO CHAIR

Preparing To Get out of Bed

All types of patients should be encouraged to get out of bed as much as possible. With patients who have had surgery, for example, getting out of bed has the advantage of reducing the chance of problems occurring after surgery. Pneumonia is one condition that can be prevented when the patient is allowed to move about on his bed. Getting out of bed increases exchanges of air and gases in the lungs and prevents the pooling of mucus secretions within the lungs.

Moving the legs while walking or getting up increases the rate of circulation in the lower extremeties and prevents the pooling of blood that needs to go back to the heart. When patients attempt to regain normal activity as quickly as possible, wounds heal better, pain is decreased, and elevated temperature may return to normal sooner.

Getting out of bed, however, should not be overdone. The condition of the patient must be the deciding factor. The very ill and the feeble, aged patient must be given every consideration. Consult the health professional for suggestions.

Getting out of bed should be done gradually. First of all, the patient should sit up in bed. A patient who has been lying down for a long period of time and has his head suddenly raised may feel dizzy, due to the lack of blood circulation in the head and other parts of the body. If the patient feels dizzy, lower his head for a few minutes. Then start raising his head again until he gets used to sitting up for longer periods of time.

The physical condition of the patient will help determine what equipment is needed, such as a chair, a wheelchair, a walker, braces, or crutches. It will also determine the type of clothing that he should wear. If the patient is going to be up for any length of time, it adds to his feeling of achievement if he can be dressed in his usual clothing rather than in nightclothes or robe. Shoes that have low heels and shoelaces and that provide support should be worn. If the patient is wearing special appliances, such as casts or braces, his clothing may have to be modified. For the patient who is able to use the bathroom or a bedside commode, clothing should be easily adjustable to meet this function. Patients in wheelchairs who cannot control bowel movements or urination will need to have clothing that is easily adjusted. Protective pads may also be needed to prevent soiling clothing and furniture or other embarrassing accidents.

After the patient can sit up in bed without dizziness, he should then be able to sit on the side of the bed. The next step involves moving from the bed to a chair. Some patients may not be able to move to the next step, which is walking with and without assistance. Those who are able to walk should be encouraged to do so.

Getting in and out of bed unassisted depends largely on the strength of the legs, arms, and back and the stomach and shoulder muscles. Muscle tone and strength become rapidly weaker at any age when a person is bedridden. Early, regular, prescribed exercises of arms and legs are essential to maintaining or regaining muscle strength.

Sitting Up in Bed Without Help

The patient's ability to come to a sitting position is basic in preparing to get out of bed. The easiest way for a bed patient to raise himself to a sitting position is to roll onto his side facing the edge of the bed. He should bend the knees and hips, then place his heels close to the edge of the bed. He should then place both hands flat on the bed, toward the edge, and push up to the side. At first, he may need some assistance at the shoulders. To lie down, he should reverse this procedure, making sure to lean forward on his hands rather than to lean back as he lies down onto his side.

When the patient is stronger and is able to get to a sitting position without assistance, he should be encouraged to do so in order to strengthen the muscles needed to sit without support. Sitting balance (the ability to sit without support) must be achieved before the patient sits in a chair, dresses himself, or performs daily living activities.

The patient may use the following procedure to sit up and lie down, using both arms:

1. Lie on the back, bend the knees, press against the mattress with the elbows, and raise the head and shoulders from the bed.

2. Slide both elbows toward the head of the bed (one at a time), thus raising the head and shoulders a little higher.
3. Push with one hand against the mattress, extending or straightening the elbow.
4. Push with the other hand, straightening that elbow, until the body is raised to a sitting position. Straighten the legs if necessary. Continue to lean on the arms for support until no longer feeling dizzy and until strong enough to sit without support.
5. When ready to lie down, reverse the procedure for sitting up. When starting to lie down, bend the head forward to help maintain balance and avoid falling backward.
6. Place the hands, palms down, on the bed alongside the hips, keeping the elbows straight.
7. Move the hands back by taking small "steps" with the hands.
8. Bend one elbow and rest it and the forearm on the bed to support the body weight. Bend the other arm and lean on both elbows.
9. Slide the elbows forward and lower the shoulders and head to the bed.

Given below is an alternate method of sitting up, especially for someone with back pain. Use an overhead trapeze or side rails if available.

1. Roll onto the side and bend the knees up toward the chest.
2. Push up on one elbow, close to the bed, while pushing with the hand of the other arm in front of the chest.
3. Gradually swing the lower leg (the one closer to the bed) off the side of the bed, then the upper leg.
4. To return to bed, raise the upper leg slowly while lowering the upper body first on both hands, then lower the elbow, then the shoulder, then the head, while raising the lower leg. When all the way down, turn onto the back.

Sitting on the Side of the Bed

When the patient is going to get out of bed, he should sit on the side of the bed with his feet and lower legs hanging over the side. To get to this position he should—

1. Move toward the side of the bed.
2. Move himself to a sitting position.
3. Slowly swing his legs over the edge of the bed and use his arms as a support while adjusting his hips.

OR—use the alternate method for sitting up.

The home nurse should remain with the patient a few minutes the first times the patient sits on the side of the bed. Signs such as dizziness, pale color, and an increasing pulse rate mean that the patient should be put back into bed. The change in circulation in the feet and legs when they are dropped to the side of the bed may cause dizziness, even in a patient who was not dizzy when sitting up in bed. There should be support under the feet (a footstool) if they do not touch the floor.

Getting out of Bed and Into a Chair

If the patient is convalescent and is not handicapped by a permanent crippling condition, the goal is to get him up and walking again as soon as possible.

The armchair that the patient will sit in when he first gets out of bed should be comfortable, strong, and high enough to allow him to rest his feet comfortably on the floor and to get up again with relative ease. If necessary, the seat may be raised by adding firm pillows or a thick foam rubber pad. The chair should have arms for comfort and security and for giving the patient support to stand up. The back of the chair should be high enough to support the head and shoulders when the patient sits back in the chair.

When a wheelchair is used, it should be of the proper size for the patient's comfort and should have the proper features for safety and easy mobility. Advice on the type of wheelchair to be rented or purchased should be given by the health professional.

When possible, it is helpful to have the mattress of the bed at about the same height as the chair seat. Both bed and chair should be stable so that they do not slip out from under the patient. It may be necessary for the home nurse to hold the chair as the patient moves into it. The casters of the bed should be removed to make the bed more stable.

When the patient is sitting in a chair, he may wish to carry out certain self-care activities such as combing his hair, shaving, or brushing his teeth. He may even wish to take a sponge bath at the sink or use a basin on a table beside the chair. He may also enjoy his meals more if they are served while he is sitting in the chair. Often, a patient will be highly motivated to get out of bed for brief periods if he can use a bedside commode instead of the bedpan. The time during which a patient is out of bed may be used by the home nurse to change the linens.

Procedure for Getting Into an Armchair

When the patient wishes to get out of bed and into an armchair—

1. Move the chair against the side of the bed at an angle facing the patient.
2. Have the patient place his arm that is closer to the chair on the far arm of the chair. He should then place the other arm, palm down, on the bed beside himself.
3. The patient should then raise his body by *pushing*, not pulling, with his hands, so that he is standing on his feet. He should then turn his body and lower himself into the chair.

If it is difficult for the patient to move from the bed into the armchair, an intermediate step may be helpful: Place a sturdy, straight chair between the bed and the armchair. Have the patient move into the straight chair first. (Steady the chair.) In a few minutes, the patient should move into the armchair.

Procedure for Getting Into a Wheelchair

When the patient wishes to get into a wheelchair—

1. Place the wheelchair against the side of the bed at an angle with the seat of the chair toward the patient. Fold the footrests up out of the way and lock the brakes.
2. If the arms of the wheelchair are removable, remove the arm nearer to the bed.
3. Have the patient move to the wheelchair using the procedure described for getting into an armchair. Steady the chair as the patient moves into it.
4. Place the patient's feet on the footrests and replace the arm of the chair if it had been removed.
5. When the patient wishes to return to bed, reverse the procedure.

WALKING

Preparing To Walk

After an illness, walking may have to be relearned. As with other activity, walking may be difficult, and progress may be slow at first. However, the patient should be encouraged to "take steps" to his independence, because walking was the goal when he began such activities as sitting up and getting in and out of bed.

Many times, the patient is so comfortable lying in bed that he may wish to avoid activity even though it is aimed at restoring him to his normal state of health. This may be more true if movement causes discomfort. However, activity such as getting out of bed and walking when able adds to the patient's physical progress as well as his mental health. The advice of the health professional and the tolerance of the patient should be used to guide the home nurse in deciding when the patient should begin to walk and how long he should be out of bed. The patient should not be pushed beyond his strength or to the point where he becomes discouraged. The stroke patient should be given special care when the home nurse is urging him to walk. The health care professional should be consulted.

For both standing and walking, the patient should wear low-heeled shoes with nonslippery soles that provide stability and give support to the feet as well. Loose-fitting shoes that may slip off, such as slippers, could cause the patient to fall and should not be worn.

Before attempting to walk, the patient should practice standing with support, to help him maintain his balance. He should also practice sitting down in a straight chair and getting up. These exercises will help him regain strength in the muscles used in walking.

The next activity should be to stand between two supports and shift the weight from side to side. A few small steps forward and back can then be taken. The backs of two heavy chairs can be used for the supports, or a chair and the footboard of the bed, or any supports that are about the same height. It is important that the supports are stable and do not move easily.

When the patient is standing, attention should be given to proper body alignment. He should stand as straight as possible, with his head up. Occasionally, he may need to be reminded to stand straight, since he may not be aware of his posture.

Helping the Patient To Walk

Normally, when a person walks, he keeps his head erect and his body in good alignment. His weight is shifted from one foot to the other evenly. His arms and legs swing forward alternately, right arm and left leg, left arm and right leg. This pattern of walking should be the goal of any person recovering from illness.

Until the patient gains strength, skill, and confidence, a helper should walk with him, being ready to provide support if it is needed.

If the patient has no disability of his legs (such as paralysis, a fracture, or an amputation) but only muscle weakness as a result of illness, it is best for him to be supported from the back, at the waist, so that his normal walking position is not changed. A belt around his waist provides a good grip for the helper.

If the patient should become dizzy, pull him back toward you and support him against your body. If he actually faints, do not attempt to hold him up but instead ease him down to the floor by sliding him down your body and legs.

The weak or apprehensive person who fears falling may at first need additional support. Walk close beside the patient, arm-in-arm, and hold his hand. Your hand should be palm-down on top of the patient's hand so that, if the patient becomes weak, you can quickly raise your upper arm into his armpit for support, and, moving your outer leg sideways to broaden your base of support, you can pull the patient against your hip for balance. If the patient should faint, you should gently ease him to the floor. This arm-in-arm method of supporting someone is an excellent method to use when assisting an elderly person who is walking. You should always hold onto the person being helped so that you will be able to hold him if he needs support.

Using Walking Aids

The use of walking aids such as crutches, canes, or walkers can sometimes give the patient the extra support he needs to walk independently. The patient's condition will be the major factor in deciding if a walking aid is indicated. It will also determine which walking aid is best for the patient.

All walking aids should be carefully fitted to the height of the person using them. If a child is growing rapidly, he will need to have his crutches lengthened from time to time. The health professional who recommended the walking aid should be able to give advice concerning proper fit.

Crutches, walkers, and canes should all have nonslip rubber suction tips on the bottom end. Inspect the tips frequently, remove dust, dirt, or mud, and replace the tips before they become badly worn. For safety, have the patient wear snug-fitting, sturdy shoes with nonslip soles and heels. Remove loose throw rugs and shift furniture as necessary to make clear paths for the patient to use when moving through the house.

Using Crutches

The purpose of using crutches is to enable the person who has lost all or partial use of one or both legs to move about in an upright position. Walking with crutches is a skill that requires both the desire and the patience to learn to walk again, as well as strength of the hands, arms, shoulders, and trunk, to support the body. The health professional may recommend exercises to strengthen the muscles needed for crutch walking. It is recommended that the patient practice standing to reestablish his balance.

There are two types of crutches: *axillary* crutches, which fit under the upper arm, and *Lofstrand,* or *Canadian,* crutches, which have a cuff that fits around the forearm. The health professional will recommend one kind or the other, depending on the patient's physical condition. Either kind must be carefully adjusted as to length and placement of hand grip.

General Principles and Points To Remember

- When using axillary crutches, the patient should hug the top of the crutch close to his body. He should bear his body weight with his hands on the hand grips, *not* on the top of the crutches. The hand grip must be adjusted so that the patient's elbows are slightly bent. There should be a space the width of two fingers between the top of each crutch and the patient's armpit when the crutch tip is placed approximately 2 inches (.8 centimeters) to the side and 2 inches ahead of the shoe toes.
- A helper should walk behind the patient when the patient is learning to use crutches. The helper should hold the patient at the waist from behind, grasping a leather belt around the patient's waist, with the other hand resting lightly on top of the patient's shoulder.
- The helper should encourage the patient to stand erect and to look ahead, not at his feet.
- Crutches should be the right length, with the hand grip adjusted properly.

Crutch Gaits

The way a person walks on crutches is called the crutch gait. The gait to be taught is determined by the nature and the extent of the patient's disability. The position of the body is called the crutch stance. To have proper body position, the patient should hold his head erect, his back straight, and his pelvis in a straight line with his head and feet; that is, his body should not be bent forward. When the patient is standing still, the crutches should always be ahead of his feet. The four crutch gaits are described below:

- *Four-point gait*—a slow, safe gait for the patient who can bear at least partial weight on each leg:
  1. Move the left crutch forward.
  2. Move the right foot forward.
  3. Move the right crutch forward.
  4. Move the left foot forward.
- *Two-point gait*—a faster gait requiring better balance and nearer-to-normal walking for the patient who can bear partial weight on each leg:
  1. Move the left crutch and the right foot forward together.
  2. Move the right crutch and the left foot forward together.
- *Three-point gait*—a gait used by the patient when one leg or foot is weak or injured and the other leg can bear full body weight:
  1. Move both crutches and the weak leg forward together.
  2. Move the strong leg forward to a point ahead of the crutch tip.
- *Swing gait*—a gait requiring a good amount of upper body strength; used by the patient with severe disability of one or both legs:
  1. Move both crutches forward together.
  2. Swing the body forward, coming down on both feet together.

Using a Cane

Canes are often used by persons with weakness on one side. There are several types of canes. Some are adjustable in length; some have handles like a shovel, a pistol grip, or a crook; some are three- or four-legged and will stand unsupported. The proper type and length for each patient will depend on the patient's disability and how much weight will be put on the cane.

The cane is usually carried in the hand on the good side. The patient moves the weaker leg and the cane forward, then bears part of his weight on the cane and part on the weak side while he moves the good leg forward.

Using a Walker

Walkers are helpful for patients who are very unsteady on their feet and would probably not attempt walking without the stability and security they receive from the walker. When considering a walker, keep it in mind that patients have a tendency to become dependent on walkers and might not relearn normal gait and balance while using them.

A walker should be adjusted so that the patient's elbows are slightly bent when he stands erect and holds the handgrips. The most common type of walker is rigid. The patient picks it up and moves it forward, then moves one foot forward, then the other. A swivel-type walker is hinged so that the two sides move independently. The patient may move the right side of the walker forward, then his left foot, then the left side of his walker, then his right foot. Or the patient may move the right side of the walker and his left foot forward at the same time, then the left side of the walker and his right foot (a faster method and more like the normal walking gait.)

Encourage the patient to stand erect and look straight ahead while using the walker. Walk behind him while he is learning to use the walker, to provide support if he needs it.

SPECIAL CONSIDERATIONS FOR THE PATIENT WITH ONE-SIDED WEAKNESS

The most common cause of one-sided weakness or incapacity is a stroke. Strokes often occur suddenly, with no major warning. The victim, who was perfectly normal before, suddenly may be unable to move his arm and leg and may have difficulty in making himself understood. The sensations or feelings that he is receiving from his own body and from the surrounding environment may have been greatly altered. These sudden changes in his body can be extremely frightening to the victim and his family and generally cause great mental distress.

The stroke victim may have to relearn many skills that were automatic before. If he is right-handed, for instance, and suddenly has right-sided paralysis, there may be a period of time during which his left hand may have to perform some of the functions previously done by his right.

An early return to activity is desirable following a stroke. When the patient must remain in bed, body positioning and exercises to prevent joint stiffness and deformities are of great importance to insure the greatest degree of recovery. Following a stroke, the involved leg and arm show increased tone. The leg extends, the arm assumes a flexed position, and the patient feels a tightness or heaviness in the limbs. For these reasons, it is particularly important to use proper positioning from the earliest stages to help prevent the increase of muscle spasms. The use of a soft hand roll for the hand, along with proper positioning, may sometimes be advisable. When a person has one-sided weakness, exercises should be done at least once a day, with particular attention to the affected side of the body.

As the patient's condition stabilizes and he is allowed to do things for himself, he should be encouraged to exercise and to use his weak arm and leg as much as possible. Holding and squeezing a rubber ball in the weak hand will increase the tone of the entire arm and shoulder, making the arm feel even heavier and making it more difficult for the patient to open the hand. Opening and closing the hand should be practiced with as little effort as possible (for example, flicking cotton balls away), with the emphasis on opening the fingers.

The frustration and discouragement about slow progress sometimes cause a patient to want to give up and not try to help himself. It is extremely important for the patient's family to provide an understanding atmosphere and to demonstrate patience as they care for him. Future use of an affected arm or leg cannot occur if joint stiffness and deformity have occurred. If the patient refuses to do his own exercises because of frustration and discouragement, it is important for the family to show support and encourage him to continue.

A patient who has one-sided weakness will require more time to do things for himself. He should be encouraged to take as much time as he needs. Help should be given, however, when the activity requires a great deal of effort. Only things that he cannot do for himself should be done for him. Doing things for himself will help improve his mental outlook. Generally, there is more than one way to do an activity. The patient should be encouraged to try various ways until he finds the one that is best for him and that requires the least effort and assistance. (See Chapter 24, "Making Your Own Equipment," and talk with the health professional about important equipment that may make self-care easier.)

Beginning Exercises for the Hemiplegic (Paralysis of One Side) Patient Lying on His Back

- With both knees bent, feet on the bed, rock the knees from side to side.
- With hands clasped, the involved thumb on top, reach the arms up toward the ceiling.
- Continue until the hands touch the bed behind the head.
- Bring the hands to the mouth, then to the forehead.

Sitting Exercise

- With the hands clasped and the involved thumb on top, raise the arms up at shoulder height in front of you, then bring the hands slowly in to the chin, then to the top of the head.

Actions When One Side Is Weak

Sitting Up in Bed

Patients who have had a stroke or a severe accident may have weakness on one side of the body. Rehabilitation of a patient with this type of problem should start as soon as possible, with the health professional's support and advice. A patient with this condition tends to lose his sense of balance. He needs to learn to balance himself in the sitting position before he is allowed to get out of bed.

Sitting Up in Bed, Rolling to the Involved Side

- Lie on the back with the affected (involved) arm on the bed, away from the body.
- Roll onto the affected side.
- Bend both hips and knees and slide the feet toward the edge of the bed.
- Place the good arm, palm down, on the bed at shoulder level.
- Roll the upper body forward, pushing up to the side to a sitting position, letting the feet slide to the floor.

Sitting Up in Bed, Rolling to the Good Side

- Clasp the hands together, raise both arms up toward the ceiling, and turn toward the good side.
- Let the affected hand rest on the bed.
- Bend both the hips and the knees and slide the feet toward the edge of the bed.

- Press the good arm or leg against the mattress, straightening the elbows and rising up to a sitting position.

The patient will find it easier to sit up when lying on his affected side.

To lie down, reverse the prodedure.

Procedure for Getting Into a Chair

- Have the patient sit on the side of the bed with his lower legs hanging down, with feet on the floor and shoes on.
- Place the chair or the wheelchair against the bed, facing the patient at an angle. It should be as close to the bed as possible. Make sure that the chair is stable and will not slip. If it is a wheelchair, *lock the brakes.*
- Have the patient slide to the edge of the bed and place his good hand on the far arm of the chair.
- Have the patient lean forward, bearing his weight equally on both legs, and stand up. He should then turn and lower himself into the chair with his head still somewhat forward. It is safer initially for the patient to lead with his good side when moving from bed to chair or from chair to bed.

Returning to Bed

- Place the chair at a 45-degree angle so that the patient's strong side is closest to the bed. Stabilize the chair so that it will not slip. The patient should—
  1. Move to the side of the chair with both feet placed evenly on the floor.
  2. Lean forward.
  3. Push down on the arm of the chair and stand up, balancing on both legs.
  4. Reach for the edge of the bed with his good arm and sit on the side of the bed.
  5. Wiggle his hips back onto the bed, keeping his head forward.
  6. Lift his weak leg onto the bed and slowly lie down onto one side, bringing the good leg onto the bed.

Points To Remember

- When the patient first begins to sit up, he should sit up for only a few minutes at a time. Gradually, as dizziness decreases, he should increase the length of time during which he is upright.

- The home nurse should stay next to the bed while the patient gets to a sitting position and until his dizziness disappears. If he should faint or feel faint, the home nurse can then ease him back onto the bed and prevent a fall. In many instances, dizziness will disappear after the patient has been sitting for 5 to 10 minutes.
- Observe changes in the patient's color, shortness of breath, increasing pulse rate, or profuse perspiration. Any of these signs indicate that the patient should be placed flat in bed again to rest.

Chapter 23

Special Nursing Measures

Special nursing measures or treatments are sometimes prescribed for a patient by the health professional for a special purpose: to relieve pain, to increase or decrease the blood supply to an affected area, to give comfort, or to promote healing. Other beneficial effects from special treatments include extra attention from the home nurse, confidence for the patient that something is being done to improve his condition, and improvement of the patient's mental outlook. All treatments are intended either to help the patient improve or to help him become more independent.

The health professional will give instructions for any treatment ordered. If the instructions are complicated, write them down. Sometimes it is necessary for the health professional to demonstrate a procedure. The home nurse should ask questions about any procedure that is unclear or whenever more information about the procedure would be helpful.

The following are points to remember for any special procedures performed at home:

- Explain to the patient all steps of the treatment to be performed and encourage him to ask questions about his care and treatments. He will then be less fearful and more ready to cooperate in the treatments.
- Explain to the patient how he can help in the treatment and encourage him to participate in the treatment as much as he is able.
- In all treatments, keep in mind the nursing basics: safety, comfort, effectiveness, neatness, and saving of energy, time, and equipment.

TREATMENTS USING HEAT

The Effects of Heat

Applying heat to an affected part of the body is a common practice because of the many benefits. Heat has a soothing effect: it relaxes muscles, eases tension, provides warmth, and often relieves pain. It promotes healing and helps the body rid itself of infection by softening discharges from open sores, increasing drainage, and relieving inflammation (soreness, redness, and swelling in an injured or infected area).

Heat applied to the outside of the body dilates (increases the inner space of) the blood vessels and brings more blood to the area. (Thus the area being treated will become red.) Heat also affects the sweat glands, causing more perspiration. If heat is used on large areas of the body, care must be taken to prevent the patient from becoming chilled after a treatment.

Always take safety precautions to prevent burning when using heat. Burns are a common side effect when the temperature of the treatment is too hot. Patients who are very young, very old, or unconscious are more likely to be burned because they are less aware of extremes of heat and cold. Since small children or unconscious persons cannot tell you when the treatment is too hot, they must be watched closely so that they can be protected from possible burns. Heat also has a drying effect; therefore, lotions and creams used on the skin are helpful in restoring moisture to the skin.

Heat treatments may be either dry or moist. For dry heat, use an electric heating pad, electric blankets or sheets, heat lamps, or hot water bottles. For moist heat, use moist compresses, tub baths, and sitz baths or soaks. (Commercial devices are also available to produce dry heat and moist heat. One is a hot-cold pack, which has effects similar to those of a hot water bottle.)

Dry Heat

Electric heating devices such as heating pads, blankets, sheets, and mattress pads are convenient and usually safe methods of applying dry heat. Whenever there is a chance that an electric heating device will be exposed to moisture, however, it is safer to use a hot water bottle or a waterproof heating pad.

Be sure that any electric heating device to be used has the Underwriters Laboratory (UL) mark of safety inspection. Do not use any device that has worn insulation, broken wires, or a control device that does not work properly. Always disconnect the device when it is not being used. Observe the following precautions when using electric heating devices:

- Never use pins to fasten a heating pad or an electric blanket in place. Pinning may damage either the heating element or any waterproof covering.
- Avoid folding or crushing the device, since such treatment might break the small wires in the heating element.
- If moist compresses are used at the same time as the heating device, or if the patient is incontinent, the only electric heating

device that would be safe to use would be a waterproof heating pad that is in good condition. (A hot water bottle would be even safer.)

- Carefully follow the manufacturer's instructions for the use and care of any electric heating device.

Electric heating pads are convenient and usually safe, if used properly. A waterproof electric heating pad is better for general use because it reduces the danger of electric shock if it should become wet. An electric heating pad usually has a removable, washable cotton flannel cover to keep the pad itself clean. Extra cloth covers may be needed if the pad is used often. Before each use, remove the cloth cover and examine the pad carefully for worn areas, holes, or exposed wiring.

Electric blankets and sheets are used to provide warmth without weight. A control device regulates the amount of heat. Carefully follow the manufacturer's instructions for washing, to avoid damage to the heating elements.

Heat lamps, through the use of a special bulb, produce infrared rays that can pass through skin and body tissues. Heat lamps have the same effect on the body as other sources of dry heat but have the advantage of placing no weight on the body. For this reason, the health professional may advise use of a heat lamp in the treatment of swollen or inflamed joints. The rays can be directed toward a small area of the body. The patient should feel warmth, but not intense heat, on the skin.

Since improper use or overuse of heat lamps can result in severe burns, observe the following precautions:

- The bulb should be placed *at least* 18 to 24 inches (45.7–70 centimeters) from the skin.
- Use the lamp for *no more than* 10 to 15 minutes at a time, unless the health professional gives other instructions.
- Always set a timer or an alarm clock to go off when the treatment time is up. The timer may be on the lamp itself, or a kitchen timer may be used. Many people have been painfully burned because they went to sleep under the lamp and other members of the family forgot about them.
- Make sure that a bell or other call signal is available to the patient.

- If the patient is very young, very old, or unconscious, keep the bulb at least 24 inches (61 centimeters) from the skin and limit treatment to 10 to 15 minutes, according to the advice of the health professional.
- Be very careful not to burn any area of the skin where the patient has little or no feeling.

Ultraviolet and sun lamps have the same effects and hazards as the rays of the sun. Ultraviolet rays are produced by electricity in electrode and mercury arc lamps. *Do not use* these lamps unless their use is prescribed by the health professional, with specific instructions for carrying out the treatment.

The dosage of ultraviolet radiation must be very carefully controlled. As with sunburn, the signs of injury from ultraviolet radiation do not appear for several hours. In the case of a severe reaction, the affected skin area is red, painful, and sometimes blistered, and usually there is swelling. Persons with fair skin are more likely to be burned than are persons with darker skin or those who are already tanned. Men can usually tolerate more exposure than women. Do not leave the patient alone because of the danger of his falling asleep and remaining under the lamp too long. To prevent damage to the eyes, both the patient and the person giving the treatment must wear dark glasses.

Hot water bottles are relatively safe and easy to use, but the water must be changed from time to time as it cools. Whether using a rubber hot water bottle or an improvised one (such as a glass bottle that will seal tightly), cover it with a soft cloth or towel to help prevent burning the patient. This is the procedure for using a hot water bottle (Figs. 108A and 108B):

Fig. 108 A

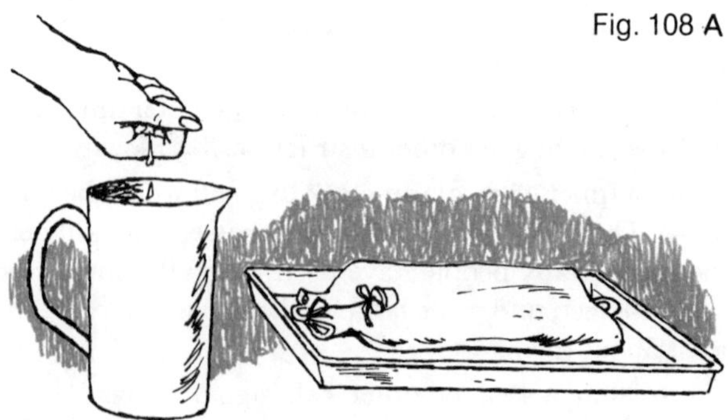

Fig. 108B

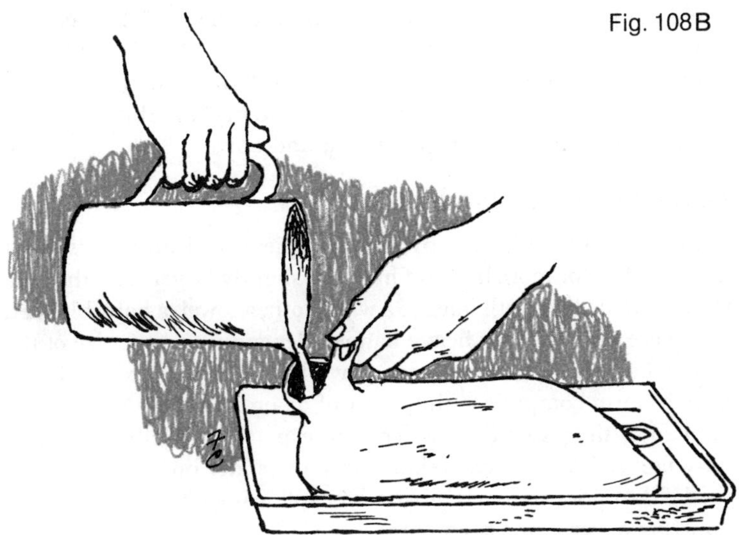

1. Test the water temperature with your hand. (The clenched fist should be able to tolerate it for a second or so.) Or test it with a thermometer. For children under 2 years of age, the temperature should be 105°–115°F (40°–46°C); for other persons, 115°–125°F (46°–51°C).
2. Fill the hot water bottle only one third to one half full, so that it will not be too heavy. Flatten it to expel air before screwing the stopper on tightly. To be sure the stopper is tight and there are no leaks, hold the bottle upside down.
3. Cover the hot water bottle with a soft cloth before placing it on the affected part.
4. Keep track of the position of the bottle. If the patient is restless, the bottle may move out of position, and the patient could be burned.
5. After use, hang the bottle mouth-down to drain and dry. After the bottle is dry, blow air into it, replace the stopper, and store the bottle in a cool, dry place.
6. Make a note on the daily record where and for how long the hot water bottle was applied and how the patient reacted to it.

Moist Heat

Moist heat is more penetrating than dry heat; therefore, there is more danger that the skin may be burned. Care must be taken to avoid temperatures that could be harmful to the skin. The average adult tolerates water at temperatures as high as 110°F, or 43°C. A child's skin is more sensitive and more easily injured. The front of the body is usually more sensitive than the back, and the feet and legs are more sensitive than the hands and arms.

Warm, Moist Compresses

A compress is a pad made by folding a piece of clean cloth so that there are four or more layers of material slightly larger than the area to be treated. The cloth may be a washcloth, a towel, a baby blanket, or a piece of blanket or heavy flannel, depending on the size of the area to be treated and the material available. To help prevent burns from a warm compress, a thin layer of oil or petroleum jelly can be applied to the patient's skin. The oil or petroleum jelly is particularly useful if the patient's skin is thin or tender but should not be used if the patient's skin is broken. The following is the procedure for applying a warm, moist compress:

1. Gather equipment:

   Two folded compresses large enough to cover the area to be treated.

   A binder (a towel or a strip of cloth to hold the compress in place). This should be lined with wax paper, aluminum foil, or other material to hold the heat.

   Safety pins to fasten the binder.

   Protective covering for the bed and the bedside table.

   A bed cradle or some device to hold the top sheet and blanket away from the body part being treated (see chapter 24 for information on an improvised bed cradle).
2. Explain to the patient the steps that will be taken.
3. Protect the bedding around the area of the body to be treated.
4. Prepare the compress: wet the compress in water that feels hot but not painful to the hand (about 115°F or 46°C) and wring it dry enough so that it will not drip. (A very large compress can be spun dry on a washing machine's spin cycle.) Compresses can be heated in the empty top of a double boiler until they are steaming, and this may take from 5 to 10 minutes.
5. Meanwhile, adjust the patient's position so that he is comfortable and in good body alignment.

6. Have the binder ready with safety pins in position so that it can be fastened as soon as the compress is applied.
7. Protect the bedside table against heat and moisture.
8. Carry the hot compresses to the bedside table in the top of the double boiler or other basin.
9. Expose the body area where the compress is to be applied.
10. Remove one of the compresses from the pan, and without unfolding it, give it two strong, quick shakes to remove steam. Apply it to the area to be treated.
11. Quickly place the binder over the compress and pin it securely in place at both ends. (The binder serves to hold in heat, keep out cold air, and protect the bedding from moisture.)
12. Place a heating device over the compress. This may be a hot water bottle filled with water of about the same temperature as the compress, a commercial hot pack, or a waterproof electric heating pad set on low heat.
13. Change the compress as often as needed to keep a constant temperature. If using a hot water bottle, refill it after about 25 minutes. How long the treatment should last and how often it should be given will depend on the advice of the health professional.
14. Remember—the compress should be comfortably warm, not so hot that it can burn the skin.

Sitz Baths and Soaks

Sitz baths and soaks are used to promote healing, to relieve pain, and to promote relaxation. A *sitz bath* is a bath taken in a sitting position. It is intended to promote healing and relieve pain, especially in the rectal and pubic genital area. (The word *sitz* is the German word for *seat.*) A *soak* means keeping a part of the body covered with water for a specific period of time. The health professional who advises these treatments will specify the temperature of the water, the length of time, how often to give the treatment, and whether any medication is to be added to the water. The water used is usually comfortably warm tap water (95°–110°F, or 35°–43°C), and the usual length of the sitz bath or soak is 15–20 minutes.

The temperature of the water should be comfortable and fairly constant, and care should be taken to avoid burning the patient. Use a thermometer to test the water temperature, because the skin can tolerate water that is hot enough to burn it. If the water seems too hot at first, the body or body part may be gradually immersed in the water; or you might start with cooler water and gradually bring it to the higher temperature by adding more hot water. When adding warm water, stir it in to prevent burning the patient. Add warm water every 5 minutes to keep the temperature constant.

A sitz bath may be taken either in a clean bathtub or with disposable sitz bath equipment, which can be purchased. If using a bathtub, first place a rubber or plastic air-filled ring on the bottom of the tub and cover it with a towel. Fill the tub with enough water to reach about to the patient's waist (usually about 6 inches, or 15.24 centimeters). Have the patient get into the tub, assisting him if necessary. Keep the upper part of his body warm by placing a bath blanket around his shoulders and on the outside of the tub, if possible. Check the water temperature every 5 minutes, adding more warm water as necessary.

When giving a sitz bath or a soak to a patient, remember the following pointers:

- Explain to the patient the steps that will be taken and what he is to do.
- Make the patient comfortable and keep his body in good alignment for any treatment.
- If the treatment is to be given in bed, protect the bedding.
- Protect the patient's body from the edge of any container used for soaking the body part.
- Take care to avoid burning the patient.

TREATMENTS USING COLD

The Effects of Cold

Applying cold to the body for limited periods of time causes the blood vessels to constrict (become smaller) and reduces the flow of blood to the exposed area. For this reason, applying cold to a *fresh* injury may slow bleeding, reduce inflammation and swelling, and prevent discoloring. Applying something cold such as an ice bag is a good first aid measure for injuries such as sprains and bruises. Immediately applying cold water to a first- or second-degree burn helps to reduce tissue damage and pain. Cooling baths and applications are often useful in controlling dangerously high fevers.

When cold is first applied, the skin tends to become pale and cool, and "goose flesh" (small bumps on the skin) may appear. Within 30 minutes after cold has been applied, however, the person begins to shiver (the body's muscle reactions to cold), the blood vessels once again dilate, and the skin becomes reddened and warm. Continued use of cold applications is no longer beneficial at this point. If cold is prolonged, it slows blood circulation, slows the activities of the cells, and may cause destruction of body tissue. For these reasons, it is generally wise to apply cold for *no more than half an hour* at a time (unless the health professional advises otherwise).

The effects of applying cold depend also upon the amount of body surface involved. The greater the area treated, the more intense is the reaction. If cold is applied to the entire body, it causes slowing of the pulse and respiration and has a sedative effect (makes the person sleepy). Persons whose bodies are less able to regulate their own temperature, such as the very young, the elderly, acutely ill persons, and persons in danger of shock, are more likely to be harmed by application of cold over large areas of the body. Treatments involving large portions of the body should be given *only* if they are ordered by the health professional.

Cold may be applied to the body by use of ice bags or commercial cold packs and by cold, wet compresses and cool baths. Moist cold, like moist heat, is more penetrating in its action, because water is a better conductor than air. Lower temperatures can be tolerated if the treatment is dry rather than moist. Whenever giving cold treatments, always observe the patient for symptoms such as skin turning blue or skin that is unevenly red. If these symptoms occur, stop the cold treatments at once.

Ice Bags and Cold Packs

Ice bags must be refilled from time to time to keep them cold, while cold packs stay colder for longer periods of time.

Fill an ice bag (or plastic bag) only one third to one half full of crushed ice. Crushed ice conforms to the shape of the body part being treated. (To make crushed ice, place several ice cubes between several layers of newspaper or towel, then break up the ice cubes with a hammer or heavy spoon.) Squeeze out excess air before closing the bag. From time to time, empty water from the bag and add more crushed ice.

Prefilled, sealed cold packs that are chilled in the freezer before use are convenient to use because they stay cold longer than ice. They are available as body packs (about the size and shape of a hot water bottle) and as child- or adult-size collars (useful after a tonsillectomy). Follow the manufacturer's directions to prepare these packs for use.

Whether you are using an ice bag or a cold pack, the cold application will be more comfortable for the patient if a soft cloth or a thin towel is placed between the ice bag or cold pack and the patient's skin. Replace the cloth if it becomes wet.

Cold, Moist Compresses

Use the same materials for a cold compress that are used to apply a warm, moist compress. The size of the area to be treated will determine whether a folded washcloth, towel, or blanket would be more appropriate.

Wet the cloth in ice water, wring it out so that it will not drip, and apply it to the area to be treated. Repeat this procedure from time to time to keep the cold constant. (If the treatment is given in bed, remember to protect the bedding with rubber sheeting or plastic.) For a longer-lasting effect, place an ice-filled bag or a piece of plastic over the moist cloth. Crushed ice in a damp washcloth can be used instead of a compress for small injured areas such as an eye or an insect sting.

Sponge Bath To Reduce Fever

A sponge bath with lukewarm water may be ordered by the health professional as an aid in reducing a dangerously high fever. The cooling action comes from the evaporation of the water from the skin surface. If the water is cold rather than lukewarm, it may cause shivering, which will increase, rather than decrease, the body temperature. Care must be taken to avoid chilling the patient.

The following is the procedure for giving a sponge bath to reduce fever:

1. Protect the bedding by placing a waterproof sheet or several towels under the patient.
2. Use water that feels slightly warm to the hands (80°–93°F or 27°–34°C).
3. To avoid chilling the patient, expose only part of his body at a

time. Placing a hot water bottle at the patient's feet can also decrease the tendency for him to become chilled and will make the patient more comfortable.

4. Bathe the patient's entire body surface, spending about 5 minutes on each arm and leg and 5 minutes on chest and back. The total time spent should be from 20 to 30 minutes, unless the health professional orders otherwise.
5. Place an ice bag or a cold compress on the patient's head to help to reduce the body temperature, if necessary.
6. Observe the patient closely for change in color and for decrease in pulse and respirations. Stop the treatment immediately if he shivers or becomes chilled. Allow the shivering to stop, then slowly continue the treatment.
7. After completing the sponge bath, dry the patient's skin and remove the waterproof sheeting or towels.
8. Replace the patient's clothing and cover him lightly with a sheet or thin blanket.
9. Make the patient as comfortable as possible.

TREATMENTS TO HELP BREATHING

The Breathing Process and What Affects It

Breathing is such an automatic process that little thought is given to it until something such as a cold, pneumonia, or some other condition of the upper respiratory tract interferes with it. When a person breathes in (inhales), air moves into the lungs, and the oxygen from the air enters the bloodstream. When he breathes out (exhales), carbon dioxide and other gases not needed by the body leave the bloodstream and lungs. Air is filtered through the nose and cleaned before it enters the lungs. If a person cannot breathe through his nose because it is stuffy, this filtering system is bypassed.

If the breathing passages and parts of the lung are filled with mucus, secretions, or other particles not common to the body, oxygen has more trouble getting into the bloodstream. Coughing and sneezing are important body defenses that help to clear out the breathing passages. The effectiveness of a cough or sneeze, however, depends on the quality of the secretions to be removed. If the secretions are extremely thick, it will be very difficult to clear the lungs. Increasing the humidity (moisture) of the air that is breathed can soften thick secretions so that they can be more easily coughed up.

A major way to increase the effectiveness of breathing is by changing the quality of the air that is inhaled. Changing the quality of the air in a stuffy room may involve opening the windows to provide fresh air. If pollution in the air is particularly bad, air conditioning can help to clean the air. A vaporizer or a humidifier can be used to add moisture to the air, thus softening secretions to be coughed up. Breathing through a warm, moist cloth can accomplish the same thing. The amount of moisture in the air has a major effect on breathing.

Vaporizers and Humidifiers

There are several different kinds of electric appliances designed to add moisture to room air. All are relatively low in cost and available at most drug, department, or appliance stores. The older type, the vaporizer, brings water to a boil and releases a flow of steam into the room. The newer type, the cool mist or cold stream humidifier, contains a pump that throws a stream of unheated water through a screen or onto a revolving wheel, breaking up water droplets into tiny particles that are blown out into the room. The cool-mist type of humidifier is safer, since there is no danger of anyone's being scalded or burned if the appliance is tipped over and water is spilled on a person.

Points to remember when using vaporizers and humidifiers:

- Place the appliance on a solid surface, below the bed level and out of the patient's reach. Protect the surface and surrounding area from moisture. Keep the electric cord safely out of the way.
- Direct the flow of moist air near the patient, but not directly into his face or onto his skin.
- If hot steam is used, see that the patient does not become overheated and then chilled when treatment is stopped. Wipe any moisture from his face and hands and see that he remains quiet and warmly covered for an hour or so after treatment ends.
- Carefully read the directions that come with any vapor appliance, especially in regard to cleaning, maintaining the water level, and the use of medications.
- Always unplug the appliance before moving it, cleaning it, or refilling it with water.

CHANGING DRESSINGS

Dressings are used to protect a wound from infection, to absorb fluids or discharge, and to apply medicines to aid healing. They are also used to apply pressure on a part of the body (such as on a wound to stop bleeding), to prevent or reduce swelling, to prevent moving of a body part, and to provide support to a weak muscle.

Dressings or bandages over wounds are either *sterile* (have no germs) or *clean* (have a minimum of germs). Sterile dressings require special care in handling to avoid getting germs on them (contamination). Often the health professional will be the one to change a sterile dressing.

Sometimes a sterile dressing becomes wet from blood or drainage from the wound. Do *not* attempt to change a sterile dressing unless the proper method of doing so has been demonstrated. Instead, tape more gauze pads to the outside of the dressing where it is wet. Then contact the health professional about the drainage and allow him to give advice or change the dressing. Report the amount of drainage and its color. Write on the patient's record when the new dressing was added and how many gauze pads were used.

When a dressing is *clean,* the home nurse may change it as follows:

1. Assemble necessary equipment: dressings, scissors, tape, any medication or solution ordered by the health professional, and a waste container or a paper bag for disposal of the old dressing.
2. Wash your hands carefully.
3. Have the new dressing ready to put in place before removing the old one.
4. Remove the tape carefully from the skin while leaving the old dressing in place. If the skin under the tape is red and inflamed, do not place new tape in the same place. (If the inflammation seems serious, discuss this fact with the health professional.)
5. Remove the dressing and observe the wound for signs of swelling, redness, drainage, or pus. Notice whether the wound is healing. Notice the amount and color of any discharge on the dressing itself. *Do not touch the wound.*
6. Discard the old dressing, being careful not to touch the area of the dressing that was next to the wound. Place the dressing in a plastic or paper bag and close the top of the bag.

7. If soaking or other treatment is needed, follow the instructions of the health professional.
8. Place the new dressing over the wound, being careful not to touch the side of the dressing that will be in contact with the wound. Tape the dressing securely in place.
9. Wash your hands thoroughly.
10. Report to the health professional any changes in the condition of the wound, the presence of pain, and the amount and color of discharges.

CARE OF STITCHES (SUTURES)

Sometimes it is necessary for a health professional to use stitches to hold skin together where it has been cut open. These stitches must stay in place for several days to keep the skin edges closed while the tissue heals and grows back together. Usually the wound will heal within a week or 10 days, and the health professional will then remove the stitches. At the time the stitches are put in, the health professional will advise you on how long a period of time it will be before they are to be removed. The health professional will also give guidelines about what activities the patient is to avoid during the healing process. The health professional will decide whether the area with stitches should be covered with a bandage or should be allowed to heal in the open air, depending on the wound and on the individual.

If the stitches are left uncovered, keep the area clean and dry. The health professional will advise whether the area should be washed or not.

If the wound is covered by a bandage, the bandage will probably not need to be changed unless it becomes soiled, wet, or soaked with drainage from the wound. If there is any question about a dressing, consult the health professional. He may give instructions for changing the dressing or may advise that the dressing be changed only by a health professional.

If the skin around the wound becomes red and swollen, or if pus and drainage begin to come out of the wound, an infection is present. If the patient develops a fever, this too could indicate the presence of infection. Report any signs of infection to the health professional, who will determine what treatment is to be given.

CARING FOR THE PERSON IN A CAST

Casts are applied to a part of the body by a health professional to keep the body part in the proper position while healing occurs. Casts are used for parts of the body such as arms or legs when a bone is broken or following some surgical procedures. Sometimes a cast is used for a large area of the body. A cast applied to the abdomen, hips, and legs is called a body cast. Casts are usually made of a plaster substance that is applied while wet over cloth (a stockinette) placed next to the patient's skin. The plaster becomes hard as it dries. The cast can be damaged if it becomes wet.

If the cast is on an arm, the patient may need help in dressing or feeding himself, depending on which arm is affected. He may need to wear an arm sling to support the cast. An arm sling may be purchased from a drug store or hospital supply store, or one can be made from materials available at home (see chapter 24).

If the cast is on a leg or a foot, the health professional may instruct that the leg be kept elevated to prevent swelling. If the patient is to be allowed to walk using crutches, the health professional will advise on how to walk. (See chapter 22 for information on the three-point gait and the swing gait.) Sometimes the health professional applies a walking cast, one with a rubber tip to provide cushioning and support.

If the patient is in a body cast, he may have to stay in bed. Because of the weight of the cast, the home nurse usually needs help to turn and position the patient. The health professional will advise on the best way to handle this type of patient, perhaps recommending the use of a hospital bed with an overhead trapeze bar so that the patient can help in moving himself. Since conditions that require a body cast often require a long time in bed, giving attention to the patient's emotional state is as important as attention to his physical needs. A positive mental outlook can speed the patient's recovery.

The following principles apply in caring for a patient in any type of cast:

- Be sure the cast is completely dry before applying pressure to any part of it. A wet cast feels cool. While drying, a cast should be exposed to the air. The use of a fan may hasten the drying time.
- Smooth any rough edges at the top or bottom of the cast. Either pull the stockinette over the edge of the cast and tape it to the cast

or place pieces of adhesive tape over the rough edges. (Use tape only when the cast is completely dry.)

- Check the circulation in the fingers or toes of any limb in a cast every few hours the first day. Squeeze a finger or toe. If it turns white when squeezed and then red when released, circulation is normal. Report immediately to the health professional any blue or white coloring of a finger or toe.
- Report to the health professional about any tingling or numbness that the patient feels, any pain from pressure of the cast, or any cold fingers or toes.
- Keep the cast dry at all times. If there is danger of the cast's becoming wet (as when the patient is bathing), use waterproof material such as a plastic bag to protect the cast.
- To improve circulation and prevent pressure sores, reach inside the cast (if possible) to massage the skin.
- To relieve itching, tap the cast over the itching area with a blunt, not sharp, object, or blow air into the cast with a bulb syringe. *Never* stick a sharp object into or under the cast.
- Use pillows to support the body part in a cast if the part is to be elevated, or to position the body properly.
- When the health professional advises exercise to strengthen the muscles of the body part in a cast, encourage the patient to tighten and then relax the muscles several times each day.
- To maintain the patient's strength generally, have him, when possible, exercise all parts of his body that are not in the cast.
- Prevent small children from placing objects in their casts, since skin irritation, pain, and infection may be caused.

ENEMAS

The usual purpose of an enema is to remove waste materials and air from the lower bowel by inserting a liquid into the rectum. This is known as a cleansing enema. Other types of enema might include drugs in solution ordered by a health professional to protect, soothe, and irrigate the mucous membrane of the lower bowel. Any enema will act to soften bowel movement (stool) and stimulate bowel action to remove the stool.

The normal, healthy child or adult will almost never need an enema. Eating a balanced diet and getting enough exercise is generally all that is needed to have normal bowel movements every 1 to 3 days. Sometimes, however, illness or the use of medicines may cause constipation that is not easily corrected by regular activity and diet. When a patient has not had a bowel movement for 3 days, use of a laxative, suppository (see chapter 19), or enema may be required to prevent fecal impaction (hard stool that cannot be passed). The health professional should advise on the best treatment for the patient.

If an enema is advisable, the health professional should recommend the type of enema to be used and the amount and type of solution. Give only the amount and kind of solution ordered. Enemas may be given by using a disposable enema unit or by using an enema bag or can and equipment to insert warm or soapy water or some other mixture advised by the health professional. An enema is given to a patient while he is lying down, and the tip of the applicator must be lubricated to avoid injury to the rectum.

Disposable enema units can be bought in drugstores. They are low in cost, easy to use, and comfortable for the patient. The enema unit is prefilled, and the applicator tip is already lubricated. The unit may be used at room temperature or may be warmed slightly by putting the entire unit in warm water shortly before using it. After use, the entire unit is discarded, and there is nothing to clean or store.

If an enema bag (usually a rubber bag) or can and equipment are used, the solution must be prepared and inserted into the bag, the applicator (nozzle) must be lubricated with petroleum jelly, and the equipment must be cleaned well before being put away.

Giving an Enema to an Adult

1. Gather the necessary equipment: a disposable enema unit *or* enema bag or can with connective tubing, clamp, enema tip or nozzle, lubricant, and solution as ordered by the health professional. (A tray may be helpful for carrying the equipment.) If the patient will remain in bed after the enema is inserted, a bedpan, toilet paper, protective covering for the bed, and a call bell will also be needed.
2. Explain to the patient the steps that will be taken and what he can do to help.
3. Place protective waterproof material under the patient's hips.
4. Position the patient comfortably: if possible, have him lie on his

left side with his upper leg bent. (This position may help the liquid flow into the bowel, because the lower bowel curves to the left.) If the patient is to give the enema to himself, he may lie on his back with his knees bent.

5. Keep the patient warm and covered to prevent chilling. Expose only the buttocks and the rectal area.
6. If using a disposable enema unit, gently insert the tip and squeeze the plastic container to force the liquid into the rectum. Be sure the liquid flows gently, without too much pressure. If only part of the solution is to be used, discard the rest of the solution.
7. If using an enema bag or can and equipment—

   Close the clamp on the tubing and fill the bag or can with 1 to 2 pints of warm water or the mixture advised by the health professional. (The temperature of the water is right if it feels lukewarm to your wrist.)

   Open the clamp and let a small amount of the solution run through the tube into the bedpan, commode, or other container. This removes the air and warms the tubing. Then close the clamp.

   Lubricate the nozzle or tip, then gently insert it 2–3 inches (5.1–7.6 centimeters) into the rectum and hold it in place. (If a hard rubber tip is used, insert it to the bulge at its base—usually about 2 inches, or 5.1 centimeters.)

   To start the flow of liquid, rotate the tip slightly but gently. If the liquid does not begin to flow, withdraw the tip and try again. If the tube becomes clogged, withdraw the tip and allow the solution to run through it, then reinsert the tip and start the fluid again.

   Hold or hang the enema bag or can about (but no more than) 2 feet (61 centimeters) above the level of the bed. (The higher the bag is above the patient, the greater the force of the fluid on the lining of the bowel. Too much force is harmful and painful and prevents retention of fluid.)

   Allow the solution to flow into the rectum slowly. When the patient has had as much as he can comfortably tolerate, close the clamp to stop the flow.
8. Remove the tip and encourage the patient to keep the enema solution in his rectum until he has a *strong* urge to have a bowel movement.

9. Help the patient to the toilet or bedside commode, or onto the bedpan. If he can be left alone, provide him with toilet paper, a call bell, and privacy.
10. If the patient is unable to cleanse himself after the bowel movement, help him. (Remember to wipe female patients from front to back to prevent infection.)
11. Help the patient off the bedpan, back to bed or to a chair when he is finished.
12. Remove the enema equipment. Discard disposable units. If an enema bag and equipment were used, wash the equipment thoroughly. Rinse the bag or can and tubing with clear water. Wash the enema tip or nozzle with hot, soapy water, using friction. Allow the equipment to dry and then store it in a cool, dark place.
13. Record the results: amount, color, and consistency (whether hard or soft) of the stool.

Giving an Enema to a Child

Give an enema to an infant or child *only* when ordered to do so by the health professional. Never use enemas to regulate bowel movements in a healthy child. When an enema is ordered for an infant or small child, use an infant enema syringe with a rubber bulb. If the child is over 2 years of age, a child-size disposable enema unit may be used.

Procedure

1. Gather the equipment: disposable enema unit *or* syringe, recommended enema solution and lubricant, waterproof pad, extra diapers.
2. If the child is old enough to understand, explain the steps that will be taken.
3. Position the child. An infant may be on his back with his legs held up. A toddler may lie on his left side with both knees drawn up to his chest. (You may need help to hold the child in the proper position.)
4. Keep the child covered, except for the buttocks and rectal area, to avoid chilling.
5. If you are using an infant syringe, lubricate the tip and squeeze the bulb to draw the enema solution into the bulb. Then, holding the tip straight up, gently squeeze the bulb to expel any air.

6. Gently insert the tip about 1 inch (2.5 centimeters) into the rectum.
7. Slowly squeeze the ordered amount of solution into the rectum. Never use more than 1–2 ounces (29.6–59.1 milliliters).
8. Remove the tip and hold the child's buttocks together for a few minutes or until the child needs to have a bowel movement. If the child is old enough, he may use the toilet or a bedpan. Otherwise, replace his diapers and change them after he has expelled the enema.
9. Record the kind of stool (consistency and color) and amount of bowel movement expelled.
10. Discard the disposable enema unit, or clean the equipment. Wash the infant syringe in warm, soapy water.

Points To Remember

- Be sure the solution flows gently, without pressure.
- Lubricate the tip well to avoid injury to the rectum.
- Give only the amount and kind of solution ordered.
- Have the patient lying down and in a comfortable position.
- Avoid chilling the patient.

Chapter 24

Making Your Own Equipment

Making a Backrest From a Cardboard Box

(See page 521 for instructions.)

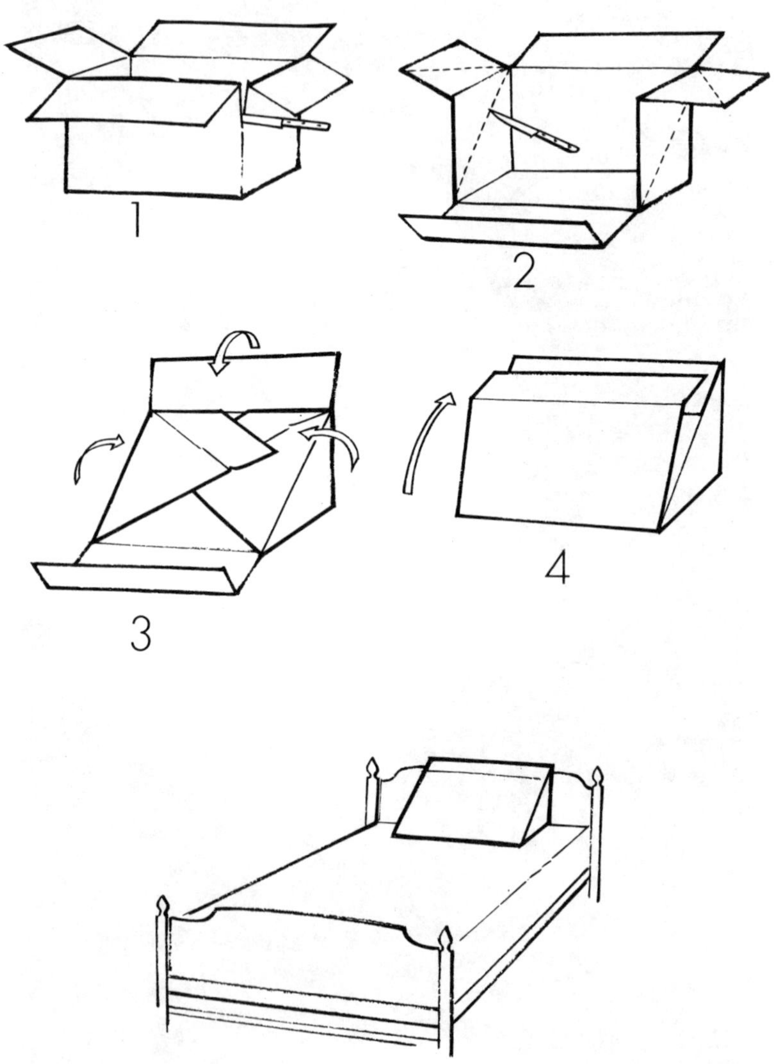

Fig. 109

When there is a sick person in the home, the right kind of equipment does much to make the patient more comfortable and to save energy, both for the patient and those who care for him. A hospital bed might be rented, or a regular bed might be raised to a height comfortable for the home nurse, and side rails might be improvised. A backrest, a bed table, a hot water bottle, and a bedpan are examples of equipment often needed by a patient. How long the illness is expected to last and the cost of the equipment are important considerations in deciding whether it would be better to buy, rent, borrow, or make the needed equipment. Although items such as bedpans are generally more satisfactory if manufactured for the specific purpose, many items can be made with materials and tools commonly found in the home. Cardboard boxes, chairs, bottles, tin cans, newspapers, and baking pans are examples of items that can be used to improvise such things as backrests, bed tables, bed rails, hot water bottles, footstools, bedpans, urinals, waste containers, and protective bed pads.

Many communities have places from which hospital-type equipment can be borrowed, rented, or purchased. The health professional can advise on ways to obtain equipment that would be helpful in caring for a patient at home. Sometimes information can be found in the Yellow Pages of the telephone book under the headings of "Rental" or "Hospital Equipment." Whenever there is a need for special equipment to care for an ill person at home, the following points should be considered:

- How long will the equipment be used? Can it be borrowed? If the needed items would have to be rented for a long period of time, would it be less expensive to buy them or to make them?
- What items could be made at home with the materials and tools available? Would they be safe, practical, and easy to use? Would they be easy to keep clean? Would they be comfortable for the patient?
- Would homemade equipment be durable enough to last as long as the patient needs it?

Instructions for making many types of equipment often needed by the patient and the home nurse are given in this chapter. Many common items can be used for purposes other than those for which they were intended. The ideas in this chapter will probably spark ideas for other ways to save money and energy while keeping the patient comfortable and safe.

EQUIPMENT FOR SAFETY AND CONVENIENCE

Bed Blocks To Elevate the Bed

Whenever the patient will require care in bed over a long period of time and does not have a hospital bed, using bed blocks to raise the bed and removing the casters to make the bed secure are desirable steps to take. Having the bed at a comfortable working height will greatly reduce the strain on the home nurse's back and shoulders and will lessen fatigue. Sometimes the health professional may recommend raising one end of the bed as a form of treatment.

The bed is at a suitable working height when the palms of the home nurse's hands can be placed flat on the mattress without either raising or lowering the shoulders, usually 30–32 inches (76.2–81.3 centimeters) from the floor, depending on the home nurse's height. To determine how many inches (or centimeters) the bed will need to be raised, first remove the casters from the bed and then measure the height of the mattress from the floor.

Blocks to elevate the bed can be bought, rented, or made, although there are also other methods of raising the bed. Commercial bed blocks may be made of sturdy plastic. Wooden bed blocks can be made at home, or some lumberyards will make them on request. The cost of making bed blocks or having them made should be compared with the cost of renting or buying them.

One method is to make four blocks of wood approximately 8 x 8 x 12 inches (20.3 x 20.3 x 30.5 centimeters) with a hole 3 or 4 inches (7.6 or 10.2 centimeters) deep in one end of each block to hold the bed leg securely.

Other methods for raising the bed include using—

- Four stacks of old magazines or folded newspapers tied securely, with a hole cut in the center of the top of each stack to hold the bed leg.
- Four large cinder or cement blocks.
- Four sturdy kitchen chairs, two under each end of the bed.
- Four large tin cans partly filled with sand. To make—

  Remove and save the tops of the cans and smooth the cut edges of the cans for safety.

Fill each can about two thirds full of sand, small pebbles, or gravel.

Place the tops of the cans on top of the sand or gravel to give the bed legs a steady base on which to rest and to prevent them from sinking.

Remove the casters from the bed and place a can under each bed leg.

Side Rails

To keep a restless or delirious patient safe, make side rails by placing kitchen chairs with their backs up against the edge of the bed. Tie the chair legs to the bedsprings or bed frame. (Old nylon stockings make good ties for this purpose.)

Bed Pads and Mattress Protectors

When a waterproof sheet is not available but is needed to prevent the mattress from getting wet or soiled, it is possible to make one from a shower curtain, a plastic tablecloth, or the back section of a plastic raincoat. If the waterproof material is not large enough to tuck well under the mattress on both sides, pieces of cloth can be sewed to both edges to prevent the plastic from wrinkling.

A bed pad or other bed protector may be placed directly under a patient to protect the bottom sheet from becoming wet or soiled during a treatment or when a wound is draining. It may also be used under a bedpan. If a patient is incontinent, waterproof bed pads will be needed. Disposable bed pads that have a waterproof plastic backing are easy to use and will save laundry expenses. If the illness will be prolonged, cloth-surfaced waterproof pads like those used for babies may be economical to use, since they can be laundered and reused.

To make a bed pad that will absorb moisture but will not be waterproof, use a piece of cloth about 26 x 36 inches (66 x 91 centimeters). Fold the cloth once to bring the ends together, then stitch along the two long sides to make a 26 x 18 inch (66 x 45.7 centimeter) case. Turn the case inside out. Place about six double sheets of newspaper inside.

To make the pad more waterproof, place a piece of plastic about the same size as the case (perhaps from an old plastic raincoat) between the newspapers and the case to help protect the bed from moisture. When using this pad, place the plastic side toward the bed and away from the patient.

Several of these pads would be needed so that some would be on hand while the soiled cloth covers are being washed and dried. After use, discard the newspapers and wash the cloth cover.

Bed Tables

A table that fits over the patient's lap while he is sitting up will be useful at mealtime, for writing letters and working puzzles, and for other activities. It is possible to buy a tray with short legs or a table that extends over the bed. These kinds of trays can also be used as "cradles" to hold blankets off the patient's feet and legs. Bed tables can also be made from materials available in most homes:

- The free end of an adjustable-height ironing board may be extended over the bed.
- A wooden box or crate, from which the two longer sides have been removed, may be placed across the patient's lap.
- The legs of a child's wooden table can be shortened to make a bed table of the right height.
- Two boards about 10 x 12 inches (25.4 x 30.5 centimeters) each can be nailed to the ends of a large board 12 x 24 inches (30.5 x 70 centimeters) to make a table 10 inches (25.4 centimeters) high.
- A sturdy cardboard box about 10 x 12 x 24 inches (25.4 x 30.5 x 70 centimeters) can be cut and made into a bed table as follows (Fig. 110):

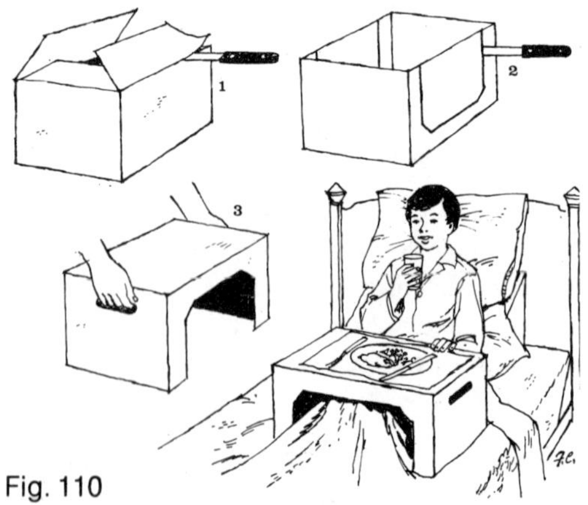

Fig. 110

Cut away the top cover flaps from the box. (For safety, always turn the knife blade away from your body when cutting.)

Cut curved pieces out of the two longest sides of the box to allow the table to fit comfortably over the patient's thighs. Leave at least 2 inches (5.1 centimeters) on each side and the top to support and strengthen the table top.

Cut narrow openings near the top on each remaining side so that fingers may be inserted to lift and carry the table.

Cover the cut edges of the box with adhesive cellophane or other gummed paper tape to strengthen the table.

Cover the table with cloth, paint, wallpaper, or adhesive-backed plastic to improve its appearance.

Cloth pockets can be attached to the sides of most of these trays to hold items used by the patient.

Before placing the table on the bed, loosen and adjust the patient's top covers to allow him to move his knees comfortably without danger of upsetting articles on the bed table.

Foot Supports

The weight and pressure of the upper sheet and blankets should be kept off the patient's feet and toes in order to maintain proper position of the feet. A foot support is used *under* the top bed covers and should keep the bedding at least 2 inches (5.1 centimeters) higher than the patient's toes. If there is a footboard on the bed, the weight of the covers can be kept off the patient's feet by putting the covers over the footboard rather than tucking them under the mattress.

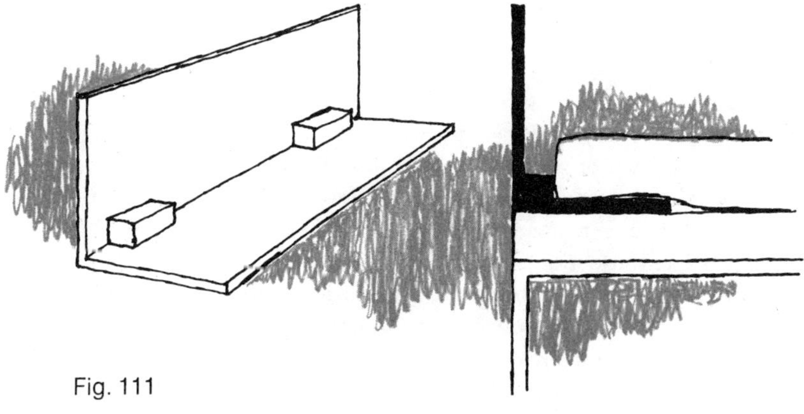

Fig. 111

Bed Cradle

A bed cradle is used to relieve pressure on the knees or some other part of the body. It can also be used to protect the upper bed covers while moist compresses are being applied to the patient. Make a bed cradle by cutting two ends out of a cardboard box or wooden crate (it will be similar to the bed table). Or make a bed cradle by bending heavy wire mesh to the shape needed, then padding the cut edges with heavy tape or strips of cloth. Or wire two coat hangers together with heavy wire.

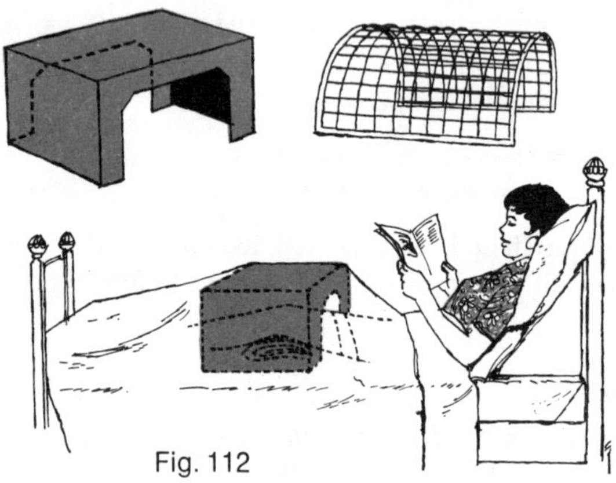

Fig. 112

Slipper Rack

A rack to hold the patient's bedroom slippers can be made by bending the ends of a wire clothes hanger. Then hang it from the springs or bed frame in a place easy for the patient to reach.

Pull Rope

If a patient had something to assist him, he could often help lift or turn himself in bed, or he could bring himself to a sitting position without the help of another person. A pull rope can be made by braiding three old nylon stockings (or pieces of other strong cloth) together. If a longer rope is needed, add more stockings. If a thicker rope is desired, use more stockings for each strand of the braid. Tie the pull rope to the foot of the bed if the patient is to use it for pulling himself up to a sitting position. If the patient needs ropes to turn himself onto his side, make shorter ropes and tie them to the sides of the bed.

Bed Trays

If a regular tray for serving meals is not available, a cookie pan, a smooth board, or a framed picture may be used. Small-size cooking pans (square or round) can be used as smaller trays for keeping medicines or other small equipment together.

Accessory Bag

Keeping things the patient uses within his reach will save time and steps for the home nurse. A cloth accessory bag that can be tucked under the mattress is very helpful for keeping small items such as a comb and scissors where the patient can reach them easily. The bag can be made from a dishtowel or other washable cloth about 12 x 28 inches (30.5 x 71 centimeters). Turn up about 6 inches (15.2 centimeters) at one end and stitch the material so as to make several pockets (these can be made to fit special items that the patient needs to have handy). At the other end, make a single pocket about 6 inches (15.2 centimeters) deep and insert a piece of cardboard 12 x 6 inches (30.5 x 15.2 centimeters). This section will be tucked under the mattress and will help keep the bag extended to its full width.

Waste Container

Paper bags from the grocery store make excellent waste containers. Small waste bags can also be made by folding newspapers as follows (Fig. 113).

1. Fold a double sheet of newspaper in half and place it on a flat surface with the fold toward you.
2. Bring the upper edge of the top half of the paper to the fold at the bottom, making a cuff to strengthen the bag.
3. Turn the paper over so that the smooth side is up, keeping the original fold at the bottom.
4. Fold the paper in thirds from the side toward the center and crease the folds well.
5. Tuck one side under the cuff of the other side to lock it in place.
6. Fold the top flap over the locked side of the cuff as a further means of locking the bag into position. The flap serves as a support when the bag is standing, as a means of fastening the bag to the side of the bed, and as a cover when the bag is to be thrown away.

Fig. 113

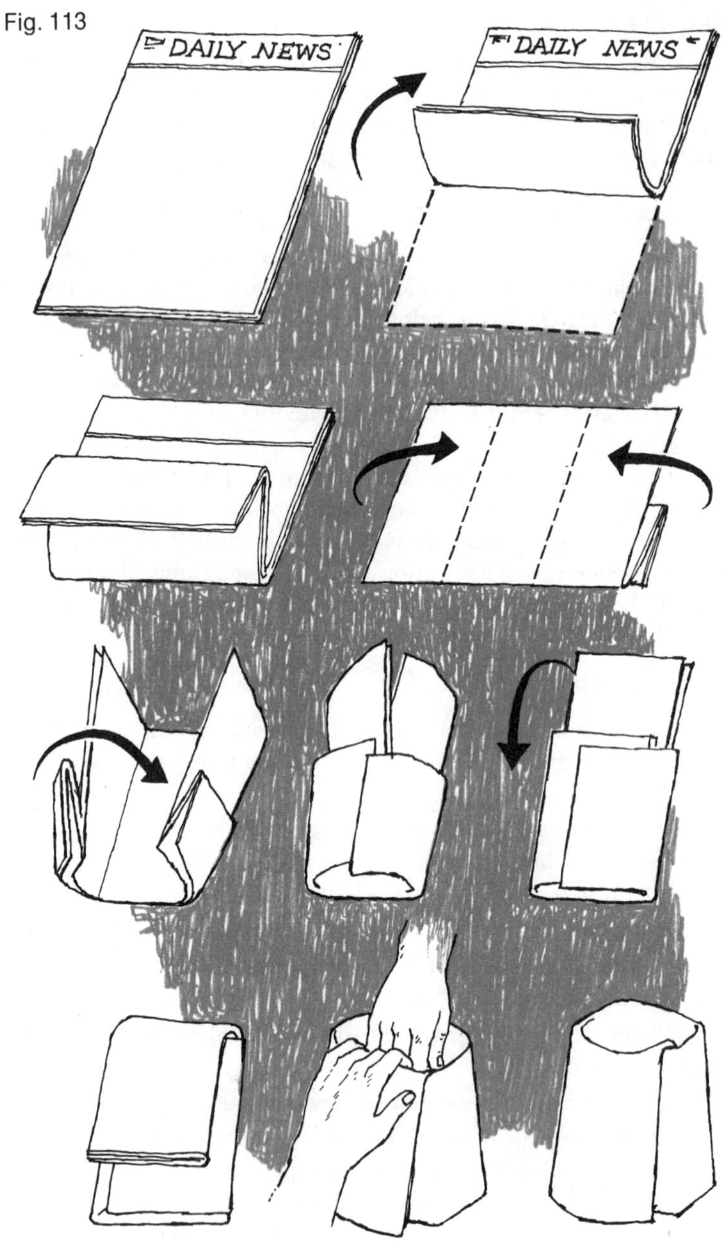

Footstool or Step Stool

A patient may be more comfortable while sitting in a chair if his feet are elevated by a footstool. A stool is also useful for getting into and out of bed. A handy and safe footstool can be made by using quart-size fruit juice cans, cardboard, and tape, as follows:

1. Place seven quart-size fruit juice cans together in a circle, with one other in the center.
2. Using adhesive tape or some other strong tape, fasten tape securely around the outside of the cans.
3. Tape thin cardboard of the proper size around the outside of the cans.
4. Cut sturdy cardboard in a circle to cover the top of the stool and tape it securely in place.

The stool can be padded on top with any soft material—old nylon stockings would serve the purpose. An adhesive paper could be used to make the stool colorful. If the stool will be used on a smooth-surface floor, place a nonskid rubber pad under it.

Backrests (See page 512.)

A backrest may be used to raise the patient's head, to provide support, and to prevent strain and fatigue for the patient when he sits up in bed. A triangle-shaped pillow or a special backrest pillow with arm rests can be purchased, but a backrest made from a sturdy cardboard box will serve just as well to support the patient's bed pillows. The box should be about 24 x 24 x 18 inches (61 x 61 x 45.8 centimeters) and is made into a backrest as follows:

1. Cut down the front side of the box at the corners and let the front side fall forward and lie flat.
2. Score the short sides of the box diagonally from top to bottom on the inside of the box.
3. Bend the sides inward along the lines of scoring. Bring the cover flap on the back of the carton forward, placing it over the folded sides.
4. Bring the front side of the box up and over the cover flap and folded sides. Fold the excess cardboard over the back of the box. Tie or tape the sides securely in place.

Backrests can also be made from any rigid object propped against the head of the bed and padded with pillows. A pastry board, a suitcase, a card table, or a pillow from an overstuffed chair might be used. Whatever is used should be tied securely in place to prevent it from slipping.

Another method of making a backrest is by placing a straight-backed chair upside down at the head of the bed and covering it with pillows.

EQUIPMENT TO PREVENT PRESSURE SORES

Pressure on any part of the body over a long period of time causes poor circulation and may destroy tissue, thus causing pressure sores. Persons who must remain in bed run a great risk of developing pressure sores unless measures are taken to relieve pressure on various parts of the body.

Foam or Sponge Rubber

Foam or sponge rubber cut to suitable shapes is often used to prevent pressure sores:

- For the hips or buttocks, cut a hole in a piece of foam rubber, 2 inches (5.1 centimeters) thick and prop the hips or buttocks over the hole.
- For elbows and heels, cut a small hole in the center of a piece of foam 1 inch (2.5 centimeters) thick.
- For the heels, make one anklet each out of a 3 x 12 inch (7.6 x 30.5 centimeters) strip of foam 1 or 2 inches (2.5 or 5.1 centimeters) thick. Tape the anklets loosely around the patient's ankles.
- Cushion the seat of a chair with a flat piece of foam 2 inches (5.1 centimeters) thick.
- Pad the top of a crutch by taping a piece of foam rubber around it.

Sheepskin

Sheepskin or synthetic sheepskin is helpful in preventing pressure sores (see chapter 17). A temporary substitute for sheepskin would be a clean, fluffy, washable nylon rug.

Waterbed

Some patients need a great deal of protection from pressure in order to avoid pressure sores. A waterbed provides a soft, pliable surface for the patient and helps to prevent points of undue pressure. A waterbed can be improvised from a camper's air mattress by filling the mattress with water rather than air.

Buy a good quality of camper's air mattress made of double-coated rubberized nylon fabric. These mattresses do not split or tear easily. If punctured by a pin or other sharp object, they will leak, but little water escapes. A repair kit for patching any leaks that do occur usually comes with the mattress.

Place the mattress on top of the regular mattress on the patient's bed before beginning to fill it. When it is full of water, it will be too heavy to move. Some form of hose (a garden hose, rubber tubing, or a portable shower hose) with an adapter for the air valve will be needed to fill the mattress with water from the nearest faucet (kitchen or bathroom). The water used should be about body temperature, 98°F (66°C).

Fill the mattress until it is about 3 inches (7.6 centimeters) thick and an adult leaning on it with both hands cannot push the top surface of the mattress against the bottom. The amount of water needed will vary somewhat according to the patient's weight. With too little water, the heavier parts of the patient's body will press the top and bottom surfaces of the mattress together. With too much water, the mattress will be too hard. If too much or too little water is used, the mattress will not be as effective as it should be.

Use a regular mattress pad and sheet over the water-filled mattress, but do not tuck the sheet in too tightly, because tightness can destroy the floating effect.

The water in the mattress will stay at the right temperature if the patient is in bed all the time. If he will be out of bed for a long period of time, place an electric blanket on top of the bed to keep the water from cooling. For safety reasons, unplug the electric blanket when the patient is in bed.

EQUIPMENT FOR BATHING AND PERSONAL CARE

Bath Blanket

It is helpful to have one lightweight blanket to use when bathing a patient. This may be a lightweight cotton blanket or a flannel sheet. If these are not available, use an old, clean bedspread, a blanket, a quilt, a cotton mattress pad, or an extra-large towel.

Denture Holder

A regular place to soak and store the patient's dentures is necessary. If the patient does not have a special container, use any plastic or glass container (a margarine or small cottage cheese container works well) and mark it clearly so that no harm comes to the dentures by accident.

Shampoo Pan

If the patient needs to have his hair washed in bed, a pan or a large piece of plastic will be needed to carry the flow of water away from the patient's head. Improvise a shampoo pan from a shallow, disposable baking pan by cutting a curved piece out at one end and removing the other end of the pan. Pad the curved end of the pan well with cloth covered by plastic so that it will be comfortable when it is used near the patient's neck. Tape a large piece of plastic to the other end of the pan. It will be used to direct soapy water into a pail or tub.

To improvise a shampoo pan with ony a piece of plastic and a pail, place one end of a large piece of plastic under the patient's head and place the other end of the plastic inside a pail or tub. Roll the edges of the plastic to form a channel that will direct the water into the pail.

Bathrobe or Bed Jacket

There are many times when the patient will need something to put over a nightgown or pajamas for warmth. If the patient does not have a bathrobe or a bed jacket, one can be made from a large bath towel or blanket:

1. Make a fold along the length of the blanket to serve as a collar. (The width of the fold will depend on the height of the patient's neck.)
2. Pull the ends forward over the patient's shoulders and fasten them with a safety pin in front.
3. Center one end of the blanket over each wrist, turning back a cuff as needed to expose the patient's hands, and pin the material so as to form sleeves.

Improvise a shawl that will serve as a bed jacket by folding a towel diagonally. Place the "V" at the back of the patient's neck and pull the ends forward over his shoulders. Fasten with a safety pin at the front.

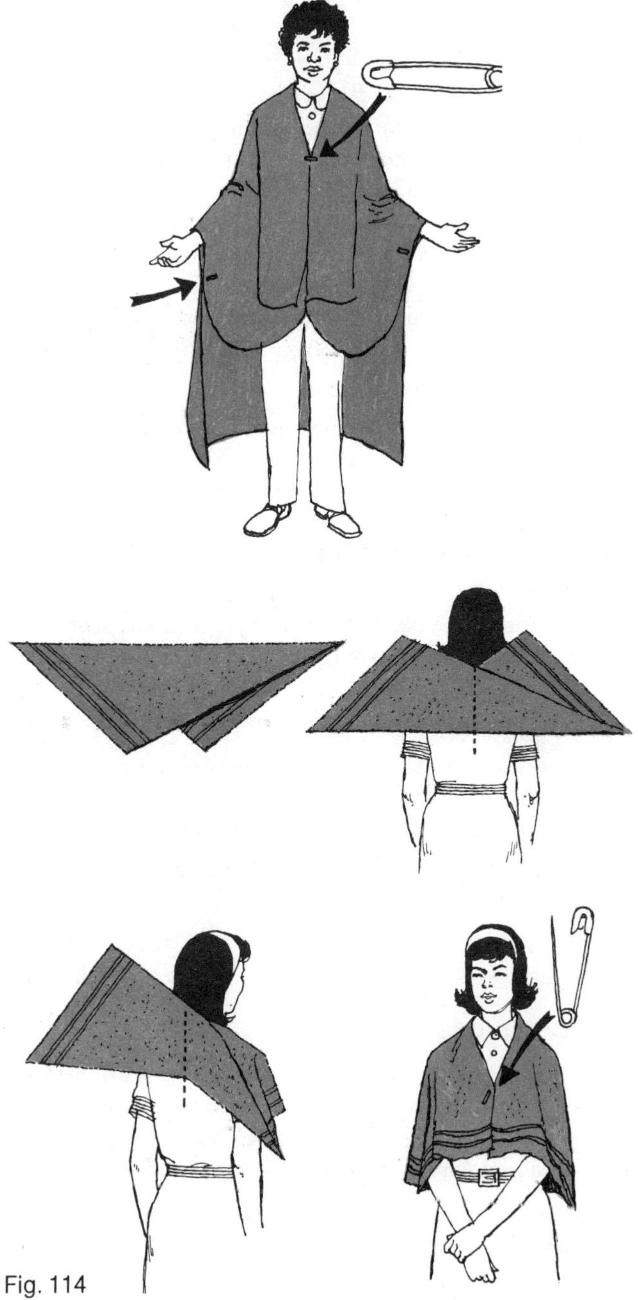

Fig. 114

EQUIPMENT FOR ELIMINATION

Bedpan

When the patient cannot get out of bed, it is necessary to provide a bedpan, a container for urine and bowel movements. It is generally better to borrow, rent, or buy a bedpan, since it is difficult to improvise one that will hold liquid and be sturdy enough for the patient. If a bedpan is not available, improvise one by using a shallow baking or dripping pan about 2 x 8 x 10 inches (5.1 x 20.3 x 25.4 centimeters) and a sturdy, flat cardboard box. Insert the pan into the cardboard box and cut an oval opening in the top surface of the box to form a seat. The pan can be removed from the box and emptied and cleaned after each use.

To make a cover for the bedpan, use an old pillowcase or fold several layers of newspaper to fit around the bedpan, and fasten them with a safety pin. A large grocery bag also serves well.

Male Urinals and Measuring Bottles

A urinal is a bottle-shaped container that is used primarily by male patients for urinating. A clear glass quart jar, a clean cardboard milk carton, or a clean plastic milk or bleach container may serve the purpose. If using a milk carton, cut off the top. If using a plastic container, cut the top back to enlarge the small opening.

Improvise a measure for urinary output by running a strip of tape or pasting a strip of paper up the outside of a clear bottle and marking ounces (milliliters) on it. Pour in two tablespoons of water and mark the level of 1 ounce (29.5 milliliters), then add two more tablespoons and mark 2 ounces (59.2 milliliters), etc.

Discard any homemade urinal or measuring bottle when it is no longer in use.

Bedside Commode

Sometimes the patient is allowed out of bed but is unable to get as far as the bathroom. Since it is always easier to have a bowel movement in the normal sitting-up position, a bedside commode—a form of chair with a removable basin or pail—may be needed.

A manufactured commode, either borrowed or rented, may be easier to keep clean and odor-free than a homemade one. When a manufactured one is not available, a commode can be improvised from items at home. Cut a hole in the seat of a sturdy wooden chair, pad and cover the seat with oilcloth, and place the chair over a large bucket or other wide-mouthed container. A piece of cloth can be tacked around the legs of the chair to prevent the bucket from being seen.

EQUIPMENT FOR SPECIAL TREATMENTS

Hot Water Bottle

There are many conditions for which the health professional recommends hot, dry treatments in order to stimulate circulation. When a hot water bottle is not available, a plastic milk container or other watertight container can be filled with warm water. Other substitutes for a hot water bottle might include a cloth bag containing heated sand, dry oatmeal that has been heated in the oven, or a heated flat stone or brick. Always test the temperature of the container to make sure the container will not burn the patient. Wrap a hot water bottle or any substitute well with a towel before placing it next to the patient.

Ice Bag

To prevent swelling in an affected area, the health professional may recommend ice bags for use, especially after a bad bruise or some dental treatments. Ice bags can be improvised by placing ice in a plastic bag that can be tightly sealed and wrapping the bag in a towel. Be careful to avoid getting the patient or the bedding wet from the melting ice. Ice may also be placed in a washcloth and held on small bruised areas.

Arm Sling

An injured arm, wrist, or hand may need to be elevated or held as immobile as possible. An arm sling to support an injured arm or hand can be made from a square of cloth 36 x 36 inches (91.4 x 91.4 centimeters). Fold the cloth diagonally to form a triangle. Place one of the most pointed corners over the patient's shoulder. Then place the injured arm over the cloth. Bring the other pointed corner over the opposite shoulder. Tie the two ends at the side of the neck. A knot can be tied in the corner at the elbow for additional support.

Steam Inhalator

Breathing in steam is often suggested for persons with hoarseness, sore throat, coughing, or difficulty in breathing. Warm, moist air has a soothing effect on the mucous membranes and tends to soften secretions. When a person is able to sit up, a steam inhalator can be improvised from a paper bag cut open at both ends and placed over a pitcher or container filled with steaming water. Place the filled pitcher or container in a basin on a sturdy table so that it cannot spill and burn the patient. Place the paper bag so that one open end is over the pitcher of water. Protect the patient's hair from the steam and be sure that the patient is warm enough. Have the patient sit comfortably near the steam, with his head at the top of the open bag so that the steam will rise to his face and be breathed in. Change the water as often as needed to provide steam for the suggested amount of time.

Incubator

Premature babies need a warm bed, called an incubator, because they do not have enough body heat. An incubator can be improvised from two cardboard boxes, one placed inside the other (see page 119). Pad the inside box for the baby and warm the incubator by placing bottles filled with hot water between the sides of the two boxes. Heated bricks or stones could be used if such bottles are not available. Refill the bottles or reheat the bricks or stones as often as necessary to maintain a constant temperature.

OTHER IMPROVISED EQUIPMENT

Baby-Bottle Brush

Baby bottles must be kept very clean. A bottle brush can be made by attaching clean rags to a stiff wire. Bend the wire slightly in order to better clean the sides and bottoms of the bottles.

Cotton Applicators

There are many uses in home nursing for cotton-tipped applicators, including moistening the lips with a glycerine and lemon juice mixture, or cleaning the mouth. Cotton-tipped applicators can be purchased in most drugstores and grocery stores at fairly low cost. When not available, they can be improvised from fresh absorbent cotton and blunt-ended wooden applicator sticks. Toothpicks may be used by cutting off the sharp ends. After thoroughly washing your hands, place the cotton, the wooden sticks, and a small glass of clean water on a clean towel. Dip the end of the stick in water and place the moist end into the center of a cotton ball. Roll the stick between the fingers of one hand, holding and shaping the cotton with the fingers of the other hand to bind it securely to the tip. Cover the end of the stick well for the patient's protection and safety. Store the applicators in a covered container with the cotton end down for cleanliness when handling.

Door Silencer

The loud noise of a door shutting is often disturbing to an ill person. A homemade door silencer can be placed over the latch, allowing the sickroom door to be closed quietly. To make a silencer, cut a strip of rubber about 3 x 10 inches (7.6 x 25.4 centimeters) from an old, leaky hot water bottle or use a strip of heavy cloth material. Cut slits in the ends to go over the doorknobs. Another method is to tie nylon stockings around the doorknobs and over the latch.

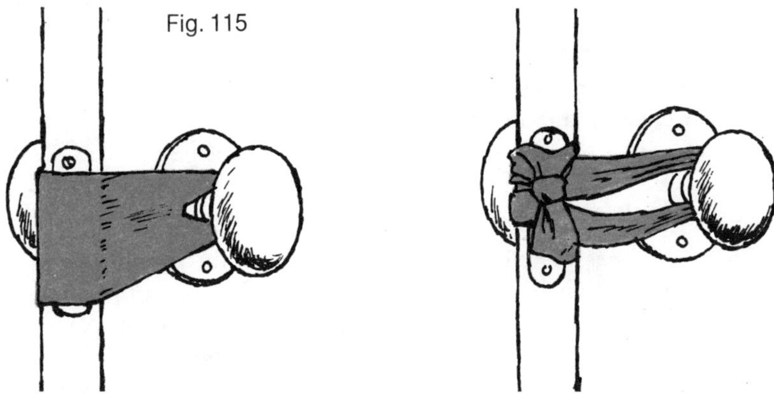

Fig. 115

Drinking Cup

There are times in emergencies, and especially in disasters, when an improvised drinking cup may be very useful. Use a piece of clean paper about 7 inches (17.8 centimeters) square and follow these steps (Fig. 116):

1. Fold the square of paper diagonally in half.
2. Place the paper with the folded edge parallel to the edge of the table.

Fig. 116

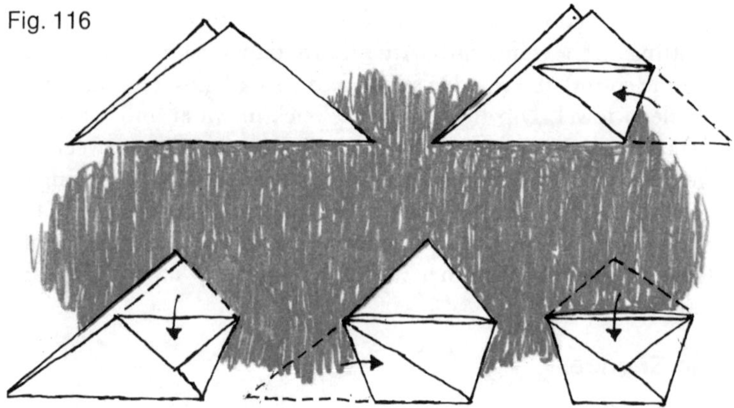

3. Fold the lower right-hand corner up toward the left until the point touches just beyond midway of the left-hand edge of the paper and make a crease.
4. Fold back the top flap of the upper corner to lock the sides and crease the edge to hold it in shape.
5. Turn the paper over from left to right. Fold the lower right-hand corner up to the left until the point touches the top corner of the left-hand edge of the paper and make a crease.
6. Fold the remaining upper corner toward the bottom to lock the side, creasing the edge to hold it in place.
7. Pick up the cup and press the sides to open it.

Face Mask

There are times when it is important to protect the patient in bed from the direct air breathed out by the home nurse and to protect the home nurse from the air breathed out by the patient. A face mask, often used for this purpose, can be improvised by using two rubber bands, two safety pins, and a paper towel. Fold the towel in thirds, then gather the ends and pin them through the rubber bands. Put the rubber bands around the ears and adjust them so that the paper towel covers the mouth and nose. A more durable mask can be made by pinning a large folded man's handkerchief in a similar manner through either rubber bands or elastic loops. Such a mask would need frequent washing to be effective.

Appendix

GLOSSARY

ABRASION—A scraping away of a portion of the skin.

ABSCESS—A localized collection of pus in any part of the body.

ACNE—A chronic inflammatory disease of the sebaceous glands and hair follicles of the skin, chiefly in adolescents. Marked by pimples, especially on the face.

ACUTE—Sharp, severe. Having rapid onset and severe symptoms and usually lasting a short period of time.

ADDICTION—State of dependence on a habit such as a drug habit.

ADOLESCENCE—The period of youth extending from puberty to maturity.

AFTERBIRTH—Placenta and membranes expelled after the birth of a child.

AIRWAY—A respiratory passage.

ALBUMIN—A protein substance found in nearly every animal or plant tissue and fluid.

ALCOHOLISM—Diseased condition due to acute or chronic excessive intake of alcoholic drinks.

ALLERGY—Hypersensitivity to a specific substance.

AMBULATORY CARE—All types of health services that are provided to persons who come to a location for care and leave the location on the same day.

ANALGESIA—A condition, usually induced by a drug, in which a patient remains conscious but is insensible to pain.

ANALGESIC—A drug that relieves pain.

ANEMIA—A condition of the blood characterized either by a reduction in the number of red cells or by a deficiency in the hemoglobin content of the cells or by both.

ANTIBODY—A substance in the body that provides immunity against substances that are foreign to the body.

ANTIDOTE—A substance that neutralizes poisons or their effects.

ANTITOXIN—An antibody capable of neutralizing a specific toxin.

ANUS—The opening to the rectum.

ANXIETY—A state of apprehension and fear, accompanied by restlessness and uncertainty.

APATHY—Indifference and dullness; being sluggish, without emotion.

APNEA—A temporary absence of breathing.

APOPLEXY—A stroke; a condition in which loss of muscular control, unconsciousness, paralysis, or death can result from the rupture of a blood vessel, causing hemorrhage in the brain or the clotting of a blood vessel in the brain.

APPETITE—Desire, natural craving, especially for food.

ARTERIOSCLEROSIS—Hardening of the arteries; a chronic disease, generally affecting middle-aged and older people, in which the walls of the arteries thicken, harden, and lose elasticity, thus preventing normal circulation of the blood.

ASPHYXIA—A lack of oxygen or excess of carbon dioxide in the body that is usually caused by interruption of breathing and that causes unconsciousness.

ASPIRATION—To withdraw fluid by suction.

AVULSION—The forcible separation or tearing of tissue from the body.

AXILLA—The armpit.

BACTERIA—A large group of typically one-celled microscopic organisms, found in air, water, soil, the bodies of living animals and plants, and dead organic matter, some of which cause disease.

BARBITURATES—Any of a group of chemical compounds produced from barbituric acid, used primarily as sedatives or to produce sleep, available legally only by a physician's prescription.

BIRTH CANAL—The cavity or canal of the pelvis through which the baby passes during labor (vagina).

BLADDER—The hollow organ of the body in which urine is stored.

BLAND DIET—Foods changed in texture, flavor, and method of preparation to reduce irritation to the digestive tract.

BLISTER—An elevation of the top layer of the skin, containing a clear, watery fluid.

BLOOD—The fluid that circulates through the heart, arteries, veins, and capillaries, carrying nourishment and oxygen to the tissues and taking away waste matter and carbon dioxide.

BLOOD CLOT—A thickened lump of blood.

BLOOD COUNT—A laboratory test in which the number of red and white blood cells within a measured sample of blood are counted and classified in order to gain information concerning a person's state of health.

BLOOD PRESSURE—The force exerted against the blood vessel walls (arteries) when the heart pumps.

BLOOD TYPE (GROUP)—Inherited patterns into which human blood may be divided for scientific or medical purposes. There are four major blood groups: A, B, AB, and O.

BODY MECHANICS—The coordinated use of the muscles, joints, ligaments, and related structures to produce motion and maintain equilibrium.

BOOSTER DOSE—The injection of a vaccine given at a suitable time following initial immunization, for the purpose of supporting and maintaining immunity.

CALORIE—A heat unit; the unit used to measure the amount of energy (heat) produced by food in the body.

CARIES—Cavity-producing decay in the teeth.

CARRIER—A normal person or one convalescing from an infectious disease who shows no signs or symptoms of the disease but who harbors and eliminates the microorganism and thus spreads the disease.

CATARACT—A diseased condition of the lens of the eye that prevents light from entering the eye and impairs vision.

CATHETER—A long, thin, flexible tube, made of rubber or other material, designed to be inserted into a body passage for the purpose of withdrawing fluid, usually urine, from a body cavity.

CERVIX—The neck or opening of the uterus.

CHILL—A sensation of cold accompanied by shivering; frequently the initial symptom of acute infection. Results from constriction of the blood vessels of the skin and is accompanied by a rise of body temperature.

CHOLESTEROL—An organic compound found in all animal fats; particularly present in bile, brain tissue, the adrenal glands, and the blood and in such foods as egg yolks, liver, milk, and some seeds and considered to be a strong contributing factor to hardening of the arteries.

CHRONIC—Lasting a long time, long drawn-out, as a chronic disease or illness (not acute).

CILIA—Tiny, hair-like structures that grow on the surface of certain cells, capable of vibratory or sweeping movements.

CIRCULATORY SYSTEM—The heart, arteries, veins, and capillaries through which the blood circulates throughout the body.

CLINICAL THERMOMETER—A thermometer used to measure the body temperature.

COLOSTRUM—The first milk from the mother's breasts after the birth of the child. It is laxative and assists in the expulsion by the newborn of the meconium (the first fecal discharge of the newborn).

COMMODE—A toilet chair with a removable waste basin, for use by the bedside.

COMMUNICABLE DISEASE—A disease that may be transmitted directly or indirectly from one individual to another.

CONCEPTION—The union of the male sperm and the ovum of the female; fertilization.

CONCUSSION—A common result of a blow to the head, or a fall on the end of the spine with transmitted force, usually causing unconsciousness, either temporary or prolonged.

CONSTIPATION—A sluggish action of the bowels.

CONTAMINATION—The presence of an infectious agent on a body surface or on or in an inanimate article or substance.

CONTRACTION (IN LABOR)—The shortening of the muscle fibers of the uterus during labor, commonly known as labor pains.

CONTRACTURE DEFORMITY—Shortening, as of muscle or scar tissue, producing distortion or deformity.

CONVALESCENCE—The restoration of health after disease; the time spent in recovery from illness.

CONVULSION—An involuntary, usually violent, general contraction or spasm of the muscles.

COPE—To struggle or deal with, successfully, certain situations of life.

CROUP—An inflammation of the respiratory passages in children, characterized by a harsh, brassy cough and raspy, difficult breathing.

CYANOSIS—A bluish tinge in the color of mucous membranes and skin, caused by lack of oxygen in the blood.

DAY-CARE CENTER—A place where persons may receive supervision during the day, with the noon meal and other activities provided. There are child day-care centers and centers for older adults and other special groups.

DECUBITUS ULCER—A bedsore; an ulceration caused by long periods of pressure on a part of the body, causing poor circulation, generally occurring in those confined to bed for long periods of time.

DEFECATION—Emptying of the bowels.

DEGENERATIVE—Having to do with the gradual deterioration and loss of function of an organ, tissues, or other body structures. Hardening of the arteries is an example of a degenerative disease.

DEHYDRATE—To deprive of water or to lose or become free of water.

DENTURE (ARTIFICIAL)—Artificial teeth of an individual, considered as a unit-complete artificial replacement of either the upper or the lower teeth.

DEPRESSANT—A drug that acts on the central nervous system, lowering the level of body activity and producing relaxation and sleep.

DEPRESSION—An emotional state of dejection, characterized by anxiety, discouragement, and a feeling of inadequacy.

DIAGNOSIS—The art or the act of determining the nature of a disease; the decision reached.

DIAGNOSTIC—A word applied to tests and other procedures that are done to help identify or diagnose diseases or other conditions.

DIALYSIS—Separation of substances in solution by passing them through a porous membrane; done naturally by the kidney and mechanically by an artificial kidney.

DIARRHEA—A common symptom of gastrointestinal disease, characterized by increased frequency and more or less fluid consistency of the stools.

DIASTOLIC—Having to do with blood pressure: the pressure in the arteries when the heart is relaxed and refilling for the next pumping action (the last sound heard when taking a blood pressure).

DIET, LIQUID—Foods in liquid form, or that have been liquefied to make them smooth in texture and easy to swallow and digest.

DIET, REGULAR—The full, well-balanced diet, without restrictions.

DIET, SOFT—Consisting of easily consumed, easily digested foods, modified to leave little residue in the digestive tract.

DILATE—To become or make larger or wider.

DISASTER—A situation, usually catastrophic in nature, in which numbers of persons are plunged into helplessness and suffering and who, as a result, may be in need of food, clothing, shelter, medical and nursing care, and other basic necessities.

DISORIENTED—Mentally confused; the loss of the ability to locate one's position in the environment.

DIVERTICULITIS—Inflammation of diverticuli—small blind pouches that form in the lining and wall of the colon.

DOUCHE—A jet or stream of water applied on or into any part of the body (for example, vaginal douche).
DYSPNEA—Difficult or labored breathing.
DYSURIA—Difficult or painful urination.

EDEMA—Dropsy; excessive accumulation of fluid in the tissue spaces.
ELIMINATION—The act or process of ridding the body of waste material.
ENEMA—The introduction of fluid into the rectum to promote removal of feces, or for providing nutrients or medicines.
EPIDEMIC—Unusual prevalence of a disease, ordinarily affecting large numbers of people or spreading over a wide area.
EPISIOTOMY—Surgery performed on the vulva or opening of the vagina to prevent tearing as the newborn emerges from the stretched vagina.
ERUPTION—Lesions on the skin, especially those of such diseases as measles or scarlet fever; a rash.
EUPHORIA—An exaggerated feeling of joy and well-being, induced by certain drugs.
EVACUATE—To expel waste materials from the body, particularly from the bowels; to have a bowel movement.
EXPIRATION—The act of breathing forth or expelling air from the lungs.

FALLOUT—The falling to earth of radioactive particles following a nuclear explosion.
FAT-SOLUBLE—Soluble, or capable of being dissolved, in fats.
FECAL IMPACTION—A hard, firm mass of stool lodged in the intestine, usually in or near the rectum. Occurs in constipation and bowel obstruction when the feces are not eliminated by normal bowel movement.
FECES—Body wastes discharged from the intestine; also called stool.
FEE FOR SERVICE—A method of charging whereby a physician, dentist, nurse, or other practitioner gives a bill or charges for each service provided (the usual method of billing patients by health professionals).
FEVER—Elevation of the body temperature above the normal.
FIRST AID—Emergency treatment given before regular medical care can be obtained in cases of accident, injury, or illness.
FLEX—To bend or move a muscle so that it contracts.

FLUORIDE—A chemical compound used as an additive to water or applied by a dentist to the teeth to reduce tooth decay.

FONTANELS—The "soft" membrane areas in the skull of the newborn that have not yet turned to bone.

FOREIGN BODY—A substance occurring in any part of the body where it is not normally found and usually introduced from without; for example, a cinder in the eye.

FORESKIN—A fold of skin that covers the end of the penis.

FRACTURE—The breaking of a bone or of cartilage.

FRIENDLY VISITOR—Usually a volunteer who visits persons in their homes or in nursing homes with the main purpose of showing interest or concern or being helpful.

FULL-TERM INFANT—An infant born at the end of the tenth lunar month of pregnancy. Not born prematurely.

FUNGI—A simple plant organism that causes an infection, such as athlete's foot.

GAMMA GLOBULIN—The part (fraction) of human blood plasma that contains disease-fighting antibodies.

GENITAL—Pertaining to the reproductive organs.

GENITALIA—The external reproductive organs; in the male, the testicles, scrotum, and penis; in the female, the labia, clitoris, the mons pubis, and the vaginal opening.

GERIATRICS—The branch of medicine dealing with diseases and problems of the aging.

GLAUCOMA—A disease of the eye that may include pain and/or blindness; usually includes an increase in inner-eye pressure.

GROUP PRACTICE—A formal association of three or more physicians or other health professionals with income from their practice pooled and redistributed to the members of the group according to some prearranged plan. (May include the same or different health or medical specialists.)

HALLUCINATION—A false sense perception; perception of objects that have no reality and of sensations that have no external cause.

HALLUCINOGENS—Drugs that have no known medical use (such as mescaline and LSD), which produce mood changes and distortion in time, space, and distance and increase the sharpness of the senses and can result in delusions, hallucinations, panic, and profound depression.

HEALTH PROFESSIONAL—A term used in this text to mean dentist, nurse, pharmacist, or physician. This term is used rather than the specific specialist title because of the rapid changes in roles and scope of authority.

HEMIPLEGIA—Paralysis of one side of the body.

HEMOGLOBIN—The red coloring matter of the red blood corpuscles, which carry oxygen from the lungs to the tissues and carbon dioxide from the tissues to the lungs.

HEMORRHAGE—Abnormal discharge of blood from the vessels, either external or internal.

HEMORRHOIDS (PILES)—Swellings of the blood vessels near the anus. Often painful.

HEREDITY—The inborn capacity of the organism to develop ancestral characteristics; the transmission from parent to child of certain characteristics, such as color of eyes and hair, bony structure, or facial resemblance.

HOME HEALTH AGENCY—An agency that provides health care in the home. To be certified under Medicare, an agency must provide skilled nursing service and at least one additional service such as physical therapy, speech therapy or occupational therapy, medical social services, or home health aide services in the home.

HOME HEALTH CARE—Health services given to an individual as needed in the home. Such services are provided to aged, disabled, or sick or convalescent individuals who do not need institutional care. Services may be provided by a visiting nurse association (VNA), home health agency, hospital, or other organized community group.

HORMONE—A chemical substance originating in an organ, gland, or in certain cells of an organ, transported by the blood or other body fluids and having a specific regulatory effect upon cells remote from its origin.

HOST—The organic body upon or in which parasites live.

HYPERTENSION—High blood pressure.

HYPODERMIC—Placed or introduced beneath the skin; the term used for a needle or syringe that introduces an injection under the skin.

IMMOBILITY—A condition in which a part of the body cannot move, either temporarily or permanently.

IMMUNITY, ACTIVE—That immunity possessed by an organism as the result of disease or of unrecognized infection or that is induced by immunization with bacteria or products of bacterial growth.

IMMUNITY, PASSIVE—Produced by actual injection of sera containing antibodies into a person to be protected.

IMMUNIZATION—The act or process of giving an individual protection against a specific disease through vaccination or inoculation.

INCISION—A cut made with a knife, especially for surgical purposes.

INCONTINENCE—Involuntary or uncontrolled evacuation of urine or feces.

INCUBATOR—Equipment in which temperature and humidity can be controlled properly for premature or other infants.

INFECTION—The communication of disease from one subject to another—a condition resulting from an infective substance.

INFLAMMATION—The reaction of the tissues to injury or infection, characterized clinically by local heat, swelling, redness, and pain.

INGESTION—The act of taking substances, especially food, into the body.

INHALANT—A gaseous substance that is or may be taken into the body by way of the nose or trachea (through the respiratory system).

INHALATION—The breathing in of air or other vapor.

INSPIRATION—The drawing in of the breath; inhalation.

INTENSIVE CARE—The special, round-the-clock care of a gravely ill patient, including careful watch of a patient's vital life signs, in a room that is set aside for this purpose and that contains sophisticated life-support equipment.

INTESTINAL TRACT—A membranous tube extending from the lower end of the stomach to the anus, including the small and large intestine.

ISOLATION—The confining of an individual with a contagious disease to a separate area to prevent the disease from spreading.

JAUNDICE—Yellowing of the white areas of the eyes or the skin and/or other tissues; caused by an excessive amount of bile pigment in the blood; a symptom, not a disease.

LABIA—The female external genital organs surrounding the vulva entrance.

LABOR—A three-stage process: the first stage lasts from onset until the cervix has thinned out (effaced) and dilated (opened) to 4 inches (10 centimeters); the second stage ends in the delivery of the baby; and the third stage ends with the expelling of the placenta and membranes (afterbirth).

LACERATION—A wound or an irregular tear of the flesh.

LACTATION—The function of secreting milk.

LARYNGITIS—Inflammation of the larynx.

LARYNX—The organ of the voice, situated between the trachea and the base of the tongue.

LAXATIVE—An agent that loosens the bowels; a mild purgative.

LAYETTE—A full outfit of garments, bedding, etc., for a newborn child.

LIFE-STYLES—Specific habits of a person that become regular and frequent, such as smoking, exercise, eating, drinking of alcoholic beverages, or religious observances.

LINEA NIGRA—A dark, pigmented line extending upward along the middle of the abdomen; found frequently in pregnant woman.

LOCHIA—A discharge from the birth canal, which occurs after childbirth.

LONG-TERM ILLNESS—Illness that is long continued or of long duration; as opposed to acute illness.

MALAISE—A general feeling of illness, sometimes accompanied by restlessness and discomfort.

MALNUTRITION—Insufficient nourishment of the body caused by a poor or unbalanced diet or the inability of the body to absorb or utilize the food ingested.

MAMMOGRAPHY—The use of X-rays in the study of the breasts.

MEALS ON WHEELS—A service of one complete hot meal and sometimes a snack, provided to eligible persons in their homes. A valuable service, especially for older persons, offered by church and other voluntary community groups such as the American Red Cross.

MECONIUM—A dark green mucus material in the intestine of the full-term fetus.

MEDICAL SOCIETY (LOCAL)—The American Medical Association includes state and local medical associations, of which most practicing physicians are members. Local associations are often referred to as the "medical society."

MENSTRUATION—A periodic discharge of blood and tissue from the uterus, occurring about every 28 days during the period of a woman's life from puberty to menopause.

METABOLISM—The sum of the chemical changes that go on in the body as food is made into body tissues, energy is produced, and bony tissue is broken down.

MICROORGANISM—An animal or plant, especially bacteria, that is so small it cannot be seen without a microscope.

MOBILITY—Having the ability to move a part of the body.

MORNING SICKNESS—Nausea and vomiting occurring sometimes during the early months of pregnancy.

MOTTLED SKIN—Spots or blotches of different colors or shades of color.

MUCOUS MEMBRANE—A mucus-secreting membrane lining body cavities (such as the mouth and throat) that connects with the external air.

MUCUS—The viscid liquid secreted by mucous glands. It consists of water, mucin, and inorganic salts, with epithelial cells, leukocytes, etc., held in suspension.

NARCOTIC—A drug that produces stupor, complete insensibility, or sleep. There are three main groups: the opium group, which produces sleep; the belladonna group, which produces illusions and delirium; and the alcohol group, which produces exhilaration and sleep.

NAUSEA—A feeling of discomfort in the region of the stomach, with aversion to food and a tendency to vomit.

NEBULIZER—A device that creates a fine spray.

NOCTURNAL EMISSIONS—Loss of fluid from the penis at night by boys; may contain spermatic fluid (contains reproductive cells) from the testes. Also called wet dreams.

NONPROFIT OR NOT-FOR-PROFIT AGENCY—An agency, usually a voluntary agency, that may receive funds from fees and other services but must not make a profit.

NOSTRIL—One of the external openings of the nose.

NUTRIENT—A nourishing food that helps to build and repair body tissue, provide heat and energy, and regulate the body processes; generally classified as proteins, carbohydrates, fats, minerals, and vitamins.

NUTRITION—The sum of the processes concerned in the growth, maintenance, and repair of the living body as a whole, or of its constituent parts as related to the consumption and utilization of food.

NUTRITIONIST—A professionally trained person who applies the science of nutrition and related subjects in research, teaching, or advisory services.

OBSESSION—An idea or an emotion that persists in an individual's mind in spite of any conscious attempts to remove it; an imperative idea, as in psychoneurosis.

ORGANIC—Relating to or coming from living organisms (as contrasted to coming from plants).

OVUM—The female reproductive germ cell; egg.

OXIDATION—Occurs when a substance combines with oxygen or loses hydrogen (burns or rusts).

PACIFIER—A device, usually nipple-shaped, used to satisfy an infant's need to suck.

PAIN THRESHOLD—The lower limit of pain capable of producing an impression upon consciousness or of arousing a response.

PALLOR—Paleness, especially of the skin and mucous membranes.

PALPATE—To examine by feeling or touching.

PARAPLEGIC—A person having the lower half of the body paralyzed.

PEDICULOSIS—A condition in which the body or the hair is infested with lice.

PENDULOUS—Drooping, hanging down.

PERINEUM—The region between the anus and the vulva in the female and between the anus and the scrotum in the male.

PERIPHERAL—The outer part or a surface of a body.

PERISTALSIS—A progressive, wavelike motion of the walls of the intestines, consisting of alternate muscular contractions and dilations that move the contents of the intestine toward the rectum.

PHENYLKETONURIA (PKU)—A liver enzyme deficiency found in the newborn.

PHYSICIAN ASSISTANT (PA)—A specially trained individual who performs tasks that might otherwise be performed by physicians themselves, under the direction of a supervising physician.

PICA—A desire for strange foods; a craving to eat strange articles, such as hair, dirt, or sand.

PLACENTA—A spongy structure that grows on the wall of the uterus to which the embryo is attached by means of the umbilical cord and through which it receives its nourishment.

PLASMA—The fluid portion of the blood in which the red cells, the white cells, and the platelets are suspended.

POISON—Any substance that when taken into the body will produce an injurious or deadly effect.

POSTMORTUM—After death.

POSTPARTUM—Taking place after childbirth; usually applies to 6 to 8 weeks after delivery (parturition).

POSTURE—Position or bearing of the body when the individual is standing, at rest, or in movement.

PREGNANCY—Being with child; the state of the woman from conception to childbirth.

PREMATURE INFANT—An infant born before the thirty-seventh to thirty-eighth week of gestation or weighing less than 5 pounds (2.27 kilograms) at birth.

PRENATAL—Existing or occurring before birth.

PRESCRIBED MEDICINE—A medicine ordered by a legally authorized health professional—a physician, a dentist, or a nurse (when it is legal for the nurse to do so).

PRESSURE SORES—See *Decubitus ulcer.*

PRIMARY HEALTH CARE PROVIDER—The health professional who serves as the person's first contact with the health care system and who assumes ongoing responsibility for the person's level of wellness in health and in illness. May be a nurse practitioner or a physician.

PROPRIETARY HEALTH AGENCY—A health care agency owned and operated for the purpose of making a profit.

PSYCHOSIS—Disturbances of such severeness that there is personality disintegration and loss of contact with reality.

PUBERTY—The period at which the organs of the body become capable of the function of reproduction.

PUBLIC HEALTH—The science and art of preventing disease, prolonging life, and promoting mental and physical health.

PULSE—The throbbing of blood vessels caused by contractions of the heart muscle as blood is forced through the arteries.

PUNCTURE WOUND—A wound produced by pricking or by a piercing instrument, weapon, or missile.

QUACK—One who pretends to have medical skills.

RABIES—An acute infectious disease of animals caused by a filtrable virus transmitted to other animals and man by the bite of an infected animal.

RADIATION, NUCLEAR—Radiant energy in the form of alpha and beta particles, gamma rays, and neutrons released by nuclear fission and atomic weapons detonations.

RADIOACTIVE—Having to do with radiation; capable of releasing radiant energy.

RANGE OF MOTION—The physical limits of the movement of the joints.

RASH—A lay term used for nearly any skin eruption, usually for acute inflammatory diseases of the skin. See *Eruption.*

RECTUM—The lower part of the large intestine opening through the anus.

REHABILITATION—The restoring of a person to optimum health.

RESISTANCE, ACQUIRED—The resistance to disease developed by frequent exposure to disease germs or by exposure to small numbers of germs over a long period of time.

RESPIRATION—The act of breathing with the lungs; taking of air into, and its expulsion from, the lungs.

RIB CAGE—The 12 pairs of long, flat, curved bones forming the semirigid wall of the chest.

ROUGHAGE—Foods rich in cellulose that contain relatively large amounts of residue, such as cereals, unpared fruits, and most vegetables.

SALIVA—The mixed secretions of the parotid, submaxillary, sublingual, and other glands of the mouth, whose functions are to moisten and lubricate the food, to dissolve certain substances, to facilitate tasting, to aid in swallowing, and to digest starches.

SEBACEOUS GLANDS—Glands in the skin that secrete oil (sebum).

SELF-MEDICATION—The administration of medication to oneself without advice or a prescription from a health professional.

SHOCK—Disruption of the circulation, which may upset all body functions.

SKILLED NURSING CARE—Refers to a government regulation that requires 24-hour nursing service and at least one registered professional nurse employed full time by the agency.

SPASM—A sudden muscular contraction.

SPERM—The male reproductive cell.

SPUTUM—Material discharged from the surface of the air passages, throat, or mouth and removed chiefly by spitting.

STERILE—Aseptic; free from living microorganisms.

STERNUM—The flat, narrow bone in the median line in the front of the chest.

STIMULANTS—Drugs, such as amphetamines, that affect the central nervous system and produce a general increase in bodily activity and that, when abused, are characterized by restlessness, confusion, irritability, aggressive behavior, etc.

STOOL—See *Feces*.

STRESS—Any condition or situation that causes strain or tension; may be physical or psychological.

STUPOR—The condition of being but partly conscious; lethargy; insensibility.

SUCROSE—Sugar found in such plants as sugar cane and sugar beets and processed for use as table sugar, unlike fructose, which is the natural sugar found in fruits such as oranges or apples.

SUPINE—Lying on the back, face upward.

SUPPOSITORY—A cone-shaped, solid medicated substance for introduction into the rectum, urethra, or vagina.

SUSCEPTIBLE—Having neither natural nor acquired immunity to a disease and for that reason being liable to contract it if exposed to it.

SYMPTOM—One of the evidences of disease that serves as an aid in diagnosis. It may be evident to others (objective) or only to the patient (subjective).

SYSTOLIC—Having to do with the blood pressure when the arterial pressure is at its maximum, the heart is contracting, and the blood is being driven into the arteries and lungs (the first sound heard when taking a blood pressure).

TENSION—See *Anxiety*.

THERAPY—Any treatment or procedure that deals with the process of healing or curing a physical disease or mental disorder.

TOXIC—Poisonous; having to do with, or caused by, poison.

TOXIN—A poisonous product of animal or vegetable cells that, on injection into animals or man, causes the formation of antibodies, called antitoxins.

TOXOID—A product formed by the treatment of toxin with physical or chemical agents. A toxoid is nontoxic but maintains the antigenic (antibody-producing) properties of the toxin. Toxoids are used for immunizations.

TRANSPLANT—Surgical technique for removing an organ from one person's body and attaching it in another person's body (for example, kidney transplant).

TRAPEZE—A short bar held by two ropes.

TRAUMA—A wound or injury. In psychiatry, an emotional shock leaving a deep psychologic impression.

TRIGLYCERIDE—A neutral fat combined from carbohydrates for storage in animal fat cells.

TRIMESTER—A period of 3 months' duration (during pregnancy).

UMBILICAL CORD—The cord that connects the baby to the placenta. It contains veins and arteries through which the fetus is nourished and through which waste products are carried away.

URINAL—A container for receiving urine.

URINALYSIS—Analysis or examination of the urine.

URINATE—To discharge urine from the bladder.

URINE—The fluid excreted by the kidneys.

UTERUS—The womb; the organ that receives and holds the fertilized ovum during the development of the fetus and that becomes the main force in its expulsion during delivery.

UVULA—The small flap of fleshy tissue that hangs down in the center and back from the roof or soft palate of the mouth.

VAGINA—The canal leading from the vulva to the uterus.

VARICOSE VEINS—Veins that are abnormally swollen, knotted or twisted, and painful, usually found in the legs or thighs. (May accompany pregnancy.)

VISITING NURSE ASSOCIATION (VNA) OR VISITING NURSE SERVICE—A voluntary, not-for-profit, health agency that provides nursing services in the home, including health supervision, education and counseling, and bedside care.

VITAL SIGNS—Signs, such as body temperature, pulse, respiration, and blood pressure, that are essential to life.

VITAL STATISTICS—Facts related to births, deaths, marriages, health, and disease.

VOID—To empty the contents of, for example, the bladder or bowels. (Usually refers to emptying the bladder.)

VOLUNTARY HEALTH AGENCY—Any nonprofit, nongovernmental agency, governed by lay and/or professional individuals, whose primary purpose is health-related. The term usually refers to agencies supported primarily by voluntary contributions from the public.

VOLUNTEER—One who offers his service freely, without salary or wages.

VOMITUS—Vomited matter.

WEANING—Having to do with the process of accustoming an infant to food other than mother's milk or the bottle.

WELFARE DEPARTMENTS—A unit of local or state government that is concerned with the basic essentials of life (for example, food, clothing, housing, or social necessities).

WELLNESS—A condition of functioning of the whole person (body, mind, and spirit) in relation to a specific environment. High-level wellness exists when the person functions at his very best capacity in a specific environment.

WOUND—An injury to the body in which the tissue is damaged.

PROFESSIONAL AND OTHER HEALTH AND WELFARE ORGANIZATIONS

American College of Nurse-Midwives, Suite 1210, 1000 Vermont Ave., N.W., Washington, DC 20005

American Dental Association, 211 East Chicago Ave., Chicago, IL 60611

American Dietetic Association, 430 North Michigan Ave., Chicago, IL 60611

American Geriatrics Society, 10 Columbus Circle, New York, NY 10019

American Home Economics Association, 2010 Massachusetts Ave., N.W., Washington, DC 20036

American Hospital Association, 840 North Lake Shore Drive, Chicago, IL 60611

American Medical Association, 535 North Dearborn St., Chicago, IL 60611

American Nurses' Association, 2420 Pershing Road, Kansas City, MO 64108

American Occupational Therapy Association, 6000 Executive Blvd., Suite 200, Rockville, MD 20852

American Optometric Association, 243 North Lindbergh Blvd., St. Louis, MO 63141

American Pharmaceutical Association, 2215 Constitution Ave., N.W., Washington, DC 20037

American Physical Therapy Association, 1156 15th St., N.W., Washington, DC 20005

American Podiatry Association, 20 Chevy Chase Circle, N.W., Washington, DC 20015

American Psychological Association, 1200 17th St., N.W., Washington, DC 20036

American Public Health Association, 1015 18th St., N.W., Washington, DC 20036

American Society of Childbirth Educators, Inc., 7113 Lynwood Dr., P.O. Box 16159, Tampa, FL 33687

Child Study Association of America, 50 Madison Ave., New York, NY 10010

Child Welfare League of America, 67 Irving Place, New York, NY 10003

Family Service Association of America, 44 East 23rd St., New York, NY 10010

International Childbirth Education Association, 11040 West Blue Mound Rd., Milwaukee, WI 53226

Maternity Center Association, 48 East 92nd St., New York, NY 10028

National Association for Practical Nurse Education and Service, 122 East 42nd St., New York, NY 10010

National Conference of Catholic Charities, 1346 Connecticut Ave., N.W., Washington, DC 20036

National Council for Homemaker–Home Health Aides Service, Inc., 67 Irving Place, New York, NY 10003

National Education Association, 1201 16th St., N.W., Washington, DC 20036

National Federation of Licensed Practical Nurses, 888 Seventh Ave., New York, NY 10019

National Health Council, Inc., 1740 Broadway, New York, NY 10019

National League for Nursing, 10 Columbus Circle, New York, NY 10019

Sex Information and Education Council for the U.S., 122 East 42nd St., New York, NY 10017

VOLUNTARY HEALTH AND WELFARE ORGANIZATIONS

Alcoholics Anonymous, General Service Board of, 468 Park Ave. S., New York, NY 10016

Allergy Foundations of America, 801 Second Ave., New York, NY 10017

American Association for Maternal and Child Health, P.O. Box 965, Los Altos, CA 94022

American Association for Rehabilitation Therapy, P.O. Box 83, North Little Rock, AR 72116

American Cancer Society, 219 East 42nd Steet, New York, NY 10017

American Diabetes Association, 1 West 48th St., New York, NY 10020

American Foundation for the Blind, 15 West 16th St., New York, NY 10019

American Health Care Association, 1200 15th St., N.W., Washington, DC 20005

American Heart Association, 7320 Greenville Ave., Dallas, TX 75231

American Kidney Fund, P.O. Box 975, Washington, DC 20044

American Lung Association, 1740 Broadway, New York, NY 10019

American Red Cross, 17th and D Sts., N.W., Washington, DC 20006

American Social Health Association, 260 Sheridan Ave., Suite 307, Palo Alto, CA 94306

American Venereal Disease Association, 401 Colley Ave., Norfolk, VA 23507

Arthritis Foundation (Rheumatic Diseases), 3400 Peachtree Rd., N.E., Atlanta, GA 30326

Continental Association of Funeral and Memorial Societies, 1828 L St., N.W., Washington, DC 20036

Cooperative for American Relief Everywhere (CARE), 660 First Ave., New York, NY 10016

Cystic Fibrosis Foundation, 3379 Peachtree Road, N.E., Atlanta, GA 30326

Division for the Blind and Physically Handicapped, Library of Congress, Taylor St., Washington, DC 20542

Epilepsy Foundation of America, 1828 L Street, N.W., Washington, DC 20036

Euthanasia Education Council, 250 West 57th St., New York, NY 10019

Group Health Association of America, 1717 Massachusetts Ave., N.W., Washington, DC 20036

La Leche League International, 9616 Minneapolis, Franklin Park, IL 60131

Leukemia Society of America, 211 East 43rd St., New York, NY 10017

Living Bank, P.O. Box 6725, Houston, TX 77005

Medic-Alert Foundation International, 1000 N. Palm St., Turlock, CA 95380

Medic-Alert Organ Donor Program, 1000 N. Palm St., Turlock, CA 95380

Muscular Dystrophy Associations of America, 810 Seventh Ave., New York, NY 10019

Myasthenia Gravis Foundation, 230 Park Ave., New York, NY 10019

National Action for Foster Children, 2047 Locust St., Philadelphia, PA 19103

National Association for Hearing and Speech Action, 814 Thayer Ave., Silver Spring, MD 20910

National Association for Retarded Citizens, 2709 Avenue E, East, Arlington, TX 76011

National Center for Voluntary Action, 1214 16th St., N.W., Washington, DC 20036

National Committee, Arts for the Handicapped, 1701 K St., N.W., Suite 801, Washington, DC 20006

National Easter Seal Society for Crippled Children and Adults, 2023 West Ogden Ave., Chicago, IL 60612

National Foster Parent Association, Suite 114, 20 South Central, St. Louis, MO 63105

National Foundation–March of Dimes, Box 1275, White Plains, NY 10605

National Hemophilia Foundation, 25 West 39th St., New York, NY 10018

National Hospice Organization, 765 Prospect St., New Haven, CT 06511

National Kidney Foundation, 116 East 27th St., New York, NY 10016

National Multiple Sclerosis Society, 205 East 42nd St., New York, NY

National Paraplegia Foundation, 333 North Michigan Ave., Chicago, IL 60601

National Retired Teachers Association, 1909 K St., N.W., Washington, DC 20049

National Safety Council, 444 North Michigan Ave., Chicago, IL 60611

National Society for Prevention of Blindness, 79 Madison Ave., New York, NY 10016

National Sudden Infant Death Syndrome Foundation, 310 South Michigan Ave., Chicago, IL 60604

National Tay-Sachs and Allied Disease Association, 122 East 42nd St., New York, NY 10017

National Urban League, 500 East 62nd St., New York, NY 10021

Pan American Health Organization, 23rd St., N.W., Washington, DC 20037

Parents Anonymous, 2280 Hawthorne Blvd., Suite 8, Torrance, CA 90505

Parkinson's Disease Foundation, William Black Medical Research Bldg., Columbia Presbyterian Medical Center, West 168th St., New York, NY 10032

Planned Parenthood World Population, 810 Seventh Avenue, New York, NY 10019

Recovery (Psychotherapy), 116 South Michigan Ave., Chicago, IL 60603

Salvation Army, 120 West 14th St., New York, NY 10011

Smithsonian Institution Programs for the Handicapped, National Air and Space Museum, Room 3566, Washington, DC 20560

Stroke Club of America, 805 12th St., Galveston, TX 77550

United Cerebral Palsy Association, 66 East 34th St., New York, NY 10016

World Health Organization (U.S. Committee for the World Health Organization–USC-WHO), 777 United Nations Plaza, New York, NY 10017

HEALTH PROFESSIONALS

(Resource: *Health Manpower and Health Facilities.* U.S. Department of Health, Education, and Welfare; Public Health Service; Health Resources Administration; National Center for Health Statistics; Rockville, MD; 1974.)

Category	Requirements and/or Brief Description of Professional Practice
Dentistry and Allied Service	
Dentist (D.D.S. or D.M.D.)	Graduating from an accredited school of dentistry and passing the state board examination for licensure are requirements to practice. Graduates of foreign dental schools are eligible as candidates for licensure examination in 15 states. Many states require written and clinical skill examinations, and some states require continuing education for relicensure and for continuing to practice. Concentration of practice: prevention, early diagnosis, and treatment of oral and dental diseases, treatment of injuries to the teeth and related structures; education of the public in proper oral hygiene and dietary counseling and early detection of systemic diseases having oral manifestations. Specialization in dentistry requires an additional 2 years of advanced study beyond the D.D.S. or D.M.D. degree in the specialty area. Specialists must limit their practice to the areas in which they announce. Certification for dental specialists is by specialty boards recognized by the American Dental Association.
Dental Specialists	
Endodontist	Treats diseases and injuries of the nerve (pulp) and root ends of teeth.
Oral surgeon	Treats injuries and defects of the mouth, teeth, gums, and face by surgery.

Category	Requirements and/or Brief Description of Professional Practice
Orthodontist	Treats all forms of malocclusion (improper coming together of teeth) and conditions of the surrounding structures.
Pedodontist	Provides dental care primarily for children.
Periodontist	Treats the tissues or gums supporting the teeth and the underlying bones.
Prosthodontist	Treats by the restoration of natural teeth and/or the replacement of missing teeth and surrounding tissues with artificial substitutes.
Public health dentist	Works toward prevention and control of dental diseases and promotion of dental health through organized community efforts.
Dental Auxiliaries	
Dental assistant	The basic requirement for a dental assistant is a high school diploma. Many dental assistants are trained on the job, and some attend an accredited dental assistant education program. Certification of dental assistants is by the Certifying Board of the American Dental Assistants Association. Assists the dentist with procedures in the office and at the dental chair; provides oral instruction.
Dental hygienist	Graduating from an accredited dental hygiene program and passing the state board examination for licensure are requirements to practice. Some states require continuing education for relicensure and to continue to practice. The dental hygienist works as a member of the dental health team, prepares diagnostic data, removes stains and deposits, applies decay-preventing agents, and promotes sound oral health habits.

Category	Requirements and/or Brief Description of Professional Practice
Medicine	
Medical Doctor (M.D.)	Graduating from an accredited medical school and passing the state board examination for licensure are requirements to practice. In more than half the states, completion of a 1-year hospital internship is also required. To qualify as a specialist, a doctor must have additional study and training in a chosen field of medicine. To be a board-certified specialist, the physician must be certified by an examining board of the particular medical specialty. A physician who does not complete the certification requirements cannot use board certification initials after his name.
General practitioner, also known as "GP," family physician, or family practitioner	Diagnoses and treats diseases, may do some minor surgery, prescribes drugs, and recommends all other accepted methods of medical care.
Medical Specialists	
Dermatologist	Diagnoses, treats, and prescribes medicine for problems and other conditions of the skin.
Internist	Diagnoses and treats diseases by medical therapy other than by surgery. The internist's specialty field may be gastrointestinal, allergy, arthritis, heart and circulatory diseases, lung diseases, or some similar area.
Obstetrician-gynecologist	Manages pregnancy and childbirth and treats diseases of the female reproductive system.

Category	Requirements and/or Brief Description of Professional Practice
Ophthalmologist	Diagnoses and treats all eye diseases and abnormal conditions including vision errors, prescribes drugs and lenses and performs surgery or other treatments to remedy conditions.
Orthopedist	Preserves and restores broken bones, impaired joints, and other related structures through surgical interventions, medications, and/or use of devices such as casts and traction.
Pediatrician	Provides consultation, diagnosis, and treatment of children's diseases.
Physical medicine and rehabilitation specialist	Helps disabled people with their disability resulting from crippling diseases and accidents, disabling chronic conditions, and loss or limitation of sight, speech, or hearing. Diagnoses and prescribes medicines and treatments by the application of heat, cold, water, and electricity, and by exercise to restore the impaired body part to useful activity.
Psychiatrist	Concerned with the treatment of persons with mental, emotional, and behavioral disturbances and with the public health aspects of mental health.
Surgeon	Surgical correction of conditions and diseases of the body, not limited to specific areas thereof. Specialty areas may include cardiovascular, gastrointestinal, and plastic surgery.
Nursing	
Registered Nurse (R.N.)	Graduating from an accredited school or college of nursing and passing the state board examination for licensure are requirements to practice. Some states require continuing education for reregistration of licensure to continue practice. Clinical practice: practice involved in helping people obtain, retain, and regain health. Regis-

Category	Requirements and/or Brief Description of Professional Practice
	tered nurses are responsible for the nature and quality of all nursing care that patients receive. Voluntary certification may be obtained through the professional nursing organizations, The American Nurses' Association, and, to a limited extent, through nursing specialty organizations. This is a peer recognition of quality of practice and is not legally required. Legal certification is required in a limited number of states where credentials above and beyond basic licensure are needed to engage in some specialized areas of practice.
Nurse Practitioners and Clinical Specialists	
Maternal-gynecological-neonatal nurse	Care of mothers and newborn infants.
Gerontological nurse	Care of older patients, well and ill.
Primary health care nurse practitioner	
Adult nurse practitioner	Primary care of adults.
Family nurse practitioner	Primary care of adults and family members.
School nurse practitioner	Primary care of children in schools.
Psychiatric and mental health nurse	Care of patients with mental and emotional disorders.

Category	Requirements and/or Brief Description of Professional Practice
Medical-surgical nurse	Care of adult patients with chronic disease and presurgical and postsurgical nursing care needs.
Pediatric nurse practitioner	Nursing care of children.
Certified nurse-midwife (C.N.M.)	Requirements are graduation from an accredited school of nursing with a license to practice nursing, successful completion of a nurse-midwifery program from a school approved by the American College of Nurse-Midwives, and successful examination for certification to use the title "certified nurse-midwife." Concentration of practice: care of women during pregnancy, labor, delivery, and the postdelivery period.
Community Health Nurse, Public Health Nurse, and Visiting Nurse	Provide nursing service for families, individuals, and groups at home, at school, and in public centers. Emphasis is on promotion of health, prevention of disease, and care of the ill at home.
General Duty Nurses	Professional nurses and practical/vocational nurses work in most direct patient care areas of hospitals, nursing homes, and other institutions that provide general and specialized care for the sick and injured and those giving birth to babies. Nursing care for patients is provided 24 hours a day, 7 days a week, in most institutions. Nurses often select a specific area of the institution in which to practice and may be referred to by the title of that area, such as pediatric nurse (care of children), emergency room nurse, or operating room nurse. Experience, rather than special preparation, is often the basis of the title used.

Category	Requirements and/or Brief Description of Professional Practice
Licensed Practical Nurse or Licensed Vocational Nurse (L.P.N. or L.V.N.)	Completing a practical/vocational nursing school program and passing a state board examination are required for state licensure to practice. Concentration of practice: provide nursing care and treatment of patients, usually under the supervision of a licensed physician or registered nurse.
Nutrition and Diet	
Nutritionist	Requirement: completion of a curriculum in home economics in a college or university with majors in food, nutrition, or institutional management. Concentration of practice: provides services in teaching people about normal nutrition and helps special groups of people such as expectant and nursing mothers and the aged to develop meal patterns and diet intake in terms of their specific needs.
Registered dietitian (R.D.)	To become a registered dietitian, a person must complete the requirements of the American Dietetic Association as well as pass the national registration examination. Basic preparation is the same as for the nutritionist. Concentration of work includes principles of nutrition and management in planning and directing food service programs in hospitals and related medical care facilities and working cooperatively with physicians to help patients needing special nutrition guidance.

Category	Requirements and/or Brief Description of Professional Practice
Occupational Therapy	
Occupational therapist	Graduating from an accredited program in occupational therapy and passing an examination conducted by the American Physical Therapy Association are required for national registration and permission to use the initials O.T.R. (occupational therapist registered). Concentration of practice: rehabilitation of physical and emotional disabilities using creative, educational, recreational, and prevocational activities.
Optometry	
Optometrist	Graduating from an accredited school of optometry and passing a state board examination are required to practice. Concentration of practice: examines eyes and related structures to determine the presence of any visual, muscular, or nerve abnormality; prescribes and adapts lenses or other optical aids.
Osteopathic Medicine	
Osteopathic Physician (D.O.)	Graduating from an accredited school of osteopathic medicine and passing the state board examination for licensure are required to practice. A 1-year hospital internship is required in most states and the District of Columbia. To qualify as a specialist, an osteopathic physician must spend additional time studying and training in a chosen branch of medicine. Board certification is awarded by specialty boards for each of the specialties.
General practitioner	Diagnoses and treats diseases, may perform some surgical procedures, prescribes drugs, and recommends all other accepted methods of medical care.

Category	Requirements and/or Brief Description of Professional Practice
Osteopathic Specialists	
Dermatologist	Diagnoses, treats, and prescribes medicines for problems and other conditions of the skin.
Internist	Diagnoses and treats diseases by medical therapy other than by surgery. The internist's specialty field may be gastrointestinal, allergy, arthritis, heart, and circulatory diseases, lung diseases, or some similar area.
Obstetrician-gynecologist	Manages pregnancy and childbirth and treats diseases of the female reproductive system.
Ophthalmologist	Diagnoses and treats all eye diseases and abnormal conditions, including vision errors; prescribes drugs and lenses and performs surgery or other treatments to remedy conditions.
Pediatrician	Provides consultation, diagnosis, and treatment of children's diseases.
Rehabilitation specialist	Helps disabled people with their disability resulting from crippling diseases and accidents, disabling chronic conditions, loss or limitation of sight, speech or hearing. Diagnoses and prescribes medicines and treatments by the application of heat, cold, water, electricity, exercise to restore impaired body part to useful activity.
Psychiatrist	Concerned with the treatment of individual patients with mental, emotional, and behavioral disturbances and with the public health aspects of mental health.
Surgeon	Surgical correction of conditions and diseases of the body, not limited to specific areas thereof. Specialty areas may include cardiovascular, gastrointestinal, plastic surgery, etc.

Category	Requirements and/or Brief Description of Professional Practice
Pharmacy	
Pharmacist	Graduating from an accredited school of pharmacy and passing the state board examination for licensure are required to practice. Concentration of practice: assures safety, efficacy, and efficiency in obtaining, storing, prescribing, dispensing, delivering, administering, and using drugs and related articles. Many community and hospital pharmacists maintain medication profiles on patients receiving prescriptions to reduce adverse reactions, allergies, and contraindicated use of drugs.
Physical Therapy	
Physical therapist	Graduating from an accredited school of physical therapy and passing the state board examination for licensure are requirements to practice. Concentration of practice: helps in the rehabilitation of people with injuries or diseases affecting muscles, joints, nerves, and bones. The therapist works under the direction of the physician to administer therapy through the use of therapeutic exercise, massage, and various applications of heat, water, light, and electricity.
Podiatry	
Podiatrist	Graduating from an accredited college of podiatric medicine and passing the state board examination for licensure are required to practice. In a few states, a period of internship or practice is also required. Concentration of practice: examines, diagnoses, treats, and provides care of conditions and functions of the human foot by medical and surgical means.

Category	Requirements and/or Brief Description of Professional Practice
Psychology	
Psychologist	Graduating from an accredited program, usually with a Ph.D., is required for practice. One year of internship or supervised clinical experience is sometimes required. All states require licensure or certification. Concentration of practice: understanding and modifying behavior, with focus on learning, perception, development, adjustment ability, and personality. Diagnoses and treats persons with mental and emotional illness in private practice or in clinics and institutions. Psychologists specialize in their practice; for example, school psychologist, clinical psychologist, child psychologist, and other areas.
Social Work	
Social Worker	A master's degree from an accredited graduate school of social work (M.S.W.) is recognized as the basic qualification for a professional social worker. Membership in the Academy of Certified Social Workers (A.C.S.W.) requires 2 years of approved clinical practice and a written examination. Some entry-level positions accept the bachelor of social work degree from an accredited undergraduate program. Licensing standards vary among those few states that license social workers. Concentration of practice: Works directly with individuals and their families who are ill, disabled, aged, or otherwise handicapped to teach them to cope with problems related to long-term illness, recovery, and rehabilitation. Social workers utilize community health agencies and other resources to assist the patient in adjustment to disability and life in the community.

COMMUNICABLE DISEASES

DISEASE	HOW SPREAD	PREVENTION	HOW LONG FROM EXPOSURE TO ONSET
Chicken pox (varicella)	From person to person by direct contact, droplet, or airborne spread; indirectly through articles freshly soiled by discharges from the vesicles and mucous membranes of infected persons.	No immunization yet available. Avoid exposure; one attack confers long immunity. Second attacks are rare. ZIG (zoster immune globulin) is recommended for high-risk individuals who have been exposed.	From 10 to 21 days; most commonly 13–17 days.
Common cold	Presumably transmission is by direct contact or by droplet spread; indirectly by handkerchiefs, eating utensils, or other articles freshly soiled by discharges from the nose and mouth of infected persons.	No specific prevention; avoid contact. Cover mouth when coughing and sneezing and dispose of nose and mouth secretions. Hand washing prevents spread.	From 12 to 72 hours, usually about 24 hours.
Diphtheria	Contact with a patient or a carrier or with articles soiled with discharges and secretions from mucous surfaces of nose and throat and from skin and other lesions.	Innoculation with diphtheria toxoid (DTP) at 2, 4, and 6 months, with boosters between 1 and 2 years and between 4 and 6 years; thereafter, boosters every 10 years.	From 2 to 5 days, sometimes longer.
Food poisoning (salmonellosis)	Contact with infected animals (often pet turtles, birds, dogs, or cats) or animal products (uncooked, unrefrigerated, undercovered, or cross-contaminated poultry, raw meat, or other foods).	Hand washing before handling food and after handling pets; proper food storage. Keep pet feeding dishes and toys away from food preparation area. Teach children to wash hands after touching pets; refrigerate foods.	From 6 to 72 hours; usually 12–36 hours.

COMMON SYMPTOMS	HOW LONG COMMUNICABLE	SOME POSSIBLE COMPLICATIONS
Acute onset, with slight fever. Small reddish pimples followed or accompanied by the disease, usually more abundant on the covered than on the exposed parts of the body, that cause itching. Disease lasts approximately 4 to 10 days.	As much as 5 days before to 6 days after last set of vesicles appears. One of the most contagious of the communicable diseases.	Complications rare. Skin lesions may become infected and may leave pitted scars.
Tickling, dry sensation in the throat; rarely fever; malaise; chilliness; cough and runny nose.	For 1 day before onset and about 5 days afterward.	Sinusitis, bronchitis, laryngitis, pneumonia, middle ear infection.
Inflammation of the nose, throat, and tonsils, with grayish-white patches in the throat; an acute infection accompanied by fever.	Variable; until the germs have disappeared from secretions and lesions; usually 2 weeks or less, seldom more than 4 weeks.	Damage to the heart; pneumonia.
Sudden onset of fever, headache, abdominal cramps, vomiting, and diarrhea, lasting a few hours or 1 to 2 days. Symptoms may be mild, often mistaken for flu.	Stools infectious for several days to several weeks after onset.	Usually none. Can be life-threatening, even fatal to infants, elderly persons, and those weakened by other illness.

DISEASE	HOW SPREAD	PREVENTION	HOW LONG FROM EXPOSURE TO ONSET
Gonorrhea	By contact with discharge from mucous membranes of infected persons during sexual activity; in the newborn, by transfer from the mother during birth.	No immunization. Avoid contact. Use prophylactic drugs in the eyes of the newborn. One attack does not protect against subsequent infection.	Usually 2 to 5 days, sometimes longer.
Hepatitis-A (infectious hepatitis)	Through intimate person-to-person contact; by contaminated water, food, and milk; by contaminated syringes and needles.	Good sanitation and personal hygiene with particular emphasis on disposal of stools; careful handling of blood-soiled needles and instruments; administration of immune serum globulin (ISG) to exposed persons.	Variable: 15 to 50 days; commonly 30 days.
Hepatitis-B (serum hepatitis)	Through transfusion of contaminated blood or blood products; sharing of contaminated needles between intravenous drug abusers, accidental skin puncture with a contaminated needle, or by improperly sterilized equipment for tattooing and ear piercing. Transmission has occurred through intimate personal contact.	Screening of blood donors and elimination of any positive donors identified; proper handling and sterilization of bloodstained needles and equipment, frequent and thorough handwashing to prevent accidental ingestion of blood. Avoid tattooing.	From 1 to 6 months, usually 3 months.
Herpes VD (venereal herpes)	By direct contact during sexual activity; or, in the newborn, by transfer from the mother during birth.	Proper use of condoms may reduce risk of spread to sexual partners.	From 2 to 20 days; about 6 is average.

COMMON SYMPTOMS	HOW LONG COMMUNICABLE	SOME POSSIBLE COMPLICATIONS
Often, symptoms are mild; discharge from mucous membranes of the genital tract or of the eyes; burning and pain on urination.	For months or years unless treated with specific drug therapy, which ends communicability.	Few complications when treated early. Can cause sterility, arthritis, heart disease, and blindness.
Fever, dark urine, loss of appetite, malaise, abdominal discomfort, usually followed by jaundice. Mild cases (especially in children) may not become jaundiced.	Stools and blood probably infectious from about 2 weeks prior to onset of jaundice until 2 weeks after onset. Lasts several months.	Relapses may occur, or the disease may become chronic, resulting in liver damage. Rarely fatal.
Same as hepatitis-A but onset is more gradual and joint pains and rash sometimes occur early. Convalescence may take longer (1 to 6 months).	Blood probably infectious from 4 to 6 weeks (or sometimes longer) before onset of jaundice until 3 months after onset. Some cases have become chronic carriers of the infection. Blood of persons with history of hepatitis-B is always considered contaminated for purposes of transfusion or when needles are used.	Same as hepatitis-A but more often fatal.
In the male, small lesions (blisters) on the penis, sometimes also infection of the urethra. In the female, lesions may appear on buttocks or near genitals. There may also be fever and headaches. Usually mild, the symptoms may not be noticed.	Unknown.	May keep recurring for several years. May be linked with cancer of cervix in women. May cause spontaneous abortion. Pregnant women may transmit infection to fetus so that child is severely ill at birth.

DISEASE	HOW SPREAD	PREVENTION	HOW LONG FROM EXPOSURE TO ONSET
Impetigo	By direct contact with moist discharges of skin lesions or indirect contact with articles recently soiled with discharges; also, contact with others whose skin, nose, or throat is contaminated or infected.	No immunization. Reinfection possible. Carry out good personal hygiene.	From 2 to 10 days, occasionally longer.
Influenza	By direct contact, through droplet spread, or by articles freshly soiled with nose and throat discharges of infected persons.	Immunity to a specific influenza virus may last for several years after attack, but because there are many strains of influenza viruses, there may be frequent attacks of the disease. Annual vaccination is recommended for the chronically ill and possibly for all aged persons, also doctors, nurses, and others who provide essential community services.	From 24 to 72 hours.
Lice (pediculosis)	Direct contact with a person who has lice; indirectly by contact with his personal belongings, especially clothing and headgear.	Avoid physical contact with infested individuals and their clothing and belongings. Wash body with warm water and soap. Launder infested clothing and bedding in hot water or dry cleaning to destroy mites and lice.	Eggs of lice hatch within 1 week, and sexual maturity is reached 2 weeks later.

COMMON SYMPTOMS	HOW LONG COMMUNICABLE	SOME POSSIBLE COMPLICATIONS
Blisters, which later become crusted, commonly on face and hands; may occur on infected insect bites, other sores.	As long as the sores are unhealed.	Occasional secondary infection of the sores.
Sudden onset; fever for 1 to 6 days; chills; headache; discomfort; aches or pains in back, legs, or shoulders; sore throat; runny nose; cough.	Probably limited to a brief period before onset and 1 week after.	Pneumonia. Deaths concentrated among the elderly and those with chronic conditions such as heart and lung disorders; diabetes mellitus and other chronic metabolic disorders.
Infestation of head and other hairy parts of body and along seams of clothing with adult lice, larvae, nits (eggs).	Until all eggs are destroyed and adult lice are dead.	None.

DISEASE	HOW SPREAD	PREVENTION	HOW LONG FROM EXPOSURE TO ONSET
Malaria	By bite of female anopheline mosquito carrying malaria organisms in malaria areas. Can spread from injection with contaminated needles or blood or from mother to unborn child.	In areas where malaria is endemic, application of long-lasting insecticides to all dwellings and surfaces where mosquitoes live; installation of wire mesh screening; nightly spraying if no long-lasting insecticides are available; use of insect repellents on skin and clothing; use of mosquito net; taking drug to decrease susceptibility; screening blood donors for history of malaria.	Most frequently 12–30 days; occasionally 8–10 months.
Measles, German or 3-day (rubella)	By droplet spread or direct contact with infected persons; indirect contact with articles freshly soiled with discharges from nose and throat.	Safe and effective vaccine is now available; recommended for all children between 1 and 12 years and for nonpregnant women shown to be susceptible by serological test. Immune serum globulin (ISG, or gamma globulin) provides irregular or unreliable protection; recommended for adult female contacts with no history of having had rubella who are within the first 4 months of pregnancy. Deliberate exposure of girls in good health before puberty is recommended by some authorities.	From 14 to 21 days, usually 18 days.

COMMON SYMPTOMS	HOW LONG COMMUNICABLE	SOME POSSIBLE COMPLICATIONS
Fever, chills, and sweating; headache; delirium; coma. With some strains there are cycles of rising fever, chills, headache, and nausea; sweating repeated every 3 to 4 days.	As long as malaria organisms are present in blood (with some strains, this is for life) of human; mosquitoes live from a few days to a month or more.	Prompt treatment usually prevents death.
Few symptoms; mild cold symptoms may be present. Slight fever; restlessness; almost always enlargement of lymph nodes behind the ears and the back of neck; rash that may resemble that of measles or scarlet fever.	From 1 week before rash appears to 4 days after.	Usually none; serious for women during first 3 months of pregnancy; may cause congenital defects in baby if mother contracts disease during early pregnancy. Arthritis, especially among adult females. Encephalitis is rare.

DISEASE	HOW SPREAD	PREVENTION	HOW LONG FROM EXPOSURE TO ONSET
Measles (rubeola)	By droplet spread or direct contact with infected persons; indirectly through articles freshly soiled with nose and throat secretion; in some instances, probably airborne. Highly communicable.	Vaccination; recommended for all children between 1 and 5 years, before going to kindergarten.	About 10 days from exposure to initial fever; about 14 days until rash appears; as long as 21 days if gamma globulin or convalescent serum has been given.
Meningitis meningococcal	By direct contact with or droplet spread from infected persons (most often not ill persons).	For use in some mass living situations, vaccine now available is effective against some strains of meningitis. Contacts of some cases may be given preventative drug therapy.	Varies from 2 to 10 days, commonly 3 to 4 days.
Mononucleosis infectious	Unknown, but believed to be from person to person by way of nose and mouth discharges.	No immunization; infection appears to give a high degree of resistance.	Unknown, seemingly varies from 2 to 6 weeks.
Mumps	By droplet spread and by direct contact with saliva of infected persons.	Vaccination. Vaccine may be given to children between 1 and 12 years. It is recommended for adolescents and adults, particularly males, who have not had mumps.	From 12 to 26 days, commonly 18 days.

COMMON SYMPTOMS	HOW LONG COMMUNICABLE	SOME POSSIBLE COMPLICATIONS
Fever, runny eyes and nose, followed by a characteristic dusky-red, blotchy rash on the face, body, and extremities. (Koplik spots in mouth may appear on third to seventh day.)	During period of runny eyes and nose until 4 days after rash appears.	Encephalitis is an uncommon but severe complication and can result in brain damage, middle ear infection, or pneumonia. Infants and children under 3 years of age are particularly susceptible.
An acute bacterial infection with sudden onset, fever, intense headache, nausea, and vomiting; frequently a rash of small, round, red-pink spots; dizziness, stiff neck, delirium, and coma.	Until germs are no longer present in discharges from nose and throat of infected persons. Usually disappears in 24 hours after appropriate treatment.	Spread of the infection to the brain tissue; pneumonia; middle ear infection; mastoiditis; chronic heart damage.
Loss of appetite; irritability, nausea, and vomiting; sleepiness; chills; fever; sore throat, enlarged lymph glands of the neck; enlarged spleen; in some cases, a rash or jaundice. Symptoms may subside in a few days or may last for several weeks.	Undetermined, but may be up to 1 year.	Prognosis is excellent; death rarely occurs. Nephritis, infected lymph glands, anemia, ruptured spleen may occur.
An acute viral infection with sudden onset of fever, and swelling and tenderness of the salivary glands.	From about 7 days before swelling of glands and persisting as much as 9 days thereafter.	Inflammation of the ovaries or testicles in adolescents and adults. Children under 12 usually are free from complications. Hearing loss or meningitis and encephalitis may occur.

DISEASE	HOW SPREAD	PREVENTION	HOW LONG FROM EXPOSURE TO ONSET
Pinworms	Ingestion of worm eggs. Eggs transferred to same or to other individuals directly by hands, food, drink, clothing, bedding, etc., contaminated by eggs.	Good sanitation and personal hygiene.	From 3 to 6 weeks. May not be recognized for months.
Polio (myelitis)—infantile paralysis	By direct contact or droplet spread of nose and throat secretions of infected persons; stools of infected persons; contaminated milk.	Oral polio vaccine (OPV) recommended at 2, 4, and 6 months of age with a booster before starting to school. (May be given together with diphtheria, tetanus, and pertussis, or DTP). At the present time, routine immunization of adults is not recommended, except in high-risk situations.	From 3 to 21 days, commonly 7 to 12 days.
Ringworm (tinea capitus, tinea corporis, athlete's foot)	Direct contact with infected persons or animals, especially dogs, cats, or cattle. Sources of infection are such materials as the backs of theater seats, barber clippers, hats, or clothing contaminated with hair from infected animals or persons.	No immunization; repeated attacks are common. Effective control of animal ringworm. Good personal hygiene and avoidance of direct contact with infected persons.	From 10 to 14 days (not known for athlete's foot).
Roundworms (ascariasis)	Eating raw vegetables grown in soil contaminated by feces of infected persons; from contaminated soil carried on shoes, hands, or clothing.	Good sanitation and personal hygiene. Teach children to wash raw vegetables before eating, to wash hands before eating and after any contact with the soil, and to not put in their mouth foods or objects that have been on the ground or floor.	From 2 to 3 months.

COMMON SYMPTOMS	HOW LONG COMMUNICABLE	SOME POSSIBLE COMPLICATIONS
Nonspecific symptoms; if severe, itching of the buttocks and anus, especially at night. Threadlike white worms, ¼ to ½ inch (.63 to 1.27 centimeters) long, may be passed in stool.	As long as worms or their eggs are present.	Usually none. Sometimes itching of buttocks.
An acute illness, with fever, malaise, gastrointestinal upset, headache, and stiffness of neck and back. Many inapparent infections occur.	From 1 day after infection (and before onset of symptoms) up to 6 weeks after infection; most commonly from 7–10 days before to 7–10 after symptoms.	Temporary or permanent paralysis of varying severity of affected parts of the body. Paralysis most often occurs in adults.
Infection begins as a small pimple and spreads outward, leaving scaly patches. Hairs break, causing baldness on the scalp. On the body, infection shows a characteristic ring-shaped lesion. On the feet, there is scaling or cracking of the skin, especially between the toes, or blisters containing a thin, watery fluid.	As long as lesions are present and live spores are present on contaminated materials.	Occasional secondary infection of the lesions.
Coughing spasms, weakness, loss of appetite, headache, disturbed sleep. Large worms (similar to earthworms) passed in stool or vomited, may be first symptom.	As long as worms or their eggs are present (in intestine or in soil).	Anemia; bronchial symptoms; blocked intestines.

DISEASE	HOW SPREAD	PREVENTION	HOW LONG FROM EXPOSURE TO ONSET
Scabies (itch)	By direct contact and from undergarments or sheets freshly contaminated by infected persons.	Avoid contact with infected persons; assure cleanliness of body, garments, and bedclothes.	From 1 to 2 days. Several days or even weeks may elapse before itching is noticed.
Scarlet fever	Direct contact with acutely ill or convalescent patients or carriers.	No immunization; avoid contact with infected persons.	Usually 1 to 3 days.
Smallpox	Contact with persons sick with the disease. Contact need not be intimate; airborne transmission may occur over short distances. Spread by nose and throat discharges or by material from skin lesions.	Vaccination recommended *only* for certain health workers and for persons traveling to certain foreign countries. Contact the state health department for travel health requirements.	From 7 to 17 days, commonly 12 days.
Strep throat (streptococcal sore throat)	Direct contact with an ill person or a carrier; rarely by indirect contact through transfer by objects or hands. May follow ingestion of contaminated milk or other food.	No immunization; avoid contact with ill persons. Persons with infections should not prepare food.	Usually 1 to 3 days.

COMMON SYMPTOMS	HOW LONG COMMUNICABLE	SOME POSSIBLE COMPLICATIONS
Penetration of the skin visible as pimples and blisters or as tiny linear burrows containing the female mite and her eggs. Primary symptom is itching at site of lesions, especially at night. Lesions commonly occur on finger webs, inner surface of wrists, the elbows, axillas, around the waist and lower portion of the buttocks.	Until mites and eggs are destroyed by treatment.	Occasional secondary infections of the lesions.
Acute onset with high fever, sore throat, strawberry tongue, nausea and vomiting; fine rash, which blanches on pressure, appears on neck and chest in about 24 hours. When the rash subsides, the skin may peel.	In untreated, uncomplicated cases, 10 to 21 days. In untreated cases, complicated from weeks to months. Adequate treatment eliminates possibility of transmission after 24 hours.	Middle ear infection; damage to the heart and kidneys. Inflammation of the glands in the neck is common.
Sudden onset with fever, chills, headache, severe backache, and prostration. Temperature falls in 3 to 4 days and rash appears, finally forming scabs that fall off in about 3 weeks.	From first symptoms to disappearance of all scabs and crusts, usually 2 to 3 weeks. Most communicable in early stage of the disease.	Secondary infection of the skin with subsequent septicemia; pneumonia; laryngitis; pleurisy; emphysema (air in tissues); middle ear infection; occasionally kidney damage.
There may be no other symptoms than a sore throat. Or there may be fever, sore throat, tonsllitis, pharymgitis, swollen glands of neck, exudate in throat.	In untreated, uncomplicated cases, 10 to 21 days. Adequate treatment eliminates possibility of transmission within 24 hours.	Rheumatic fever; acute glomunclonephritis.

DISEASE	HOW SPREAD	PREVENTION	HOW LONG FROM EXPOSURE TO ONSET
Syphilis	By direct contact (fondling of children, sexual activity, kissing), during primary and secondary syphilis. Source of infection is discharge from early lesions of skin or mucous membrane of infected persons. An infected woman may transmit syphilis to her unborn child.	No immunization; one attack does not confer immunity. Best measures are health and sex education, preparation for marriage, premarital and prenatal examinations as part of a general physical examination.	10 to 90 days, usually 3 weeks.
Tetanus (lockjaw)	Tetanus spores, found in soil, street dust, and animal and human feces, enter the body through injury, usually a puncture wound. These spores may also enter the body through burns and trivial or unnoticed wounds.	Vaccination. Tetanus toxoid (in DTP) at 2, 4, and 6 months of age with boosters every 10 years; or upon injury if no booster given within 3 years; tetanus immune globulin (TIG) provides protection to the injured person.	Commonly from 4 days to 3 weeks.
Tuberculosis (TB; pulmonary tuberculosis)	Infection usually results from continued and intimate exposure to infected persons with active disease. Coughing or sneezing by a patient whose sputum contains the tubercle bacillus releases a cloud of highly infectious droplets. Bovine tuberculosis is transmitted by ingestion of unpasteurized dairy products from infected cows.	Periodic chest X-ray of persons with positive tuberculosis tests; treatment of infectious cases; prompt examination of contacts and treatment when indicated; preventive therapy with isoniazid for high risk infected persons; pasteurization of milk products and the elimination of tuberculosis among dairy cattle; BCG vaccination for uninfected persons exposed to untreated cases is unreliable.	From infection to primary phase lesions, several weeks. Progression or dissemination may occur early, within months of initial infection or years later. First 6 to 12 months are most hazardous.

COMMON SYMPTOMS	HOW LONG COMMUNICABLE	SOME POSSIBLE COMPLICATIONS
Primary lesion (chancre) at the point of contact, which will heal without treatment; a secondary eruption involving skin and mucous membranes. Latent period may last for years, with occasional relapses and appearance of lesions. In congenital syphilis, only the late manifestations, such as the listed complications, occur.	Most contagious during primary and secondary stages (first 2 or 3 months). Rarely infectious after first year except for pregnant woman who can infect unborn child while in latent stage.	Sterility, abortion or miscarriage, damage to the heart, blindness, deafness, paralysis, insanity.
Painful muscular contractions of neck, jaw, and trunk muscles. Stiffness increases until jaws become locked; the head is drawn backward. Slight stimulation of patient causes convulsions and extreme pain.	Not directly transmissible from person to person.	Rare under proper treatment and prevention; probably fatal if not treated promptly.
Primary infection usually goes undetected but may resemble the common cold. Course of disease varies widely. Most common symptoms of progressive disease are persistent cough, sputum production, fatigue, weight loss, loss of appetite, fever.	For weeks or months before diagnosis and start of treatment, and for a few weeks after treatment begins.	Pleurisy, with or without effusion; meningitis; infection of gastrointestinal tract when sputum is swallowed; infection of the lymph system; rectal fistulae and abscesses; tuberculosis of bones and joints.

DISEASE	HOW SPREAD	PREVENTION	HOW LONG FROM EXPOSURE TO ONSET
Typhoid fever	Direct or indirect contact with infected persons or carriers. Principal vehicles of spread are water and food contaminated with feces or urine of infected persons. Contamination is usually by hands of a carrier or of an undiagnosed case. Flies may also play a part in the spread.	Vaccination recommended only for persons known to have been exposed, in epidemic situations, and for persons traveling to some foreign countries. Good sanitation should be carried out.	Variable; usual range 1 to 3 weeks.
Whooping cough (pertussis)	By direct contact with infected persons, by droplet spread, or indirectly by contact with articles freshly soiled with discharges from the nose and throat.	Vaccination. Pertussis vaccine (in DTP) at ages of 2, 4, and 6 months, with boosters between 1 and 2 and between 4 and 6 years of age.	Commonly 7 days; almost uniformly within 10 days and not exceeding 21 days.

COMMON SYMPTOMS	HOW LONG COMMUNICABLE	SOME POSSIBLE COMPLICATIONS
Continued nonsweating fever; headache; loss of appetite; constipation more common than diarrhea; abdominal tenderness and distention; rose spots on the trunk; respiratory symptoms, including bronchitis and pneumonia.	As long as typhoid bacilli appear in excreta; usually from second week throughout convalescence; thereafter variable. From 2 to 5 percent of patients become permanent carriers.	Hemorrhage or perforation of the intestine; peritonitis; early heart failure.
Acute bacterial infection involving the respiratory tract and characterized by irritating cough, which gradually becomes a typical "whooping" cough, lasting 1 to 2 months. Beginning symptoms are like those of the common cold.	From 7 days after exposure to 3 weeks after onset of typical paroxysmal cough. If antibiotics are given, communicability ceases after 5 to 7 days.	Pneumonia is usually the chief cause of death from this disease. Bronchiectasis; emphysema; middle ear disease; brain damage; hernia; convulsions.

REFERENCES

Health and Wellness

Dental Care

Cleaning Your Teeth and Gums. Chicago: American Dental Association. 1977.

Happiness Is a Healthy Mouth. Chicago: American Dental Association. 1976.

They're Your Teeth—You Can Keep Them. Chicago: American Dental Association. 1976.

Foot Care

Feet First: A Booklet About Foot Care, prepared by Nursing Research Field Center, Division of Nursing. Washington, DC: U.S. Department of Health, Education, and Welfare. 1970. Stock No. 017-011-00011-8.*

Foot Care for the Diabetic Patient. Washington, DC: U.S. Department of Health, Education, and Welfare. 1977. Stock No. 017-001-00026-4.*

Light on Your Feet, by Jules Saltman. New York: Public Affairs Pamphlets. Public Affairs Pamphlet No. 345A. June 1973.

Personal and Family Health

Family Health Care, by Debra P. Hymovich and Martha Underwood Barnard. New York: McGraw-Hill, Inc. 1973.

Health: Man in a Changing Environment, by Benjamin A. Kogan. New York: Harcourt Brace Jovanovich, Inc. Revised 1974.

High-Level Wellness, by Donald B. Ardell. Emmaus, PA: Rodale Press. 1977.

Take Care of Yourself: A Consumer's Guide to Medical Care, by Donald M. Vickery and James F. Fries. Reading, MA: Addison-Wesley Publishing Company, Inc. 1976.

Washington Consumers' Checkbook: Health, A Guide to Health Care in the Metropolitan Area. Washington, DC: Washington Center for the Study of Services. Vol. 1, No. 1. 1976.

*Contact Superintendent of Documents, U.S. Government Printing Office, Washington, DC 20402. Request information on cost of single or multiple copies. Always identify material by title and Stock No.

Periodicals

American Health Care Association Journal. Bimonthly magazine published by American Health Care Association, 1200 Fifteenth St., N.W., Washington, DC 20005.

Family Health. Monthly magazine published by Family Media, Inc., Portland Place, Boulder, CO 80302.

Health. Bimonthly publication published by the American Osteopathic Association, 212 E. Ohio St., Chicago, IL 60611.

Health Values: Achieving High-Level Wellness. Bimonthly publication published by Charles B. Slack, Inc., 6900 Grove Rd., Thorofare, NJ 08086.

Urban Health. Magazine published 10 times a year by Urban Publishing Co., 3079 Campbellton Road, S.W., Atlanta, GA 30311.

Food and Nutrition

Baking for People With Food Allergies, by Lois Fulton and Carole Davis, Consumer and Food Economics Institute, Agricultural Research Service. Washington, DC: U.S. Department of Agriculture. Home and Garden Bulletin No. 147. Revised 1975. Stock No. 001-000-03362-0; Catalog No. A 1.77:147/2.*

The Complete Gourmet Nutrition Cookbook: How To Change Your Eating for the Better and Enjoy It!, by Margaret C. Dean. Washington, DC: Acropolis Books, Ltd. 1978.

Cultural Food Patterns in the U.S.A., by Marion Mason. Chicago: The American Dietetic Association. Revised 1976.

Family Fare: A Guide to Good Nutrition, prepared by Consumer and Food Economics Institute, Agricultural Research Service. Washington, DC: U.S. Department of Agriculture. Home and Garden Bulletin No. 1. Revised 1977. Stock No. 001-000-03280-1.*

Food and Your Weight, by Louise Page and Nancy Raper, Consumer and Food Economics Institute, Agricultural Research Service. Washington, DC: U.S. Department of Agriculture. Home and Garden Bulletin No. 74. Revised 1977. Stock No. 001-000-03735-8.*

Food for Today, by Helen Kowtaluk and Alice Orphanos Kopan. Peoria, IL: Chas. A. Bennett Company, Inc. 1977.

---

*Contact Superintendent of Documents, U.S. Government Printing Office, Washington, DC 20402. Request information on cost of single or multiple copies. Always identify material by title and Stock No.

List of Available Publications of the United States Department of Agriculture, prepared by Publications Division, Office of Communication. Washington, DC: U.S. Department of Agriculture. List No. 11. 1978. Stock No. 001-003-00033-0.*

Living Nutrition, by Fredrick J. Stare and Margaret McWilliams. New York: John Wiley & Sons, Inc. 1977.

Living With High Blood Pressure: The Hypertension Diet Cookbook, by Joyce Daly Margie and James C. Hunt. Bloomfield, NJ: HLS Press, Inc. 1978.

Nutrition Labeling: How It Can Work for You, by National Nutrition Consortium, Inc., with Ronald M. Deutsch. Bethesda, MD: The National Nutrition Consortium, Inc. 1975.

Nutritive Value of Foods, Prepared by Agricultural Research Service. Washington, DC: U.S. Department of Agriculture. Home and Garden Bulletin No. 72. Revised 1977. Stock No. 001-000-03667-0.*

Periodicals

Food and Nutrition. Magazine published six times a year by the Food and Nutrition Service, U.S. Department of Agriculture, Washington, DC 20250.

Nutrition Action. Monthly publication published by Center for Science in the Public Interest, 1755 S St., N.W., Washington, DC 20009.

Growth and Development

Childhood and Society, by Erik H. Erikson. New York: W. W. Norton & Company, Inc. Revised 1963.

Family Development, by Evelyn Millis Duvall. Philadelphia: J. B. Lippincott Co. Revised 1971.

Human Development, by Diane E. Papalia and Sally Wendkos Olds. New York: McGraw-Hill, Inc. 1978.

Learning About Sex: The Contemporary Guide for Young Adults, by Gary F. Kelly. Woodbury, NY: Barron's Educational Series, Inc. 1976.

Study Guide To Accompany Human Development, prepared by Danuta Bukatko and John W. Hullett for P.S. Associates. New York: McGraw-Hill, Inc. 1978

*Contact Superintendent of Documents, U.S. Government Printing Office, Washington, DC 20402. Request information on cost of single or multiple copies. Always identify material by title and Stock No.

Pregnancy

Be Good to Your Baby Before It Is Born: A New Look at What To Do and What To Expect During Pregnancy. White Plains, NY: The National Foundation–March of Dimes. 1977.

From Conception to Birth: The Drama of Life's Beginnings, by Roberts Rugh and Landrum B. Shettles, with Richard Einhorn. New York: Harper & Row, Publishers, Inc. 1971.

Guide for Expectant Parents, by Maternity Center Association. New York: Grosset & Dunlap. 1969.

Methods of Childbirth: A Complete Guide to Childbirth Classes and Maternity Care, by Constance A. Bean. Garden City, NY: Dolphin Books. 1974.

Unmarried and Pregnant: What Now? by Ida Critelli and Tom Schick. Cincinnati, OH: St. Anthony Messenger Press, 1977.

Periodicals

Birth and the Family Journal. Quarterly publication sponsored by the International Childbirth Education Association (ICEA) and by the American Society for Psychoprophylaxis in Obstetrics (ASPO), 110 El Camino Real, Berkeley, CA 94705.

Briefs. Official publication of Maternity Center Association. Published by Charles B. Slack, Inc., 6900 Grove Road, Thorofare, NJ 08086. Ten issues per year.

Infancy and Childhood

Books That Help Children Deal With a Hospital Experience, by Anne Altshuler. Rockville, MD: U.S. Department of Health, Education, and Welfare. 1976. Stock No. 017-031-00013-9.*

The Children's Charter. A pamphlet stating the rights of the child. New York: American Social Health Association.

How To Discipline With Love, by Fitzhugh Dodson. New York: New American Library. 1978.

How To Father, by Fitzhugh Dodson. New York: New American Library. 1973.

---

*Contact Superintendent of Documents, U.S. Government Printing Office, Washington, DC 20402. Request information on cost of single or multiple copies. Always identify material by title and Stock No.

How To Parent, by Fitzhugh Dodson. New York: New American Library. 1973.

Infants and Mothers, by T. Berry Brazelton. New York: Dell Publishing Company, Inc. 1972.

Older Children Need Love Too, by Jacqueline Neilson. Washington, DC: U.S. Department of Health, Education, and Welfare. 1973. Stock No. 1791-00184.*

The Parent Test: How To Measure and Develop Your Talent for Parenthood, by Ellen Peck and William Granzig. New York: G. P. Putnam's Sons. 1978.

Parenting: A Guide for Young People, by Sol Gordon and Mina McD. Wollin. New York: Oxford Book Company, Inc. 1975.

The Parenting Advisor, by the Princeton Center for Infancy, edited by Frank Caplan. Garden City, NY: Anchor Press/Doubleday. 1977.

Parents' Yellow Pages, by the Princeton Center for Infancy, edited by Frank Caplan. Information about the whole range of problems that face all parents during their children's first 8 years of life. Garden City, NY: Anchor Press/Doubleday. 1978.

Preparing for Parenthood, by Lee Salk. New York: Bantam Books, Inc. 1975.

Textbook of Pediatric Nursing, by Dorothy R. Marlow. Philadelphia: W. B. Saunders Co. Revised 1977.

Toddlers and Parents, by T. Berry Brazelton. New York: Dell Publishing Company, Inc. 1976.

What Every Child Would Like His Parents To Know, by Lee Salk. New York: Warner Books, Inc. 1973.

Periodicals

American Baby Magazine. Monthly publication by American Baby, Inc., 575 Lexington Ave., New York, NY 10022.

Baby Talk. Monthly publication by Leam Corporation, 66 East 34th St., New York, NY 10016.

Children Today. Bimonthly publication by the Children's Bureau, Administration for Children, Youth and Families, Office of Human Development Services.*

*Contact Superintendent of Documents, U.S. Government Printing Office, Washington, DC 20402. Request information on cost of single or multiple copies. Always identify material by title and Stock No.

MCN: The American Journal of Maternal Child Nursing. Bimonthly magazine published by the American Journal of Nursing Co., 10 Columbus Circle, New York, NY 10019.

The Adult Years

After 65: Resources for Self-Reliance, by Theodore Irwin. New York: Public Affairs Pamphlets. Public Affairs Pamphlet No. 501. December 1973.

A Full Life After 65, by Edith M. Stern. New York: Public Affairs Pamphlets. Public Affairs Pamphlet No. 347A. Revised January 1976.

Growing Old in the Country of the Young, by Charles H. Percy. New York: McGraw-Hill, Inc. 1974.

Male "Menopause": Crisis in the Middle Years, by Theodore Irwin. New York: Public Affairs Pamphlets. Public Affairs Pamphlet No. 526. August 1975.

Why Survive?: Being Old in America, by Robert N. Butler. New York: Harper & Row, Publishers, Inc. 1975.

Periodicals

Aging. Official bimonthly publication of the U.S. Department of Health, Education, and Welfare, Administration on Aging.*

Dynamic Years. Official bimonthly publication of Action for Independent Maturity (AIM), 215 Long Beach Blvd., Long Beach, CA 90801. Available to members of AIM only.

Modern Maturity. Bimonthly publication of the American Association of Retired Persons, 1909 K St., N.W., Washington, DC 20049.

Death and Dying

A Death in the Family, by Elizabeth Ogg. New York: Public Affairs Pamphlets. Public Affairs Pamphlet No. 542. December 1976.

Death: The Final Stage of Growth, by Elisabeth Kübler-Ross. Englewood Cliffs, NJ: Prentice-Hall, Inc. 1975.

The Dying Child, by Jo-Eileen Gyulay. New York: McGraw-Hill, Inc. 1978.

*Contact Superintendent of Documents, U.S. Government Printing Office, Washington, DC 20402. Request information on cost of single or multiple copies. Always identify material by title and Stock No.

The Dying Person and the Family, by Nancy Doyle. New York: Public Affairs Pamphlets. Public Affairs Pamphlet No. 485. November 1972.

New Meanings of Death, by Herman Feifel. New York: McGraw-Hill, Inc. 1977.

On Death and Dying, by Elisabeth Kübler-Ross. New York: Macmillan Publishing Co. 1969.

"Using Children's Stories To Teach 'Something We Don't Talk About' (Death Education)," by Judith K. Scheer and Clay Williams. *Health Values: Achieving High-Level Wellness.* Thorofare, NJ: Charles B. Slack, Inc. Vol. 1, No. 3. May-June 1977. pp. 120–126.

Nursing Homes

How To Choose a Nursing Home: A Shopping and Rating Guide, prepared by Citizens for Better Care, Detroit, MI; The Institute of Gerentology, The University of Michigan, Ann Arbor, MI; and Wayne State University, Detroit, MI. 1974.

Nursing Home Care, by Office for Consumer Services, Medical Services Administration. Washington, DC: U.S. Department of Health, Education, and Welfare. Revised 1977. Stock No. 017-061-00040-2.*

First Aid and Safety

Advanced First Aid and Emergency Care, by the American Red Cross. New York: Doubleday & Co., Inc. 1973.

Emergency Action Principles: Red Cross First Aid Module. Washington, DC: American Red Cross, 1977.

First Aid for Burns: Red Cross First Aid Module. Washington, DC: American Red Cross. 1977.

First Aid for Wounds: Red Cross First Aid Module. Washington, DC: American Red Cross. 1977.

Home Accident Facts. Chicago: National Safety Council, 1976.

Standard First Aid and Personal Safety, by the American Red Cross. New York: Doubleday & Co., Inc. 1973.

*Contact Superintendent of Documents, U.S. Government Printing Office, Washington, DC 20402. Request information on cost of single or multiple copies. Always identify material by title and Stock No.

Nursing Care and Techniques

Community Health Nursing, by Kathleen M. Leahy, Marguerite M. Cobb, and Mary C. Jones. New York: McGraw-Hill, Inc. Revised 1977.

Community Health Nursing Practice, by Ruth B. Freeman. Philadelphia: W. B. Saunders Co. 1970.

Illustrated Manual of Nursing Techniques, by Eunice M. King, Lynn Wieck, and Marilyn Dyer. Philadelphia: J. B. Lippincott Co. 1977.

Introduction to Patient Care: A Comprehensive Approach to Nursing, by Beverly Witter DuGas. Philadelphia: W. B. Saunders Co. Revised 1977.

Nursing Skills for Allied Health Services, edited by Lucile A. Wood and Beverly J. Rambo. Philadelphia: W. B. Saunders Co. Vols. I and II. 1977.

"Taking Adult Temperatures," by Glennadee A. Nichols and Delores H. Kucha. *American Journal of Nursing.* June 1972. No. 6, pp. 1091–1095.

Vital Signs Module I: Temperature, Pulse, and Respiration. Washington, DC: American Red Cross. 1976.

Vital Signs Module II: Blood Pressure. Washington, DC: American Red Cross. 1976.

Rehabilitation

Basic Rehabilitation Techniques: A Self-Instructional Guide, edited by Robert D. Sine, Shelly E. Liss, Robert E. Roush, and J. David Holcomb, MD: Aspen Systems Corp. 1977.

Caring for and Caring About Elderly People: A Guide to the Rehabilitative Approach, edited by Janet Long. Philadelphia: J. B. Lippincott Co. 1972.

Handling the Handicapped: A Guide to Lifting and Movement of Disabled People, by The Chartered Society of Physiotherapy. New York: Springer Publishing Company, Inc. 1977.

Independent Living for the Handicapped and the Elderly, by Elizabeth Eckhardt May, Neva R. Waggoner, and Eleanor Boettke Hotte. Boston: Houghton Mifflin Co. 1974.

---

*Contact Superintendent of Documents, U.S. Government Printing Office, Washington, DC 20402. Request information on cost of single or multiple copies. Always identify material by title and Stock No.

Strike Back at Stroke. Dallas: American Heart Association. 1972.

Up and Around: A Booklet To Aid the Stroke Patient in Activities of Daily Living. Dallas: American Heart Association. 1976.

Periodicals

American Rehabilitation. Official bimonthly publication of the U.S. Department of Health, Education, and Welfare, Rehabilitation Services Administration.*

General

Alcohol and Drugs

Alcohol and Drugs at Work, by Sibyl Cline. Washington, DC: Drug Abuse Council, Inc. 1975.

Facts About Alcohol and Alcoholism, prepared by Leonard C. Hall, National Institute on Alcohol Abuse and Alcoholism. Washington, DC: U.S. Department of Health, Education, and Welfare. DHEW Publication No. (ADM) 74-31. 1974. Stock No. 1724-00351.*

Go Ask Alice. Author anonymous. Englewood Cliffs, NJ: Prentice-Hall, Inc. 1971.

Questions and Answers About Drug Abuse, by Anne MacLeod, Jean McMillen, Carol Marcus, and Joshua Hammond. Washington, DC: Special Action Office for Drug Abuse Prevention. 1975.*

What You Should Know About Drug Abuse, by Jules Saltman. New York: Public Affairs Pamphlets. Public Affairs Pamphlet No. 550. September 1977.

The Woman Alcoholic, by Vera Lindbeck. New York: Public Affairs Pamphlets. Public Affairs Pamphlet No. 529. October 1975.

You and Your Alcoholic Parent, by Edith Lynn Hornik. New York: Public Affairs Pamphlets. Public Affairs Pamphlet No. 506. April 1974.

Communicable Diseases

Control of Communicable Diseases in Man, edited by Abram S. Benenson. Washington, DC: American Public Health Association. Revised 1975.

---

*Contact Superintendent of Documents, U.S. Government Printing Office, Washington, DC 20402. Request information on cost of single or multiple copies. Always identify material by title and Stock No.

Other

An Adolescent in Your Home. Washington, DC: U.S. Department of Health, Education, and Welfare. 1975.*

Annual Report of the Director 1976. Washington, DC: Pan American Health Organization. Official Document No. 150. August 1977.

1977 Cancer Facts and Figures. New York: American Cancer Society, Inc. 1976.

Diabetic Guide for Nurses. Atlanta, GA: U.S. Department of Health, Education, and Welfare, Center for Disease Control. Revised 1969.*

Living With a Heart Ailment, by Theodore Irwin. New York: Public Affairs Pamphlets. Public Affairs Pamphlet No. 521. April 1975.

The VD Book: Venereal Disease Update, by Joseph A. Chiappa and Joseph J. Forish. Atlanta, GA: Holt, Rinehart and Winston. 1976.

Periodicals

American Journal of Nursing. Official monthly publication of the American Nurses' Association. Published by American Journal of Nursing Company, 10 Columbus Circle, New York, NY 10019.

American Journal of Public Health. Official monthly publication of the American Public Health Association, 1015 Eighteenth St., N.W., Washington, DC 20036.

The Journal of Practical Nursing. Monthly publication of the National Association for Practical Nurse Education and Service, Inc., 122 East 42nd St., New York, NY 10017.

Occupational Outlook Quarterly. Magazine published quarterly by U.S. Department of Labor, Bureau of Labor Statistics, Washington, DC 20212.*

Public Health Reports. Bimonthly magazine published by the U.S. Department of Health, Education, and Welfare, Health Resources Administration, Hyattsville, MD 20782.*

R.N. Monthly magazine published by Medical Economics Company, Oradell, NJ 07649.

---

*Contact Superintendent of Documents, U.S. Government Printing Office, Washington, DC 20402. Request information on cost of single or multiple copies. Always identify material by title and Stock No.

INDEX